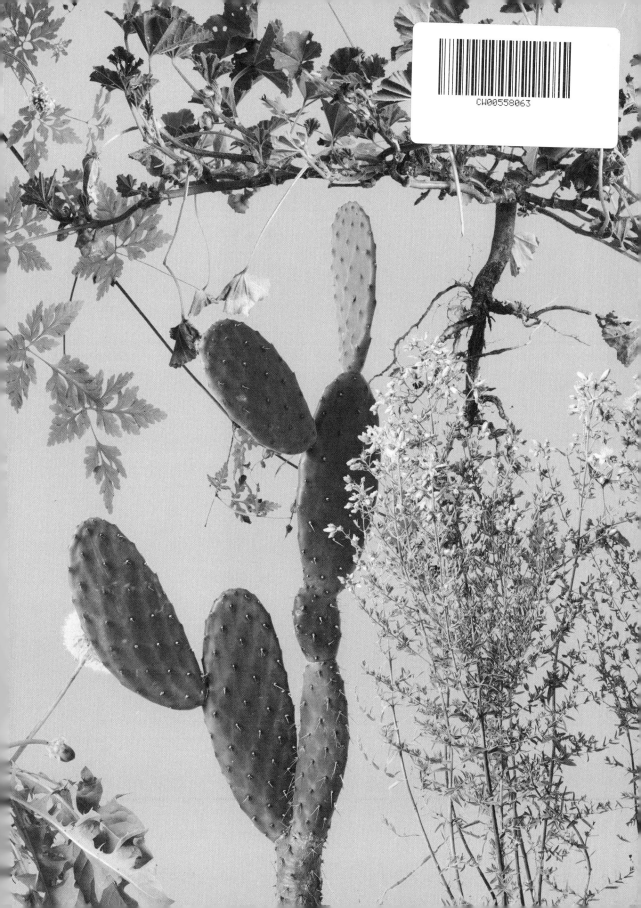

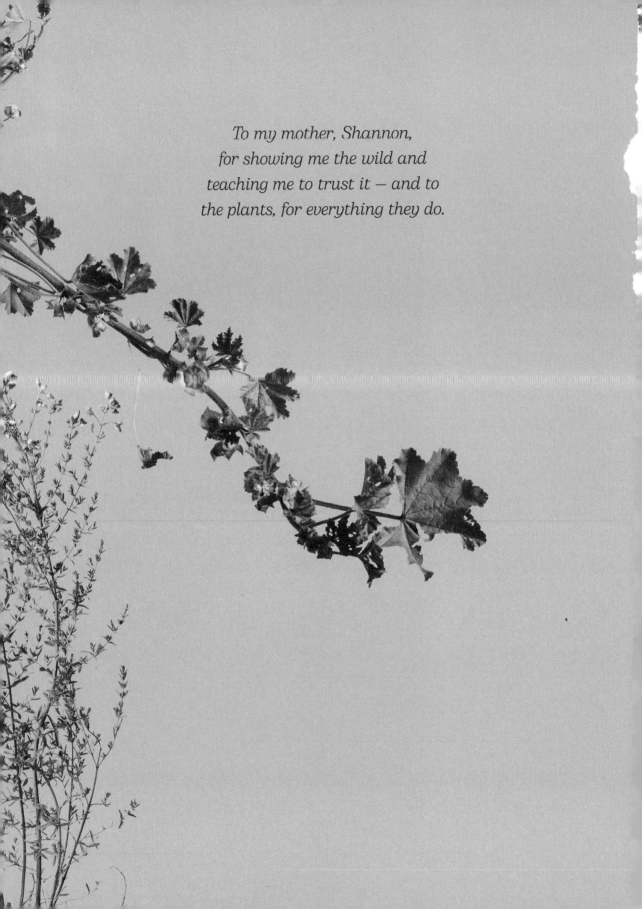

To my mother, Shannon,
for showing me the wild and
teaching me to trust it — and to
the plants, for everything they do.

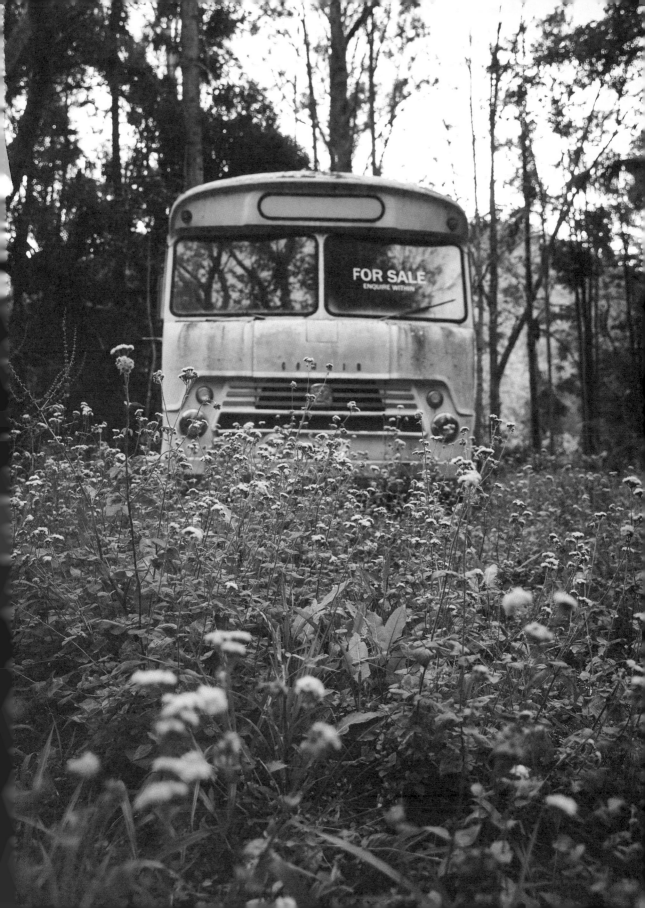

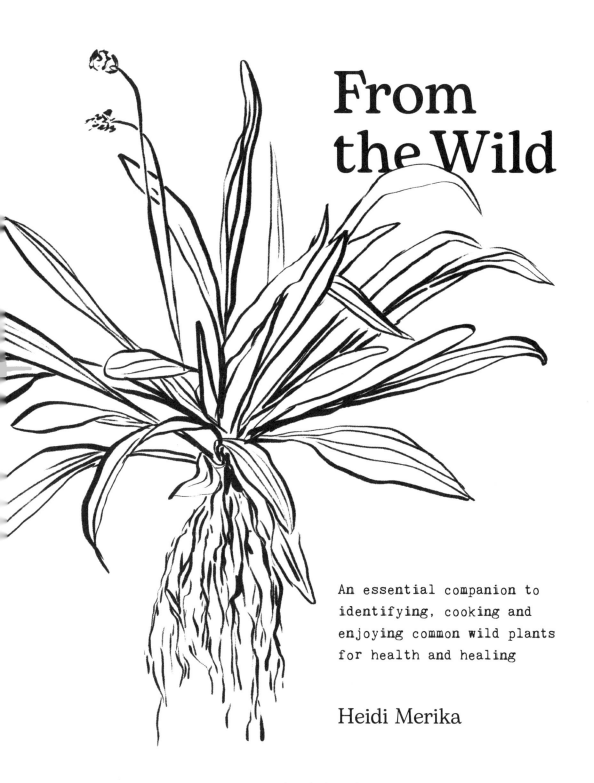

From the Wild

An essential companion to
identifying, cooking and
enjoying common wild plants
for health and healing

Heidi Merika

murdoch books

Sydney | London

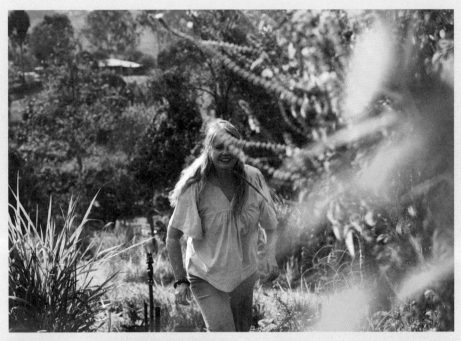
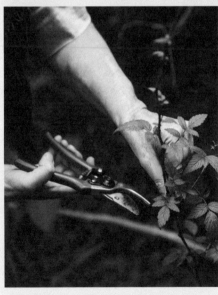
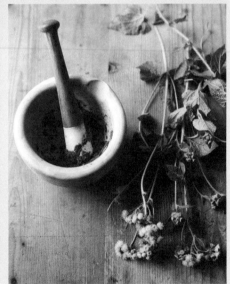

Contents

INTRODUCTION 6

PART 1: WILDCRAFTING 12
Welcome to wildcrafting 14

PART 2: USING WILD PLANTS FOR FOOD & HERBAL MEDICINE 18
Herbal medicine-making fundamentals 20
Herb guide 26
Equipment 44
Ingredients & raw materials 46

PART 3: RECIPES 52
Amaranth 54
Asthma weed 64
Blackberry nightshade 72
Blue top 82
Broadleaf plantain 92
Cat's ear 102
Chickweed 110
Chinese mugwort 120
Cleavers 128
Clover, white 136
Cobbler's pegs 144
Dandelion 152

Dock 162
Fat hen 174
Fennel 184
Gotu kola 192
Herb robert 200
Lantana 208
Mallow 214
Nasturtium 222
Nettle 230
Nodding top 242
Oxalis 250
Prickly pear 256
Purslane 264
Ribwort 272
Sow thistle 282
St John's wort 290
Tropical chickweed 298
Wild raspberry 306

REFERENCES 314

ACKNOWLEDGEMENTS 323

INDEX 325

Introduction

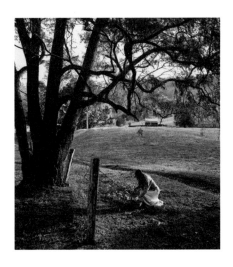

'Here, go give this to the farmer,' says Mum, holding out a soggy ball of muslin containing a fist-sized ball of cottage cheese. She'd made it from milk from the dairy cows owned by the farmer whose paddock we are camping in. She'd boiled the milk in the billy, added lemon juice, then hung it up in a cheesecloth-wrapped ball from a tree. It's her way of thanking the farmer for the milk, and for letting us camp on his property. It's the mid-1970s and we are somewhere in northern New South Wales.

My sister and I, only a year apart, are four or five. We don't want to take the cheese to the farmer, but Mum told us to, so we head off towards the farmhouse. I feel sick in my stomach from nervousness. We don't know the farmer, but he represents something to my sister and me. We know that in the farmhouse they are 'normal'. There are things in the farmhouse like Tip Top white bread and Meadow Lea margarine and Vegemite and Arnott's assorted cream biscuits in a tin in the cupboard and cups of tea with milk and sugar and a television in a lounge room with a couch in it and a car in the driveway ... because this is what is in 'normal' houses in Australia.

Somehow, this ball of cottage cheese shows the farmer that we have none of those things. All we have is a tent in his paddock and a billy and a bag of apples and this bloody ball of stinking cottage cheese. We are ashamed of the cheese.

My sister carries the cheese. Being a year older, she bears the brunt of the responsibility. As we near the edge the paddock, out of Mum's sight, she does the unthinkable. She throws the cottage cheese into the grass and says, 'Run!'

We run like the ball of cottage cheese is a grenade about to explode. We can't get away from it fast enough.

I can't remember where we ran to, or what we said when we got back, but we spent the afternoon catching yabbies from the creek where we swam most of the day, completely naked — no hat, no sunscreen, no shoes. Those things belonged to an era that hadn't arrived yet. The yabbies in the creeks were big then, with blue or green shells. We'd catch them in the billy and boil them on the fire.

Mum walked with us about the paddock to collect thistles. She said the hard part at the base of the flowers was like artichoke, but the flowers were mainly just fluff and prickles. We ate some of their hard parts, though, with our yabbies and cottage cheese and apples.

Eventually Mum came across the cottage cheese, bright white against the green grass at the edge of the paddock. She was dumbfounded. Why would we do something like that? The shame of that ball of cheese came back for another swing in the look on her face.

I would never have imagined then that, forty-five years later, I would be writing a book encouraging people to live the kind of life we were living back then. Sometimes it takes a lifetime to see things clearly, to have had enough life experience to contrast the good against the bad, and to realise that nothing is black and white.

We're always swinging between the extremes of habits, good and bad. Junk food still has its way with us from time to time, with its promises of cheap thrills that come with a side of shame.

About five years after the cottage cheese incident, when my sister and I were around eight or nine, we moved to Tasmania, camping on an island off the coast. You weren't allowed to stay long term, but the ranger was kind and probably lonely, so he let us stay for a few months. We caught fish from the ocean and collected dandelions, cleavers and bracken shoots, and the ranger would buy us food when he went to town on the ferry.

Sometimes it takes a lifetime to see things clearly, to have had enough life experience to contrast the good against the bad, and to realise that nothing is black and white.

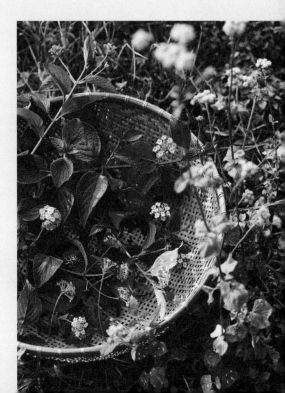

It was on this island that my sister and I discovered a nearly empty tube of sweetened condensed milk at one of the campsites recently vacated by weekend tourists. Being used to foraging, we were deeply fascinated by what was in the tube. Very hesitantly, we tried a bit on the tip of our finger — and fireworks in our brains exploded in delight. It was the best thing we had ever tasted. We squeezed every single drop from that tube, then hacked at the tube with a sharp rock until we split it open. (The tubes were aluminium back then, not plastic like they are now.) We managed to tear it apart and licked every last drop off. We were like bears that go crazy after eating human food and start ripping people's cars apart, looking for more food.

Months later, when we got back to the city, we saved up enough money to buy a *full* tube of sweetened condensed milk from the shop — and discovered you could buy a whole tin of it. So that's exactly what we did. We got two spoons and ate the lot! We felt sick after doing it, but that didn't stop us from doing it again. And again. And again.

Years later when I studied biology and physiology, I learned about how our brains are designed to seek out foods high in complex sugars and starches as a survival mechanism — to forage for foods like berries and yams that are high in complex fruit sugars and starches. But when pure refined sugar and highly processed oily carbs hit our biology, the chemical zapping that ensues rewires our brains. We start screaming for more, and a cycle of addiction can set in.

I didn't know back then that our foraged food and nature connection was making us healthier and more adaptable to life, and that the 'normal' food and couch and television like the farmer had, or the sweetened condensed milk the camper had, were going to make them sick and fat and tired. I just thought they were lucky, and we were poor, and that was that.

This is the same physiological and psychological trap experienced by 'undeveloped' communities all over the world. When communities that have lived for thousands of years in harmony with nature, eating and living off the land, come into contact with the highly processed Western fast food diet, they eventually become addicted to excessively sugary, salty, fat-laden, chemically adulterated foods and begin to think of them as 'normal'.

This dietary conversion has spread like a disease across the planet, perpetuated by the addictive physiological chemistry in our brains.

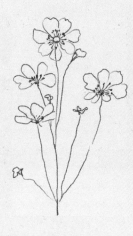

I've had the physical experiences of living on whole foods and foraged plants, as well as having had my share of 'normal' food and junk food, and it's obvious to me how different my body feels on these two diets. The effect it has on my behaviour is also profound, with junk food causing addictive eating patterns, lethargy and irritability.

Having spent the past twenty years studying human and plant biology and chemistry, it is clear to me that a whole-food, plant-based diet is optimal for the physical and spiritual health of humans, food animals and the Earth we live on.

A wholefood, plant-based diet is optimal for the physical and spiritual health of humans, food animals and the Earth we live on.

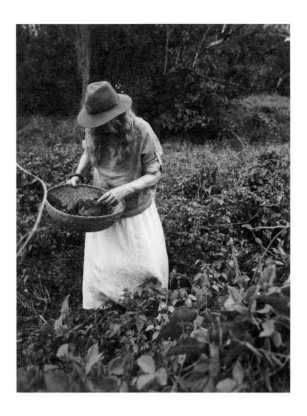

For the past decade I have been on a journey into wildcrafting — gathering wild plants as they grow in nature, steadily learning about the plants that grow literally in my own back yard, as well as back yards all over the planet.

As a kid, I felt like a weirdo for living an unconventional life and eating whole food off the land. That's also how I felt when I started running my first wildcraft courses. All my colleagues were focused on running successful naturopathy clinics with big dispensaries full of lots of products and patients — while I was heading out into the paddocks where I first learned plants as a kid, telling people, 'Look! The herbal medicine is here. It's free and it's yours.' Once again, I was the strange kid in the paddock.

Understanding these plants and running my wildcrafting workshops has taken me more and more towards using what is available in my environment, rather than what I can buy from a manufacturer.

The material for my first book, *Wildcraft*, was born out of the course guide for my two-day Wildcrafting and Medicine Making Course. The book that you are now holding in your hands introduces the botanical, medicinal and spiritual qualities of 30 different common plants, their use in folk and modern medicine, and which bits to harvest, showing you how to make your own herbal remedies from them — along with plenty of plant-based recipes to cook and enjoy.

The plants in this book were chosen because they were the ones in my immediate environment. Working with local plants, the ones in your back yard and the streets around you, is a beautiful way to connect to place. Beyond the physical benefits of increased nutrition and options for home healing, this approach also offers profound psychological and spiritual benefits.

Furthermore, the plants in this book are also found in human settlements across all major continents. When I teach people about these plants, I often get messages from students who have travelled to other countries telling me they have just found chickweed, dandelion or ribwort on the other side of the world. It is truly like meeting old friends in new places. Not every plant will be available in every place, depending on your climate, but the ones featured in the following pages are some of the most widely used plants around the world.

With medicine making, I have also had to find a unique path. While most herbalists use beeswax and alcohol in their preparations, in my life and my work I strive to live by two principles:

- ahimsa — *Refrain from harming any living being.*
- the Hippocratic oath — *First, do no harm.*

In this book, I have chosen to incorporate these principles as much as possible by making my preparations mostly vegan and alcohol free.

Sadly, this does not make them perfect. I still have issues with the sustainability of certain products. Some waxes, and even glycerine, cause me concern. I encourage you to try to source them as sustainably as possible, always seeking newer and healthier ingredients and encouraging suppliers to produce sustainably.

Some preparations in this book have a shorter shelf life than remedies in other herbals. I have chosen recipes that are fresher and have more life force, for optimal effects on both the physiology and the subtle energetics of the body. They are designed to help us reach our full potential for health and vitality, and minimise the impacts of living in a sick culture on a planet in crisis. We need to optimise our health in every way we can to face the period of transition we are in right now.

I want to share these recipes with you so that we can create a new 'normal' — one that encourages us to share our resources, to make things from scratch, to find food in our environment, to eat less, to have less, and to spend less money and more time in nature. A normal that is kinder and softer and more trusting of the gifts of the natural world.

I want to encourage a type of normal that says 'no thank you' to the commercialisation of foods and medicines made with ingredients that do not serve us or the planet. That says no thank you to artificial products with long shelf lives, that can be sold in larger quantities, for longer periods, simply to make more money. I want to encourage a type of normal that respects simple living, for the good of all beings, in harmony with nature. Please come join me.

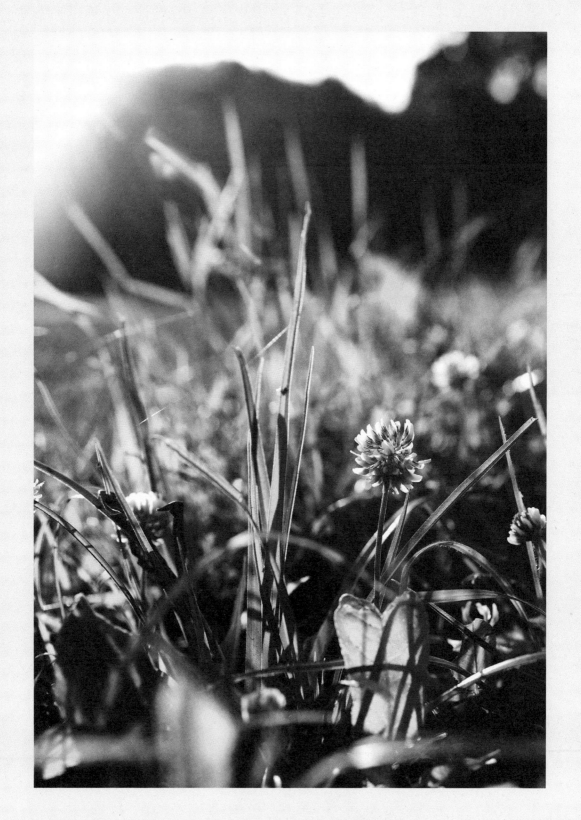

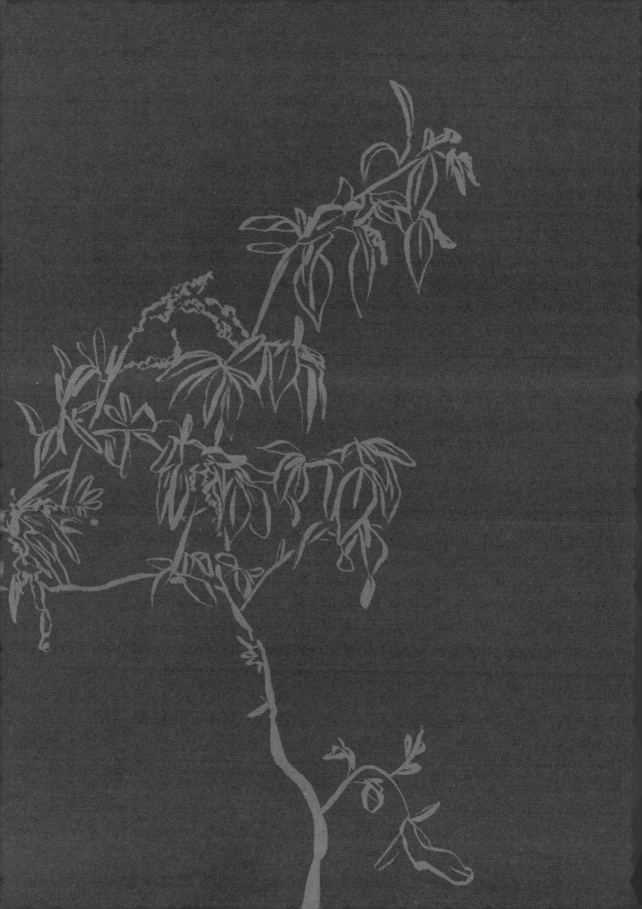

PART 1

Wildcrafting

Welcome to wildcrafting

Wild plants contribute to people's health and food security across the globe. Every culture has a rich history of wild plant recipes that have been passed down for generations. It is only in recent times in Western countries that we have become disconnected from our wild plants, thanks to the rise of supermarkets as our primary food supplier.

Across the world, wild plants are still an essential and widely used source of food — especially in developing countries, where poverty forces reliance on natural resources. Approximately one billion people use wild foods (mostly from plants) on a daily basis.

Wild plants can be incredibly invaluable during seasonal food shortages and famines caused by climate catastrophes (such as droughts, floods and fires), socioeconomic catastrophes such as recessions and market crashes, and health catastrophes such as pandemics and lockdowns.

Wildcrafted food — superior nutrition

Wild herbs generally contain many more vitamins and minerals, and much more protein, than cultivated vegetables (see table below). The plant foods with the densest energy profile are nuts, seeds, roots, tubers and inner shoots.

Nutrition in raw leaves of common vegetables and wild plants per 100 g

	Protein	Magnesium	Calcium	Iron	Vitamin C	Beta-carotene (Vitamin A)
Raw vegetables						
Cabbage, white	1.3 g	12 mg	40 mg	0.5 mg	37 mg	98 IU
Carrots	0.9 g	12 mg	33 mg	0.3 mg	5.9 mg	16,705 IU
Green beans	1.8 g	25 mg	37 mg	1 mg	16 mg	690 IU
Kale	3.3 g	34 mg	135 mg	1.7 mg	120 mg	15,376 IU
Lettuce, iceberg	0.9 g	7 mg	18 mg	0.4 mg	2.8 mg	502 IU
Spinach	2.9 g	79 mg	99 mg	2.7 mg	28 mg	9376 IU
Tomatoes	0.9 g	11 mg	10 mg	0.3 mg	13 mg	833 IU
Wild herbs						
Amaranth	2.5 g	55 mg	215 mg	2.3 mg	43.3 mg	2917 IU
Chickweed	1.5 g	39 mg	80 mg	8.4 mg	37.4 mg	63,8330 IU
Cobbler's pegs	24 g	0.23 mg	1721 mg	15 mg	63 mg	19,999 IU
Dandelion	3.3 g	23 mg	50 mg	1.2 mg	35 mg	26,423 IU
Fat hen	4.3 g	93 mg	310 mg	3 mg	5.6 mg	113 IU
Nettles	5.9 g	71 mg	630 mg	7.8 mg	333 mg	1,233,328 IU
Nodding top	3.2 g	–	260 mg	0.056 mg	9.17 mg	–
Purslane	1.3 g	68 mg	65 mg	2 mg	21 mg	1320 IU

Health benefits

Not only are wild plants a better source of nutrition than cultivated plants, they also contain active constituents known as phytochemicals ('plant chemicals'). Many of these naturally occurring phytochemicals have strong tastes that are bitter, sour or spicy (pungent). Cultivated vegetables have been genetically bred to be more palatable, with milder and sweeter flavours. In the process of doing this, we have inadvertently bred out the very compounds that provide the most nutritional and medicinal value. This, coupled with over-cultivated soils and monocrops, has led to a sharp decrease in the nutritional profile of cultivated vegetables.

The phytochemicals in wild plants may help contribute to less inflammation in the body, and a reduced risk of diabetes and heart disease, as well as a host of other common diseases. While caution should always be exercised when starting to learn about wild plants, we only need to learn a few plants in our local area, from a trusted educator, to dramatically boost the nutrient profile of our day-to-day diet.

Wildcrafting challenges

Wildcrafting in this day and age is not without its challenges, with the following concerns being the greatest barriers to people using foraged foods.

Private property
It can be hard to wildcraft widely without trespassing on private property. I have found, however, that if you knock on people's doors and ask to do some 'weeding', people are often happy for you to do so.

Loss of knowledge
Colonisation has devastated Indigenous food preparation knowledge globally. Humanity's most nutrient-dense wild foods (nuts and seeds) are difficult to harvest and prepare, requiring sharp tools, cooking and a degree of know-how to make them edible. Acorns, wattle seeds, bunya nuts and pandanus nuts, for example, all require persistence and patience to access their hidden stores of fat and protein. Loss of this know-how is a major barrier to wild foraging.

Pollution
Even for people who have sought out knowledge of wild plants, contamination from herbicides and pesticides, along with pollution from traffic and industry, is a major deterrent to wild harvesting. Edible plants are common and abundant along inner-city walking paths, parks and gardens — however, the risk of contamination from dog urine and faeces, and toxic weed spraying by local councils, means much of this abundance is rendered unusable.

Community gardens and designated spray-free inner-city wild spaces offer a solution to this problem in urban areas.

Safe wildcrafting

Identify your plant

To go wildcrafting, you will need some good plant identification books — and preferably an experienced guide who can show you where to go and what to look for. **Importantly, do not eat any plant unless you are confident you have identified it correctly.** There are now many excellent foraging groups on social media where you can share pictures of plants you have found to confirm identification. Rather than trusting the first response, I recommend waiting for several responses. Once several people agree, the plant's identification will be more reliable.

Pick the correct part of the plant

Wild plants do not taste anything like salad mixes from the shop. They are bursting with valuable phytochemicals that give them their amazing nutritional and medicinal properties — but these also contribute strong flavours that you may need to get used to.

Be mindful that plants are less bitter before flowering, and stems can be tough and unpleasant. Generally, pick fresh young leaves or perfectly ripe berries. Roots are best collected after winter, when they are the most nutrient dense.

You can research online or in herbal medicine textbooks the best part of each plant to use.

Avoid contaminated areas

You can eat and use most wild herbs and weeds as long as:

- you are confident no one has used toxic chemicals on them
- they aren't next to a highway or in a highly polluted urban area
- they aren't in close proximity to neighbours who use lawn chemicals
- they are unlikely to be contaminated with animal faeces.

A strip of dead vegetation with green vegetation on either side indicates the use of herbicides and/or pesticides. I call this 'the line of death' and avoid collecting plants anywhere near it.

Do not collect plants that look sickly or are a strange colour. Generally, if plants look healthy, they are. Use common sense.

Many people prefer to wash their wild plants before use to make sure they are free from bugs and air-borne pollutants or allergens. Personally, I often don't wash plants, although I do check them for insects and so on. If a plant is really healthy and vibrant, and collected from a location I know is safe, then I love eating directly from nature, with the fresh dew or sunlight on a plant. You can feel the energy of the environment, and as soon as you wash it, something essential is gone. But this requires a degree of familiarity with both the plants and the environment they are growing in — so if you are new to foraging, it's safer to wash your plants before using them.

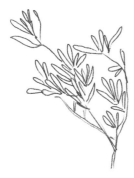

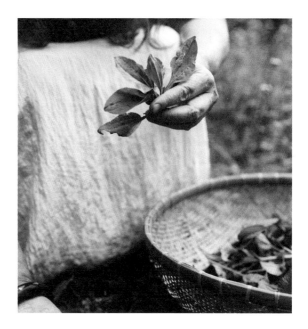

Guidelines for sustainable wildcrafting

- Only ever take as much of a plant as you can realistically use.
- If the plant is rare or there is only a small amount, can you use a more common plant instead?
- If harvesting a plant for its roots, make sure there is a large enough population of roots left in the ground to sustain the population.
- After taking roots, fill in holes, replace root crowns and leave the leaves there to compost.
- When harvesting a plant with seeds, drop seeds back onto the site to regrow in that area.
- Leave the oldest and strongest-looking plants, so they can replenish the species with their good genetics.
- As often as possible, try to harvest so that you can't tell you have been there. This means finding a large enough population of plants, then harvesting from throughout the group of plants rather than just clearing an area.
- Be mindful of animals or insects that depend on this plant for food or shelter. Are there enough plants left for them?
- What is the environmental impact of your presence in an area? Are you trampling plants that are trying to grow, or clearing paths, destabilising riverbanks or slopes that depend on plants to keep them in place? Try to have the most minimal impact as you move through the landscape.
- Create 'wild' gardens so that you can take from them, rather than having to upset delicate wild populations and ecosystems.

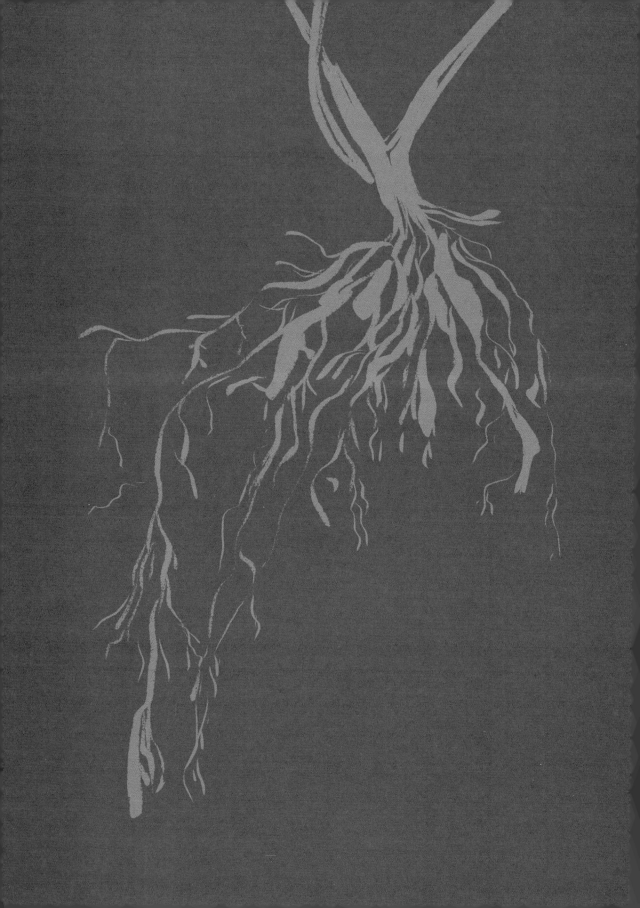

PART 2

Using wild plants for food & herbal medicine

Herbal medicine-making fundamentals

This chapter covers everything you need to get started on your journey into making herbal remedies at home — including the importance of sterilising your bottles and jars; tips for harvesting and storing your herbs; how to make herbal teas, powders and capsules, glycetracts, gels, creams, ointments, salves and balms; and dosage information.

It also contains a section on meditating and connecting with plants and making flower essences, to help deal with emotional, psychological and spiritual issues.

Note: the information contained in this book is not intended to treat or cure any medical condition. It is for general interest only. If you require medical advice, please contact a qualified healthcare professional.

Harvesting & drying herbs

There are few things as satisfying as harvesting and drying your own herbs, whether they are grown in your back yard, or foraged on wilderness adventures.

Harvesting

Home-grown herbs are most often harvested according to need, rather than under optimal harvesting conditions. However, knowing when to harvest a plant can optimise its medicinal properties. Below are some general guidelines for harvesting according to season.

Roots: Late autumn to early spring, when nutrients are concentrated in the root.

Barks: Late autumn and early winter.

Leaves: Spring or summer, before flowering.

Flowers: Spring or summer, before midday.

Fruit: When ripe and mature, and the fruit drops easily from the plant.

You'll find more detailed information about individual herbs from a range of books and online resources. I recommend:

Southern hemisphere plants
Jekka McVicar, *The Complete Book of Herbs in Australia*

Northern hemisphere plants
Mrs M. Grieve, *A Modern Herbal*

Collecting seeds

Seeds can be collected by hanging the flower heads of a herb over a bowl and letting the seeds fall into it — or placing a paper bag over the flower head, tying the end and hanging the plant upside down so the seeds will fall into the bag.

Once you've collected your seeds, any husks can often be blown off with a gentle breath, or loosened in a 'winnowing' motion (gentle shaking) in a light breeze.

Drying herbs

You can dry your own herbs at home using the following methods. You'll know they are sufficiently dried if they crumble when crunched between your fingers, and they still have a vibrant colour and strong smell. Once they lose colour and smell, they are no longer suitable to use in herbal remedies.

Hanging bunches: Small bunches of herbs can be tied and hung in a well-ventilated space out of direct light. They are best to the side of a window rather than directly in front of it. Check them regularly to see when they are dry and to make sure there is no mould forming in the bunch. They should only be left to hang for 5–10 days before storing.

Drying racks: You can make simple drying racks out of fly screen, fine mesh or dehydrator trays. These can be placed into racks or on a clothes horse to allow for the air to circulate around them. A clothes horse is good because it can be moved around the house and garden to maximise low light and good breeze and minimise harsh direct sunlight, and can be brought inside if it starts to rain or gets too damp.

Dehydrator: A temperature-controlled dehydrator that can be set to around 35°C (95°F) is a good way to dry herbs quickly and prevent them going mouldy in humid climates. Herbs can be dehydrated for 12–24 hours, depending on their moisture content and thickness.

Cardboard boxes: You can place fresh herbs in cardboard boxes that have ventilation holes cut into them. Different herbs can be stacked in separate boxes on top of each other. Make sure the herbs are well spread out, and only one layer thick. Densely packed herbs are likely to go mouldy. Herbs can be moved around the house to maximise good air flow and low humidity. Leave for 3–5 days.

Garbling (cleaning up the dried material)

When the herb is dry and crispy and crumbles easily in your hand, you can strip off any twigs or stems and discard any brown or unsightly parts of the plant to improve the overall quality of your dried herb. In herbal medicine, this process is known as garbling.

Storing

Dried herbs can be stored in clean airtight jars or snap-lock bags. They are best stored out of direct sunlight, with air exposure minimised as much as possible. If storing in plastic snap-lock bags, squeeze the air out before sealing them. Label your herbs with their common name, Latin name, harvesting date and expiry date (1–3 years).

Powders & capsules

Dried herbs can easily be ground into a powder, which can be a great way to use dried herbs that have a bitter taste. Simply place a handful of dried herbs in a coffee grinder and grind them until you get a fine powder. This powder can be stored in a sterilised glass jar, or used to fill capsules.

Vegetable-based capsules can be bought online, or from a health food shop or health products distributor. If you want to make large batches, you may want to get a product called a Cap-em-Quick or another manual capsule maker. These can be used to make lots of capsules quickly and are cheap to buy online.

Capsules offer many benefits. They can deliver high-potency herbs without the hassle of preparing infusions and decoctions. They don't contain the alcohol associated with tinctures, they have no taste, and they can be stored for long periods of time. The dried herbs also contain important prebiotics that help maintain a healthy microbiome in the gut, and are the closest we can come to ingesting the preserved herbs in their 'whole' form.

Using self-harvested herbs and making your own powders is incredibly satisfying on a good day and somewhat tedious on a bad day. One of the drawbacks is that you will never be as exactly sure of the strength of your medicine as you are when using manufactured herbs.

However, over time, your sense of sight, smell and taste ('organoleptic' testing) can become quite refined, and you will develop a sense of how strong the plants you are working with are.

Calculating the dose for capsules

Check the recommended daily dose of a dried herb, then assess how much fits your chosen capsule size, using a trusted reference source, such as the following books.

Books

Michael Thomsen, *Phytotherapy Desk Reference*

Kerry Bone, *The Ultimate Herbal Compendium*

Matthew Wood, *The Earthwise Herbal* (two volumes)

David Hoffmann, *The New Holistic Herbal*

Capsule sizes and weight of dried herbs (1000 mg = 1g)

Size 000:	800–1600 mg
Size 00:	600–1100 mg
Size 0:	400–800 mg
Size 1:	300–600 mg
Size 2:	200–400 mg
Size 3:	150–300 mg
Size 4:	120–240 mg

The recommended dose for dried dandelion root, for example, is 2–6 g per day, so you would take 3–4 capsules per day if using 000 capsules.

Infusions & decoctions

Fresh or dried herbs can be made into infusions (using leaves, flowers and seeds) or decoctions (from roots and barks). Unlike tinctures, teas contain no alcohol, making them a suitable way to administer an infused herb to those who need to avoid alcohol for religious, lifestyle or health reasons, such as pregnancy, liver disease, kidney infection or kidney stones.

Drinking a hot tea infused with diaphoretic herbs (those that make you sweat), such as yarrow, enhances their effect. This is useful when you are trying to promote sweating.

With mucilaginous herbs such as marshmallow, mucilage is more soluble in water than alcohol. It is useful to reduce inflammation throughout the body and help expel mucus from the lungs.

Infusions

An infusion can be made very simply by pouring boiling water over the leaves, flowers or seeds of fresh or dried herbs and letting them steep for 10–15 minutes, or even overnight. It is best if the vessel is covered during infusing, to avoid losing essential oils through steam, and to keep out uninvited bugs.

Dried herbs are stronger and more concentrated than fresh ones, due to their lower water content. The standard dose for an infused, decocted or fermented tea is 30 g (1 oz) dried herb to 600 ml (21 fl oz) water daily, taken in three or more doses across the day.

Fermented herbal teas

Fermented herbal teas have more flavour, and are richer and darker than non-fermented herbal teas. Some herbs ferment better than others without going mouldy. Fermenting also works best with herbs that do not have a high oil content — so herbs like rosemary and lavender do not ferment well. Fruity herbs such as blackberry, raspberry and mulberry leaves work well as a fermented herbal tea.

Normal black tea made from *Camellia sinensis* is made via a process of oxidation in which the tea is exposed to air, which causes it to darken, but it's not truly fermented. Fermentation requires the introduction of bacteria, which you can get from simply rolling the herbs in your hands.

To ferment leaves for teas, harvest fresh leaves and, if needed, wash and dry them. Place in a big bowl, removing the stems. Roll the leaves into marble-sized balls in the palms of your hands, squeezing and crushing them a bit to break down the cell walls. Once you've rolled and crushed the whole amount, break up the balls with your fingers to allow the air to get to all the crushed leaves.

Place back in the bowl, cover the bowl with a wet tea towel (not touching the leaves), then cover the wet towel with a dry one. The leaves will be fermented within 5–7 days. They will have changed in colour from green to dark brown, and have a nice strong smell, but will not smell off or look or smell mouldy.

Remove the cloth and dry the fermented leaves, either in a cardboard box for 3–5 days, or overnight in a dehydrator. When fully dry, store in an airtight container.

Decoctions

Decoctions are made by boiling the hard woody stems, barks and roots of herbs. Usually they are simmered for 10–20 minutes, then left to infuse for another 10–15 minutes or even overnight.

Start by adding 30 g (1 oz) of the herb components to 700–900 ml (24–31 fl oz) cold water. Bring to the boil, then reduce the heat to a rapid simmer and let the liquid reduce down to 600 ml (21 fl oz).

It can be beneficial to let the herbs infuse in cold water for up to 12 hours before heating in order to extract compounds that are more soluble in cold water. Mucilaginous herbs such as marshmallow and liquorice are better extracted in cold water before boiling.

Dosage guide

For more accurate herbal tea dosages, refer to the Dosage Chart on pages 26–29. Remember, dosages vary a lot depending on the individual herb, its quality and preparation, as well a person's age, body weight and the condition being treated. These dosages are a basic starting point for using your herbs safely.

Glycetracts

Also called glycerites, glycetracts use glycerine (see page 49) instead of alcohol for the extraction and preservation of herbs, making them suitable for people who need to totally avoid any alcohol,

Sterilising bottles & jars

When storing your herbal medicines, it is important to use bottles and jars that have been sterilised to prevent the growth of bacteria and mould. There are a few simple ways to do this in your kitchen. Start by washing your bottles, jars and lids in hot soapy water, making sure they are clean to the eye, then rinse each item well and sterilise using one of the following methods.

Dishwasher: Simply place your bottles or jars, with the lids off, in the dishwasher, and wash them on the pots and pans setting. Metal and hard plastic lids can go in as well, but should be separated from the bottles or jars, so each item gets washed thoroughly. Once the wash cycle is complete, leave them in there to dry — or allow to cool, then place on a clean tea towel until completely dry.

Oven: While they're still wet from being washed by hand, stand the jars and metal lids upside down on a roasting tray and dry in a preheated 160–180°C (315–350°F) oven for about 15 minutes. Turn the oven off and let the jars and lids cool in the oven until they are cool enough to handle.

Boiling: Place bottles, jars and metal lids in a pot of water with enough water to cover them. Boil for 10–15 minutes. Use tongs to remove them and place them on a bench on a clean tea towel or tray to cool and air-dry.

Note

If you don't have a dishwasher, it's better to use jars with metal lids. Hard plastic lids will melt in an oven — and while some will survive boiling, it is hit and miss, often leading to lids that don't seal properly. Generally, I have come to avoid jars with plastic lids for storing medicines. Trust me, I know this from experience!

whether for health or lifestyle reasons. However, adding a small amount of alcohol can extend the shelf life of a glycetract.

I use a food-grade, vegetable-sourced glycerine (rather than glycerine made from pork fat). Although it is very sweet, glycerine is generally safe for diabetics because it is metabolised as a fat rather than a sugar. It is an effective solvent for mucilaginous herbs such as liquorice and marshmallow, and has a soothing action on inflamed tissues. It is an emollient on the skin, helping trap moisture, keeping skin and tissues soft and supple. It can have a drawing action on the lungs that promotes expectoration of mucus. When used in suppositories, it has a laxative effect.

To improve its solvent action, glycerine can be added to alcohol or vinegar to draw out different plant constituents.

For the home herbalist, glycetracts offer a safe and effective alternative to the potent alcoholic tinctures used by trained herbalists. Home-made glycetracts will last for 6–12 months.

RATIOS FOR A DRIED HERB GLYCETRACT

1 part dried herb
2 parts distilled or purified water
3 parts glycerine

FOR EXAMPLE:

50 g dried herb
100 ml distilled or purified water
150 ml glycerine

Universal solvent
(glycerine, vinegar & distilled water)

In the scientific community, plain water is generally referred to as the 'universal solvent', but it's also the name given to this recipe by folk herbalists in the 1970s. It fell out of favour when alcohol tinctures became increasingly popular in the 1980s as herbal medicine attracted more scientific interest and investigation and underwent a rapid process of commercialisation.

My experience has shown the following combination of glycerine, vinegar and water to be a wonderfully safe and effective solvent for

home herbalists. Combining the three solvents is more potent and extracts a broader range of constituents than using any of them on their own or in pairs. For more information on using universal solvents with fresh and dried plants, see *In Touch with the Earth: Pat's Herbal Recipes*, by Australian herbalist Pat Collins.

UNIVERSAL SOLVENT (100 ML)

25 g dried or fresh herbs, coarsely chopped
50 ml apple cider vinegar
25 ml glycerine
25 ml purified water

Sterilise a small glass jar and its lid by washing in a dishwasher or boiling (see page 23).

Add the herbs to the jar, then the remaining ingredients. Place greaseproof paper over the top of the jar to stop the vinegar interacting with the metal in the lid, then seal with the lid.

Label the jar with the name and part of the plants used, the solvents used (glycerine, vinegar and water) and the date it will be ready, which will be 2 weeks from the day of making.

Leave in a cool, dark place and shake regularly for 14 days.

Strain into a bowl, through a sieve lined with muslin (cheesecloth), then pour into an amber glass bottle. Label the bottle with the name and part of the plant used, the solvents used and an expiry date of 6 months, even though your glycetract can potentially last much longer.

Store in the fridge or a dark cupboard.

Dosage: For glycetract dosages, refer to the Dosage Chart on pages 26–29. Remember, dosages vary a lot depending on the individual herb, its quality and preparation, as well a person's age, body weight and the condition being treated. These dosages are a basic starting point for using your herbs safely.

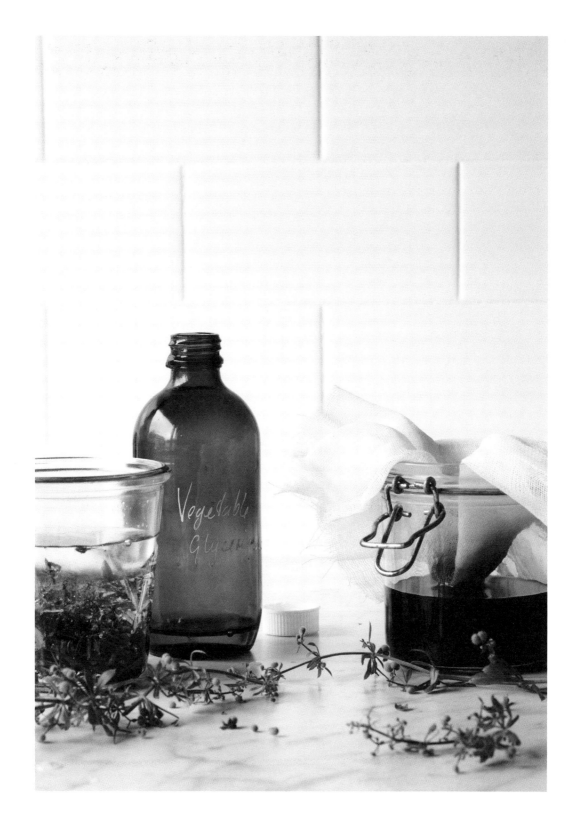

Herb name	Considered useful for	Cautions / Contraindications	Part used	Dry herb dose	Glycetract dose
Amaranth *Amaranthus* spp.	Nutrient-rich leaf and seed; source of antioxidants. Antibiotic, laxative.	Some species can cause allergies. Large quantities can build toxic levels of nitrates and oxalates. Cooking reduces this effect.	Leaves, stems, seeds	Seeds can be soaked and cooked as a grain, or ground into flour. Leaves can be eaten raw as a salad or pot herb, or cooked.	Used as a food
Asthma weed *Euphorbia hirta*	Respiratory conditions including cough, bronchitis, asthma. Anti-inflammatory effects. Also, hypertension and oedema.	No contraindications identified. Rare side effects include nausea and gastrointestinal upset. Use low dose.	Whole plant	1–6 g per day ¼–1 teaspoon 1–3 times per day (for short-term use only, 1–2 weeks)	Start at 10 drops; if well tolerated, you can increase by 10 drops per day, up to 4 ml per day
Blackberry nightshade *Solanum nigrum*	Pain, inflammation, fever, constipation (juice), liver protective, neuroprotective (berries). Externally for cold sores, herpes, neuralgia, eczema, psoriasis.	Green fruit associated with gastrointestinal upset, headache, dizziness, loss of speech, fever, sweating, heart palpitations, pupil dilation. Ripe fruit and leaves safe. Solanaceae family associated with increased joint pain in people with arthritis. Not to be used in pregnancy. Avoid if allergic to Solanaceae family.	Leaves, stems, ripe berries	6–12 g per day 1–2 teaspoons 1–3 times per day	Safest cooked or taken as a tea, to reduce levels of solanine (the slightly toxic compound found in the Solanaceae family, e.g. green potatoes)
Blue top *Ageratum* spp.	Reduces pain and swelling of bites. Array of antibacterial effects. Anti-allergic, antioxidant and anti-inflammatory, blood sugar regulation. Externally for wound healing, eczema, dandruff.	Not to be used in pregnancy or by those with liver disease, due to the plant's pyrrolizidine alkaloids. Toxicity studies show it is safe in relatively high concentrations.	Whole plant	6–12 g per day 1–2 teaspoons 1–3 times per day	4 ml per day
Broadleaf plantain *Plantago major*	Cystitis with haematuria (blood in the urine). Haemorrhoids, especially with bleeding. Mouth ulcers. Soothing for coughs, mild bronchitis. Array of antibacterial effects. Antiviral and immune-modulating. Topically for slow-healing wounds.	None known.	Leaves, seeds	6–12 g per day 1–2 teaspoons 1–3 times per day	4 ml per day
Cat's ear *Hypochoeris radicata*	Antioxidant, antibacterial and antifungal properties. Traditionally for urinary and liver conditions; wound healing and skin infections.	Caution if allergic to Asteraceae family.	Whole plant	6–12 g per day 1–2 teaspoons 1–3 times per day	4 ml per day
Chickweed *Stellaria media*	Inflammation and ulceration. Gastrointestinal disorders, including ulcers. Cleansing and tonifying for liver, kidneys, lymph. Topically for inflamed and itchy skin disorders including eczema, ulcers, abscesses.	Caution with allergy or sensitivity to chickweed.	Leaves, stems	12–30 g per day 2–6 teaspoons 1–3 times per day	15 ml per day Can also use fresh juice
Chinese mugwort *Artemisia verlotiorum*	Used for moxa in traditional Chinese medicine and acupuncture. Also, smudge sticks for energetic clearing. Relaxant for respiratory, circulatory digestive and nervous systems. Similar to common mugwort, infused oil assists with sleep and dreaming. Applied externally for fungal skin infections.	Avoid in pregnancy. High doses can be toxic due to essential oils. Can cause rash and hay fever in sensitive individuals.	Leaves	1–6 g 1 teaspoon 1–2 times per day (for short-term use only, 1–3 days)	Used as a tea

* spp. means there are several different common species

Herb name	Considered useful for	Cautions / Contraindications	Part used	Dry herb dose	Glycetract dose
Cleavers *Galium aparine*	Assists elimination in lymphatic system, especially where lymph glands enlarged. Supports kidneys and urinary system. Skin eruptions and dry skin, including psoriasis. Externally for ulcers, wounds, burns, bites, stings.	None known.	Leaves, stems	6–12 g per day 1–2 teaspoons 1–3 times per day	6 ml per day Can also use fresh juice
Clover, white *Trifolium* spp.	Wounds, sores, ulcers and boils; chronic skin conditions, acne, eczema, psoriasis. Also, colds, coughs, bronchitis.	Use with caution in pregnancy. Limit or avoid in oestrogen-dominant hormonal conditions and cancers.	Flowers, leaves	6–12 g per day 1–2 teaspoons 1–3 times per day	6 ml per day
Cobbler's pegs *Bidens pilosa*	Digestive complaints including constipation, diarrhoea; gastrointestinal inflammation and bacterial infections; worms, haemorrhoids. Respiratory conditions; asthma, sore throat, colds, flu, cough, earache. Antimicrobial against acute infections including hepatitis, conjunctivitis, renal infections. Supports immune system, cases of inflammation, allergies. Externally for cuts, burns, wounds, nose bleeds.	Avoid where grown in soil with high levels of silica and cadmium, as it can accumulate these minerals.	Leaves, stems	5–15 g per day 1–2 teaspoons 1–3 times per day	6 ml per day Can also use fresh juice
Dandelion *Taraxacum officinale*	Nutrient-rich leaf and root; source of minerals, vitamins and protein. Disorders of liver, gallbladder and kidneys. Supports weak digestions, stimulates bile flow and increases appetite. Improves liver function and helps prevent gallstones. Mineral-balanced diuretic.	Do not use during pregnancy without professional supervision. Contraindicated in those with known allergy to Asteraceae family.	Whole plant	Root: 6–8 g per day 1–2 teaspoons 1–3 times per day Leaf: 4–10 g per day 1–2 teaspoons 1–3 times per day	Leaf 6 ml per day Root 6 ml per day
Dock *Rumex crispus*	Assists elimination and detoxification, stimulating liver, gallbladder and bowel. Strengthens and tones bowel, relieving colitis, diarrhoea and constipation. These detoxification actions support the skin where digestion is sluggish, for eczema, psoriasis and acne.	Stimulant laxative, not for prolonged use or at high doses. Griping pain common. Do not use in pregnancy or lactation, or on children. Avoid in intestinal obstruction or inflammation.	Root	6–12 g per day 1–2 teaspoons 1–3 times per day	4 ml per day
Fat hen *Chenopodium album*	Nutrient rich; protein, fibre, minerals, vitamins. Liver and gastrointestinal protective. Bacterial and viral infections. Expels parasites. Anti-inflammatory, analgesic, antioxidant.	Contains oxalates that accumulate with prolonged consumption. Sensitive people may experience asthma and rashes.	Leaves	Can be eaten as a pot herb, raw or cooked	Used as a pot herb
Fennel *Foeniculum vulgare*	Eases digestive discomfort, bloating, nausea, flatulence, indigestion, intestinal spasms, irritable bowel syndrome; encourages appetite. Seed relieves bronchial symptoms, asthma, coughs, congestion. Slight oestrogenic effect, promoting menstruation. Supports breast milk production. Antibacterial, antifungal.	Essential oil and alcoholic extracts not to be used in pregnancy or lactation; tea safe under supervision. Essential oil not to be given to infants and young children. Essential oil irritates digestive tract. Avoid with allergies to Apiaceae family.	Leaves, seeds	2–3 g seeds per day ¼–1 teaspoon 1–3 times per day	6 ml per day (seeds)
Gotu kola *Centella asiatica*	Supports nervous system, vitality, enhances cognition and memory. Enhances endurance, energy and mood. Assists venous insufficiency and flow, alleviating varicose veins, restless legs. Reduces scars and stretch marks. Topically for mild wound healing, ulcers, burns, psoriasis, varicose veins.	High saponin content. Avoid in cases of coeliac disease, fat malabsorption, deficiencies in vitamins A, D, E, K, upper respiratory irritations. Do not use on open wounds, unless using a tincture. Can cause gastric irritation and reflux.	Leaves	1–12 g per day ½–1 teaspoon 1–3 times per day	6 ml per day

Herb name	Considered useful for	Cautions / Contraindications	Part used	Dry herb dose	Glycetract dose
Herb robert *Geranium robertianum*	Traditionally for wounds, ulcers. Diarrhoea and inflammatory or ulcerative gastrointestinal presentations. Toothaches and gingivitis. Influenza, exhaustion after influenza. Antimicrobial actions. Supports immunity.	May cause allergic rash in those with sensitivities. Avoid in pregnancy.	Leaves	1.5 g per day ½–1 teaspoon 1–3 times per day	4 ml per day
Lantana *Lantana spp.*	Seeds and leaves both rich in protein and minerals. Mosquito repellent; may reduce cattle ticks. Traditionally for ulcers, tumours, asthma, respiratory infections, catarrh, rheumatism. Also, gastrointestinal diseases, eczema. Research indicates strong antibacterial and antioxidant activity.	Red-flowering species considered more toxic to both humans and animals. Use pink or yellow species. Cooking reduces volatile oils, tannins and oxalates, thus reducing toxicity. Cooking also reduces anti-nutrients that can inhibit absorption of other nutrients if eaten raw. Avoid in pregnancy.	Flowers, leaves, seeds	2–6 g per day ½–1 teaspoon 1–3 times per day (for short term use only, 3–5 days)	Safest cooked as tea
Mallow *Malva spp.*	Relieves irritation and inflammation through entire digestive tract, used in both constipation and diarrhoea. Additionally for respiratory tract, urinary tract and reproductive organ irritation and inflammation. Externally for wounds, boils, bites, burns, rashes.	Generally safe. Use with caution in pregnancy.	Leaves, root	6–12 g per day 1–2 teaspoons 1–3 times per day	6 ml per day
Nasturtium *Tropaeolum majus*	High in protein, minerals, vitamin C, antioxidants, with flowers the highest plant source of lutein. Antibiotic and antimicrobial effects across respiratory and urinary systems, bronchitis, sinusitis, rhinitis, colds, flu. Externally for muscular aches, bacterial infections, minor wounds.	Contains volatile mustard oil, which may cause skin irritation. Avoid in pregnancy and lactation. Avoid in kidney disease and ulceration of stomach or intestinal tract.	Flowers, leaves, seeds	Flowers + leaves 2–6 g per day 1–2 teaspoons 1–3 times per day	6 ml per day
Nettle *Urtica spp.*	Traditionally a blood-building tonic, rich in minerals, vitamins, protein. Nourishing, strengthening and supporting whole body. All parts of plant support kidneys and urinary system. Leaf relieves arthritis and rheumatic conditions, eczema and gout. Root used for prostate and urinary conditions.	Fresh herb hairs sting, causing stinging pain, rash, itching. Avoid if known allergy to stings. Avoid in pregnancy and lactation.	Whole plant	Leaf: 9–18 g per day Root: 2–4 g per day 1–2 teaspoons 1–3 times per day	Leaf: 6 ml per day Root: 8 ml per day
Nodding top *Crassocephalum crepidioides*	Indigestion, headaches, fresh wounds, nosebleeds. Roots to treat swollen lips. Leaves for indigestion. Leaf sap in upset stomach. Decoctions of whole plant for colds, fevers, gastroenteritis, urinary tract infections. Externally, leaf sap for fresh wounds. Dried leaf powder as snuff to halt nose bleeds.	Caution in cases of liver disease, as it may contain pyrrolizidine alkaloids, but also has liver-protective effects. Use in liver conditions should be monitored by a medical professional. Not to be used in pregnancy.	Leaves	6–12 g per day 1–2 teaspoons 1–3 times per day per day	4 ml per day
Oxalis *Oxalis spp.*	Rich source of vitamin C. Traditionally to alleviate mouth sores and sore throat, to relieve cramps, fever and nausea. Weak digestion and appetite, and to stop vomiting. Antibacterial and antifungal properties. Topically for wound healing, reduces swelling and inflammation.	High in oxalic acid. Avoid in cases of gout, rheumatism, arthritis, hyperacidity, kidney stones.	Flowers, leaves	6–12 g per day 1–2 teaspoons 1–3 times per day	1–2 ml per day
Prickly pear *Opuntia stricta*	Oxidative stress, including in cases of diabetes, obesity, rheumatism, asthma, high cholesterol, hypertension.	Caution in handling as prickles cause painful, irritating stings.	Fruit, prickly pear pads, seeds	Fruit and prickly pear pads can be eaten cooked or raw	Fruit and prickly pear pads can be eaten cooked or raw

Herb name	Considered useful for	Cautions / Contraindications	Part used	Dry herb dose	Glycetract dose
Purslane *Portulaca oleracea*	High in alpha-linolenic acid (an omega-3 essential fatty acid), antioxidants, vitamins and minerals. Burns, headaches, disease of liver, stomach and intestines. For coughs, shortness of breath, purgative, cardiac tonic, emollient, muscle relaxant. Reduces inflammation in arthritis, psoriasis. Traditionally, reduces bleeding, clears heat, resolves toxins, fever, diarrhoea, eczema. Topically for wounds, possibly anti-inflammatory effect.	High in oxalic acid. Avoid in cases of gout, rheumatism, arthritis, hyperacidity, kidney stones. Caution in pregnancy. Those with 'underactive' stomachs suggested to concurrently use warming spices for ingestion.	Leaves, seeds	9–15 g per day 2–3 teaspoons 1–3 times per day	6 ml per day Can also use fresh juice
Ribwort *Plantago lanceolata*	All types of coughs, supports mucous membranes of respiratory tract, for catarrh, rhinitis, sinusitis, laryngitis. Haemorrhoids and bladder infections. Topically for slow healing wounds, inflamed skin, insect bites.	Use under supervision in pregnancy and lactation.	Leaves, seeds	6–12 g per day 1–2 teaspoons 1–3 times per day	6 ml per day
Sow thistle *Sonchus oleraceus*	Mineral rich and nutritive. Supports liver and digestive system; traditionally used as a cathartic laxative. General tonic, also for headaches, general pain, hepatitis, infections, inflammation, rheumatism. Infused leaves for delayed menstruation. Topically for cleaning and healing ulcers, treating warts, inflammatory swellings.	Avoid during pregnancy.	Leaves, stems	6–12 g per day 1–2 teaspoons 1–3 times per day	4 ml per day
St John's wort *Hypericum perforatum*	Anxiety and depression, exhaustion and fatigue. Menopausal depression. Nervousness. Externally for minor cuts, burns, skin ulcers, viral infections including cold sores (herpes), bites. Eases fibrositis, sciatica, neuralgia.	Not to be used in pregnancy and lactation. May cause photosensitivity; avoid excessive direct sunlight. Contraindicated for numerous pharmaceutical drugs, including contraceptive pill, antidepressants (SSRIs). In such cases, use only under clinical supervision, check with interactions for ALL medications you are on. Discontinue 7 days before general anaesthesia.	Flowers, leaves	1–3 g per day ¼–1 teaspoon 1–3 times per day	6 ml per day
Tropical chickweed *Drymaria cordata*	Nutritive. Sore joints, eye infections, fevers, coughs, sinusitis, acute colds, bronchitis, laxative, diuretic, increases appetite. Antibacterial action. Topically for wounds, burns, eczema, dermatitis.	May cause skin sensitivity. Avoid internal use in pregnancy.	Flowers, leaves, stems	10 g per day 2 teaspoons in 1 litre of hot boiled water, drunk throughout the day	Used as a tea or steam
Wild raspberry *Rubus* spp.	Nutritive, source of antioxidants, vitamins and minerals. May help prepare uterus for childbirth and facilitate labour, ease afterbirth pains, stimulate breastmilk production. Eases heavy menstrual bleeding and period pain. Relieves diarrhoea and constipation where there is reduced bowel tone. Also for sore throats, mouths, eyes, especially with inflammation and pus or mucus discharge.	Not to be used in first trimester of pregnancy. Avoid in constipation due to dehydration and tightness. Use with caution in iron-deficiency anaemia and malnutrition (or take 2 hours before or after food and supplements). Use cautiously with increased inflammation in ulcerative conditions of gastrointestinal tract.	Fruit, leaves	2–6 g per day 1–2 teaspoons 1–3 times per day	6 ml per day

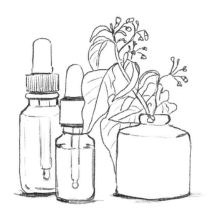

Infused oils

Infused oils are simply neutral carrier oils in which herbs have been soaked long enough for their constituents to infuse into the oil. Infused oils are different from essential oils, which are made using steam distillation and are much more concentrated.

It's a good idea to make up a basic set of infused oils to have on hand, because they can take 2 weeks to infuse, and are needed as an ingredient in many balms, salves and ointments — and balms, salves and ointments are often needed quickly.

Usually, it is best if infused oils are made using low heat from the sun or a nearby heat source like a fireplace or heater; around 40°C (105°F) is recommended. If warming in the sun, cover the jar with a paper bag to prevent light damage.

The infused oils can be used either on their own, or as a base oil for making medicinal creams and ointments. Oil is a good base or solvent for extracting herbs rich in essential oils and resins, because the oil is a carrier for these fat-soluble compounds.

Olive oil is most commonly used as it is widely available, and has its own beneficial properties for skin healing. My personal favourite is **rice bran oil**, as it is very pale and odourless, so you can judge how much colour and smell has come into the oil from the plant. It is also cheap to buy in large quantities, and the vitamin E it contains acts as a preservative and is beneficial to the skin. **Sweet almond oil** is also good for small batches, but is expensive. **Coconut oil** can be used if you keep it warm enough so it stays liquid and doesn't set solid, but it is erratic in how it performs depending on the brand used.

How long to leave your oils to infuse depends on a few factors, including the quality and type of herb you are infusing. Some plants are more easily extracted than others. It also depends on how warm the infusion stays. If it is cold, the extraction process will take longer, so it is best kept near a warm window, heater or fireplace. You want it warm, but not hot enough to damage the oil. You don't want to leave it too long; usually 1–2 weeks is ideal, but you can stretch it to 4 weeks if it's taking a while.

When I infuse herbs in a jar of oil, I always label the jar with a 'ready' date of 2 weeks from when the herbs went in. Sometimes you might decide to take the herbs out sooner, or leave them in longer, but 2 weeks is a good guide. You can decide if it's ready by how much it has changed colour and/or absorbed the smell of the herb.

Many medicinal plants can be made into infused oils for topical use.

Making a slow-infused oil with dried herbs
Place your dried herbs in a sterilised jar and pour in enough of your chosen oil (e.g. olive, rice bran, almond) to cover your herbs by about 3 cm (1¼ inches), leaving some space at the top of the jar so the herbs have room to expand. Stir well and seal the jar tightly.

Place the jar near a fireplace or hot water heater, or on a warm, sunny windowsill with a paper bag over it to keep the light off it. Let it sit for 2 weeks, shaking the jar every now and then.

Strain the herbs into a bowl through a sieve lined with muslin (cheesecloth), squeezing the herbs through the muslin. Discard the plant material into the garden or compost.

Pour your infused oil into a sterilised amber bottle (see page 23) and label it with the ingredients and date made. Herbs made with this method are more shelf stable and can last 1–2 years if stored in a cool, dark place.

Infusing an oil with fresh herbs

It is more common to use dried herbs for infused oils, as the moisture in fresh herbs can make the oil go cloudy or rancid. The exception to this is **St John's wort** (*Hypericum perforatum*) flowers, which are best infused as fresh as possible.

If using other fresh plants, let them wilt for a day to release some of their water content. Oils infused from fresh plants require constant care and monitoring to make sure they don't go mouldy. If using fresh herbs, chop them roughly and infuse as directed for the dried herbs above.

Fast-infused oil

Sometimes you want an infused oil quickly — for example, you may need an ointment for someone's injury. In this case, you can speed up the process in several ways, using 1 cup of dried herbs or 2 cups of fresh herbs to 1 cup of oil. Leave the mixture to infuse in:

- a yoghurt maker for about 12 hours
- a slow cooker on a very low setting for 4–6 hours
- a jar or bowl in a dehydrator set at 40°C (105°F) for 12 hours.

Fast-infused oil with fresh herbs

Add your fresh herbs to a saucepan with the oil and stir gently over medium heat. Tiny bubbles will form on the sides of the pan, and steam will rise as water from the herbs evaporates. Just before boiling point, there is a moment when the tiny bubbles on the side of the pan disappear and the steam stops. Immediately take the pan off the heat when the bubbles stop forming; if the oil reaches boiling, the herbs will burn. Once you've done this a few times, it becomes obvious when you reach the point between a simmer and boil.

Strain your infused herbs into a bowl through a sieve lined with muslin (cheesecloth). Wrap the muslin around the herbs and squeeze as hard as you can to get all the oil out. (If the oil is hot, let it cool first, or press it though the sieve with a wooden spoon.) Pour the strained oil into a sterilised amber glass bottle (see page 23), then seal and label with the date made and ingredients.

Store the oil in a cool dark cupboard. The expiry date is 12 months, but can be much longer if stored well.

FOR ALCOHOL-INFUSED OILS

Adding a little bit of alcohol, such as vodka, to a dried herb can also greatly speed up the extraction process, reducing it from 2 weeks to the next day. There are pros and cons to this method. The pros are that it's superfast, more shelf stable and tends to produce oils with a nice rich colour. The cons are that the alcohol can cause drying of the skin, and can sometimes affect the emulsification of creams and ointments.

30 g dried herbs
20 ml alcohol
250 ml oil

Grind the dried herbs to a coarse powder. Place in a jar and mix in half the alcohol (10 ml). The consistency here is important: you want the herb moist but not wet, so it forms a clump. You do not want the herb soaking in liquid — just enough to dampen the herbs, so carefully add only as much of the remaining 10 ml of alcohol as needed to dampen the herb; you may not need the full amount. Mix it in, then leave the herb to soak in the alcohol overnight.

The next day, add the herb to 1 cup (250 ml) oil and place in a blender. Whiz for 3–5 minutes, stopping to scrape down the sides after a minute or two.

Pour the mixture into a bowl through a sieve lined with muslin (cheesecloth), squeezing the herbs through the muslin. Discard the plant material into the garden or compost.

Bottle your infused oil and label it with the ingredients and date made. Herbs made with this method are more shelf stable than other infused oils and can last 1–2 years if stored in a cool, dark place.

Balms, salves & ointments

Balms, salves and ointments are all topical applications made from a combination of waxes and oils. As mentioned in the infused oils section above, slow-infused oils will need to be made at least 2 weeks ahead, and fast-infused oils 1–2 days before making the balms.

The terms 'balm', 'salve' and 'ointment' are used somewhat interchangeably, but typically they refer to texture, with balms being the firmest, most stable and long lasting — followed by salves, then ointments, which are the softest. The ratios of wax to oil tend to be:

- hard balms 1:3
- regular salves 1:4 or 1:5
- ointments 1:6 to 1:8.

For example, for a hard balm you would use 5 g wax to 15 ml infused oil. A regular salve would be 5 g wax to 20 ml oil, and an ointment 5 g wax to 30 ml oil.

Balms & salves

Balms provide a protective barrier in areas that are exposed to constant moisture, such as the lips.

Due to their high wax content, they stay on the skin longer without sinking in, making them an effective carrier for essential oils (which do soak in).

Typically, you'll see balm recipes used for lip balms, chest rubs and muscle pain balms such as Tiger Balm. Below are some of the common ingredients used in each.

Lip balms: Beeswax, candelilla wax, carnauba wax, sunflower wax, honey, glycerine, hempseed oil, coconut oil, shea butter, cocoa butter, citrus essential oils, vanilla extract, peppermint essential oil, beetroot powder and alkanet powder (for colouring).

Chest rub balms: Beeswax, candelilla wax, carnauba wax, sunflower wax, eucalyptus essential oils, lemon myrtle essential oil, peppermint essential oil.

Muscle pain balms: Beeswax, candelilla wax, carnauba wax, sunflower wax. Essential oils of eucalyptus, peppermint, wintergreen, cinnamon and cloves. Tinctures or infused oils of prickly ash bark, peppermint, rosemary, chilli and ginger.

VEGAN BASE BALM (30 ML)

Below is the base balm recipe I have come to prefer, using Ecocert-certified sunflower wax as my hard wax instead of beeswax. I have added castor oil because sunflower wax is harder than beeswax; the castor oil softens it, stops it cracking, and has many benefits of its own for the skin, including being antiviral, antibacterial, moisturising and pain relieving.

20 ml infused oil
5 ml castor oil
5 g sunflower wax
5 drops of essential oil (optional)

Add the infused oil, castor oil and sunflower wax to a Pyrex or other heatproof glass jug.

Place the jug in a saucepan, then pour about 5 cm (2 inches) water into the pan to make a water bath.

Bring the water to a slow boil, then reduce the heat to a simmer. Stir the mixture in the jug until the wax has melted, about 8–10 minutes.

Take off the heat and stir in the essential oil, if using.

Pour into a sterilised amber glass jar (page 23), or recycled lip balm pot. Allow to set.

Seal with the lid, then label with the ingredients, date made, and an expiry date of 12 months. If making multiple batches, add a batch number. (I generally put a 12-month expiry date on balms to be conservative, but they will often last much longer than this, especially if they contain essential oils.)

Store in a cool dark cupboard.

15 ml infused oil

5 g beeswax

5 drops of essential oil (optional)

Add the infused oil and beeswax to a Pyrex or other heatproof glass jug, then follow the method for the vegan base balm opposite.

Ointments & salves

Like balms, ointments and salves are designed to create a protective barrier on the skin. This makes them ideal for preventing irritation from contact with moisture, and also provides a barrier against infection. They tend to have a longer action on the skin surface than creams, as they are not absorbed readily into the lower layers of the skin like a cream.

Essential oils added to ointments will, however, penetrate into the skin, making an ointment a good carrier for essential oils. They are particularly useful where the surface of the skin is dry, cracked or damaged, but the underlying layers of the dermis are intact.

Ointments tend to be long lasting; if stored in sterilised amber glass jars out of direct sunlight, they will often last for up to 3 years. As with balms, when adding expiry dates, I tend to be conservative and put 1 year from the date made, but they will often last much longer than this.

The basic ingredients of an ointment are waxes and oils. The most commonly used wax is beeswax; I use vegan waxes such as candelilla, carnauba, olivem 1000 (from olives), rice bran wax — and, my favourite, sunflower wax.

Ointments have also traditionally been made using lanolin, Vaseline or animal or vegetable lard. Moisturising butters such as cocoa butter, shea butter or mango butter can also be added to ointments, both for their moisturising effects, and for softening the texture of the ointment.

Using herb-infused oils such as calendula, comfrey, rosemary, cayenne, arnica and lavender is a perfect way to add herbs to ointments. Any herb with a high resin or essential oil content can be made into a successful infused oil.

Other herbs commonly incorporated into ointments are burdock, ginger, golden seal, marshmallow, mullein, nettle, plantain, St John's wort, yarrow and poke root.

Any essential oil can also be added to an ointment or salve to boost its medicinal actions — especially its antibiotic and anti-inflammatory effects — and to provide heating, cooling or soothing effects on the skin. Essential oils also act as preservatives, extending the shelf life of the remedy.

Below is the base ointment recipe I have come to prefer, using Ecocert-certified sunflower wax as my hard wax to replace beeswax. I have added shea butter to soften the ointment, because sunflower wax is harder than beeswax, and the shea makes it feel softer and smoother and prevents it cracking. Shea butter also has its own benefits on the skin, being anti-inflammatory, moisturising, sun protective and rich in vitamins A and E.

This is a soft, easily spreadable ointment with a nice skin feel. If making it in on a hot day, you could reduce the infused oil to 40 ml to give a slightly firmer ointment, but the version below works well in most climates.

VEGAN BASE OINTMENT (60 G)

50 ml infused oil

5 g shea butter

5 g sunflower wax

5–10 drops of essential oil (optional)

Add the infused oil, shea butter and sunflower wax to a Pyrex or other heatproof glass jug.

Place the jug in a saucepan, then pour about 5 cm (2 inches) water into the pan to make a water bath.

Bring the water to a slow boil, then reduce the heat to a simmer. Stir the mixture in the jug until the wax has melted, about 8–10 minutes.

Take off the heat. If using the essential oil, stir in only half the amount until incorporated. Test the strength of the mixture by dabbing a small amount on the inside of your wrist, then add more essential oil if desired.

Pour into a sterilised amber jar. Allow to set.

Seal with the lid, then label with the ingredients, date made, and an expiry date of 12 months. If making multiple batches, add a batch number.

Store in a cool dark cupboard.

BEESWAX BASE OINTMENT OPTION (60 G)

50 ml tablespoons infused oil
5 g beeswax
5 g shea butter (optional)
5–10 drops of essential oils (optional)

Add the infused oil, beeswax and shea butter, if using, to a Pyrex or other heatproof glass jug, then follow the method for the vegan base ointment on the previous page.

Creams

In herbal manufacturing, creams are one of the most challenging things to make, but also one of the most satisfying when you do it well. Creams are made from a combination of infusions, infused or plain oils and waxes. The challenge lies in combining water and oil, which famously do not like to mix — which is why one of the most essential ingredients in a cream is an emulsifier.

An emulsifier helps to bind the water and oil molecules to keep them together in the suspension, so your cream does not separate. If your emulsifier is too weak, it may hold for a short time, then separate after a few days or weeks. A good emulsifier will hold indefinitely; an emulsifying wax is best for this.

As infused oils are one of the main ingredients of a cream, you need to think well ahead, because it takes 2–4 weeks to make your infused oil — unless you use the 'fast' methods detailed on page 31. I try to keep a store of key infused oils in the cupboard, ready for cream making. My essentials are oils infused with calendula and St John's wort; rosemary, comfrey, arnica, lavender and rose are also staples.

Below are the ingredients commonly used when making creams.

Emulsifying wax

Emulsifying wax is traditionally made from a waxy substance — usually coconut or palm oil, and sometimes a petroleum-based wax, so check the source for sustainability. Because of environmental issues, new emulsifying waxes made from olive oil (olivem 1000), and/or sunflower wax have recently come on the market.

Emulsifying wax is treated with a detergent, which enables the oil and water in it to bind together to create a smooth emulsion, usually in the form of white waxy pellets or flakes. Emulsifying wax is by far the most effective wax to use in your cream.

Natural emulsifiers

Due to issues with the sustainability and production of some emulsifying waxes, many people prefer to use natural emulsifiers such as beeswax, lanolin, lecithin or glycerine. A teaspoon of these can be added to the emulsifying wax for their added emulsifying, preservative and skin-healing properties.

These emulsifiers are not usually sufficient for large batches, or for batches of cream requiring a long shelf life, but can work well enough in small home batches, sometimes … if you're lucky.

Infused & plain oils

Using infused oils made from high-quality herbs is the best way to make strongly medicinal creams. Some of the most popular infused oils used in creams are calendula, St John's wort, rosemary, arnica, lavender, comfrey, plantain, chickweed and rose. (See the section on infused oils on pages 30–31.)

If you don't have an infused oil to hand, you can still make your cream with plain oils such as olive, rice bran, coconut, wheatgerm or sweet almond oil.

Essential oils

Essential oils are often used in creams for added medicinal value, to improve the fragrance and for their preservative effects.

Infusions & decoctions with fresh or dried herbs

All creams have a herbal infusion or decoction as the foundation of their water component. Just about any medicinal herb can be used topically to make a cream. Dried herbs tend to create creams that are more concentrated in herbal constituents and less likely to go mouldy.

You can make your infusions or decoctions for your cream from fresh or dried herbs that have first been decocted for 15 minutes on a slow boil, or infused for 2–12 hours. If you're feeling impatient you can just infuse them for 15 minutes, but this will give you a weaker cream. Often, I will do the 12-hour infusion by letting it sit overnight before making the cream the next day. Sometimes I also blend the infusion with a stick blender to extract more of the chlorophyll and other plant constituents, then strain the infusion before using. This tends to give the cream a brighter colour.

Preservatives

I have found creams to be far less stable and more prone to spoilage than ointments, due to their water and herb content — so it's a good idea to add a natural preservative such as tincture of benzoin, made from the resin of the plant *Styrax benzoin*, or citricidal, made from citrus seed extract. An Essential Therapeutics product called Amiox, made from rosemary extract, can also be used as an antioxidant. Vitamin E oil is another popular antioxidant used in creams.

Tinctures

Tinctures are often added to creams to make a strong topical application. However, I have found that adding tinctures can cause your cream to 'split' or 'separate' (also known as cracking). To minimise this risk, use low-alcohol tinctures and add them a tiny bit at a time. Try not to go over 10% or 10 ml in 100 g of cream.

Nutritional substances

You can also add nutrients to you creams, such as vitamin E oil, vitamin A or beta-carotene, vitamin C (or vitamin C–rich powders such as Kakadu plum or camu camu), rosehip oil or powder, as well as a range of B vitamins.

Colours

You can colour your cream with various natural colouring agents.

Blue: butterfly pea
Yellow: turmeric
Green: chlorophyll
Red or pink: beetroot powder, alkanet root powder

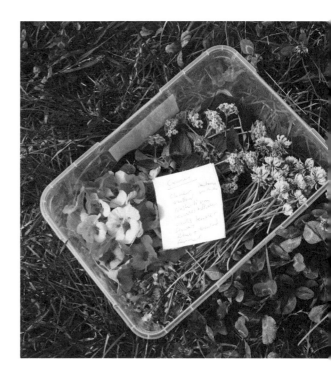

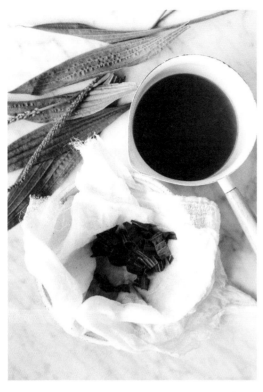
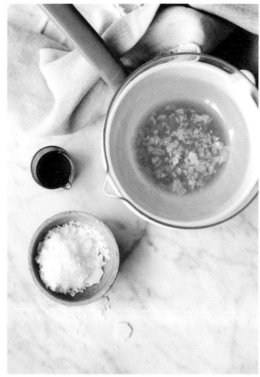
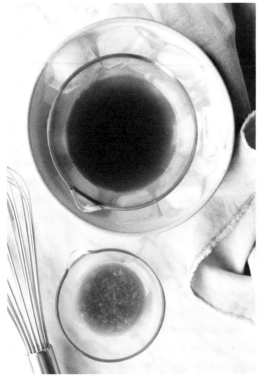
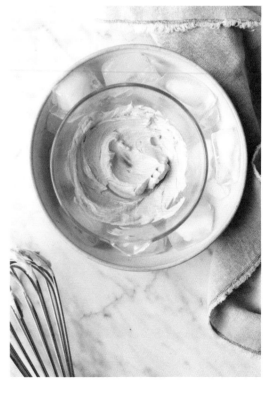

USING WILD PLANTS FOR FOOD & HERBAL MEDICINE

When things go wrong … as they often do when making creams

I have had some very spectacular and public failures when making creams, and have at one point or another made ALL of the following mistakes, resulting in a sloppy or gritty mess. But when it works, oh my, it is truly a glorious thing! There are few things as satisfying as the moment your cream forms its first stiff peak and you see all the ingredients transform into something smooth and silky and fluffy. Then it's all air punches and 'Woo hoo!'

So you can learn from my mistakes, here are some of the most common pitfalls of cream making.

The cream splits, and the oil and water separate

There are several reasons this might happen:

- The cream was over-whipped. To avoid this, stop whipping as soon as it reaches a consistency with peaks.

- There was too much alcohol or glycerine added. This can result in blobs of congealed wax sitting in puddles of liquid.

- You used too much preservative. You need to get the amounts just right, especially if using citricidal. For citricidal, use a dropper bottle, so you can measure small drops. It is very thick and viscous, so it's easy to drop in big blobs that might seem like one drop, but is actually 10 drops!

The cream didn't set

- The emulsifier wasn't strong enough, or you didn't use enough of it. Try making the cream again and increasing the amount of emulsifier by one-quarter or one-third.

- The emulsifier was too old. If your wax is too old, sometimes it just won't set, no matter how long you stir it.

Gritty cream

Gritty cream can happen when there is a big temperature difference between your oil and water elements. This is why you reheat the infusion before adding it to your wax. If you don't, you will get a gritty cream, because the cool infusion will harden the wax too quickly.

Mouldy cream

If your cream goes mouldy after a few days or weeks, this is generally because the jar was not sterile, or there was not enough preservative (citricidal, tincture of benzoin or essential oils).

Healing a split cream

You can sometimes heal a split by adding about 1 tablespoon lecithin per 100 g cream. This works about half the time, depending on what the problem was. You need to gently heat the lecithin and the cream to incorporate the lecithin.

VEGAN HERBAL BASE CREAM (125 ML)

This recipe (pictured opposite) combines several great herbal cream recipes from my favourite herbalists. In the original versions, most used beeswax and several used honey. I use this recipe as the base for most of my creams, as it can be adapted to incorporate many variations of infused oils, essential oils, herbal tinctures and infusions.

Equipment

2 saucepans
a heatproof jug
a large bowl of iced water (optional)
a whisk or fork
a stick blender (if making large batches)

Ingredients

2 tablespoons dried herb or 1 cup fresh herb
3 tablespoons infused oil
1½ tablespoons olivem 1000
1 teaspoon vegetable glycerine
12 drops of citricidal (citrus seed extract), or 12 drops of tincture of benzoin
5–10 drops of essential oil (optional)

Infuse the dried or fresh herbs in ½ cup (125 ml) hot boiled water overnight, or for a minimum of 30 minutes. Sometimes I blend the infusion with a stick blender while the herbs are infusing, to release the chlorophyll and plant constituents to get a stronger and more colourful cream.

Strain and compost the herbs, then pour the infusion into a small saucepan, but leave it off the heat.

Pop some ice cubes in a large bowl half filled with water, to have an ice bath ready for when you are mixing your cream. (You can leave the ice bath in the fridge or freezer until needed.)

In a Pyrex or other heatproof glass jug, combine the infused oil, olivem 1000 and glycerine. Place the jug in a separate saucepan, then pour about 5 cm (2 inches) water into the pan to make a water bath. Bring the water to the boil, then reduce the heat to a slow boil. Stir the ingredients in the jug frequently until the wax has melted, about 8–10 minutes.

Add the citricidal or tincture of benzoin to your herb infusion in the other pan. Heat the infusion until close to boiling point — but take it off the heat as soon as bubbles form.

The oil mixture and the infusion need to be as close as possible to the same temperature to incorporate smoothly and avoid a gritty cream, so as soon as the wax has melted and the infusion is near boiling, pour the melted oil mixture into the infusion, place the saucepan in the ice bath (this will help the mixture thicken much more quickly) and start mixing with a fork or whisk. (If making a large batch, a stick blender will be much faster.)

When the cream has cooled but is not stiff, add the essential oil, if using, and keep mixing to incorporate.

Stop mixing when the mixture forms nice stiff peaks like whipped cream.

Spoon into sterilised amber glass jars (see page 23) and label with ingredients, date made and an expiry date of 3 months.

Best stored in a dark, cool cupboard or drawer, or in the fridge.

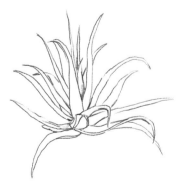

Herbal gels

Herbal gels are used when you want to cool the skin, as heat can be trapped or exacerbated by oily creams and ointments. Their cooling, soothing nature make gels ideal for burns, bites, stings, pain, redness and swelling of the skin. They are also good for painful arthritis or hot eczema characterised by heat and redness.

Laponite gel

Laponite is a clear synthetic clay mineral that is often used in scientific labs because it is very good at maintaining substances in suspension. It is stable and inert and is excellent for a wide range of topical applications of tinctures, fresh plant juices, essential oils and herb-infused vegetable oils. It has an excellent 'skin feel' when applied, as it is non-sticky and dries matte. It has its own cooling and soothing properties that can be enhanced by adding anti-inflammatory herbs. It lasts and holds its shape and consistency for up to 3 months in the fridge.

Aloe vera gel

Aloe vera can be used directly from the fresh plant. The gel is highly moisturising and great for sunburns, bug bites and minor cuts or wounds. It is also easy to make at home, from the leaves of an aloe plant, but it's best to only use one or two leaves at a time, as the gel only lasts about 1 week. If you plan to keep it longer, you need to freeze it.

If buying aloe vera gel, look for ones with minimal preservatives and additives.

FRESH ALOE VERA GEL

Cut off one of the outer leaves from the base of the plant. Wash it to remove any dirt, then stand it upright in a cup or bowl for 10–15 minutes, to allow the yellow-tinted resin to drain out of the leaf. (The resin contains latex, which can irritate the skin, so it's best to soak it out.)

Using a small knife, cut the spikes off both edges of the leaf, then cut just below the surface of the skin of the front and back.

Peel off the thick skin (using the knife or a vegetable peeler) to expose the natural aloe vera gel.

Put the gel in a blender, being careful not to include any skin. Blend the gel for a few seconds, until it's frothy and liquefied.

Add 6 drops of citricidal (citrus seed extract) as a preservative per 100 g gel.

Refrigerate in an airtight jar or container, labelled with the name of the plant, the citricidal, the date made and an expiry date of 3–5 days.

To preserve the gel for up to 6 months, freeze it in small batches in an ice cube tray.

Personal lubricants

Water-based personal lubricants can be used as a base for fresh herbs and tinctures. They are the most expensive of the gel options, but can be useful when obtaining laponite gel or aloe vera is difficult. They tend to have a more slippery and slimy consistency, but can be quite soothing on inflamed tissue, especially in areas where chafing can happen, such as armpits or thighs, or when there is eczema or prickly heat in these areas. They are also useful if wanting to use herbs for vaginal infections or inflammation.

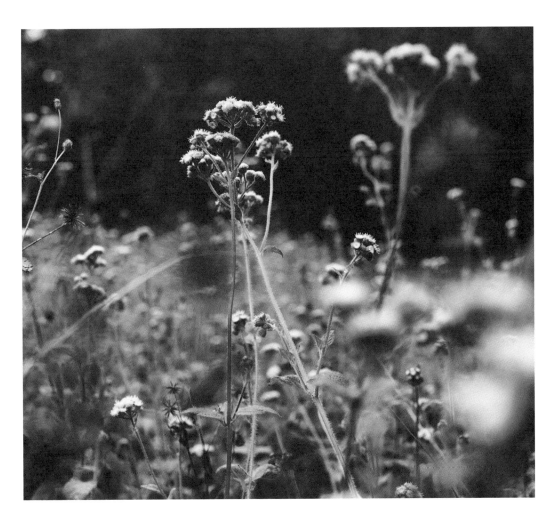

Plant awareness & communication

Working with plant spirit energies is about learning to feel the sensations you receive from the plant. The sensations will bring up an emotional response that can guide you in your relationship. The sensations are the doorway by which we enter into the realm of the spirit. When working with plant energies, we need an attitude of humble reverence and respect as we reach out with our intention, calling them to us, and asking for their assistance.

Observe the plant with all your senses

Find a quiet place in nature and allow your focus to shift to a particular plant. Something about it will attract you. It could be a physical attraction: you find it beautiful in some way. It could be an emotional pull, or a flash of recognition or knowing, like meeting an old friend. Approach the plant and ask if you can work together. You could offer a small gift as a physical symbol of your good will.

Sight

Spend time observing the plant, becoming aware of what that observation brings up in you. Is it a plant that likes the sun or the shade? Sun-loving plants, such as sage and rosemary, tend to be warming and drying, whereas plants that like moist shady environments, like mints, gotu kola and lemon balm, tend to be more cooling.

Observe which plants tend to grow near each other, so you will know who to look for when you come across similar groups of plants. For example, dock and nettle often grow near each other, and dock can be used to treat nettle stings.

By observing the colour of plants and flowers, you may get insight into the chakras they might have an affinity with — and some of the issues a person needing this plant might be working with.

Sounds and intuition

Do plants swish or rustle, or make no sound at all? Energetically, each plant will play its own tune (telepathically) — which, if you are lucky to be gifted with it, you can 'hear' with your heart or inner listening. It could be a tune, a song or a message. This is spoken about regularly in the literature of Indigenous peoples.

Touch

Come closer and touch the plant. Is the plant soft or prickly? Observe your emotional response. Do you want to rub it on your body because it is so soft and nurturing, like lamb's ear (*Stachys byzantina*), or do you need to wear gloves to hold it because it stings like nettle? What do these qualities bring to mind, both in terms of actions and emotions?

Smell

Hold it to your nose and inhale its aroma. Smell can give you an immediate indication of whether a plant contains volatile oils. Smelling plants can trigger many associations, emotions and memories, both from this life and past lives. Smells have an immediate effect on your physical, mental and emotional state.

Meditate with the plant

When you have finished observing the plant with your physical senses, take several deep breaths and relax your body. Allow your mental chatter to pass through your mind without any attachment to it. Bring your awareness to your heart and allow a sensation of love and gratitude to arise there. If it helps, you can think of a loved one to get the sensation started, then allow it to expand to include all beings and all of nature.

From this space, ask with a feeling of reverence for the assistance of the plant spirits. Be aware of your connection with the plant via your breath. Know that every breath you take in has been breathed out by the plants around you. It is an exchange of more than just gases. It is also an exchange of energy and frequency. It is evidence of your absolute interconnectedness.

You may want to either close your eyes and go into a meditative or relaxed state, or hold the plant in your gaze with a soft focus. Observe any of the following things that might arise.

Feelings: You may experience a sudden strong emotion that was not there before and that seems to be triggered by asking the plant for communication.

Knowing: This can be a thought, a feeling or both. You just suddenly 'know' something from a very deep place. There is no doubt or confusion. It is an absolute knowing.

Thoughts: You might get thoughts that pop into your mind that have a quality to them that you know is not your own. There might be a very clear instruction or a single word or some gentle reassurance. You may even be lovingly chastised in some way for inadvertently harming or offending the plant devas.

Images: You might go into a state of daydreaming with your eyes open or closed. From this state you may see images that lead you on a journey, or you may see a being that has come to give you a message or make a connection.

Sensations: You might simply begin to feel strong sensations in your body like heat or cold, buzzing, tingling or prickling. You might feel pulling or spinning sensations in certain parts of your body. These are the sensations associated with the activation of your chakras and meridians.

As you tune in to the plant energies, the energy in your body begins to shift in response, moving into a state of higher frequency as you move into higher bodies or planes. Allow any experience to unfold without judgement.

You may want to keep a journal recording your experiences, as it is very common for synchronicities and experiences to keep unfolding over days, weeks or years.

Imagination is the doorway

When people begin working with plants in this way, they try not to use their imagination for fear that they might 'make things up'. It's actually vitally important to allow your imagination free rein in this process, because you are working with energy, and it is your imagination that will give this energy form and meaning. The experience you have will be a combined experience coming from the energy field and imagination of both you and the plant.

Your imagination is the door you need to walk through to have access to non-physical experience. You will know if something is 'real' or significant because you will be affected by it. Physically, mentally or emotionally, you will feel an effect. This will be all the proof needed.

It can feel awkward when you first start working with plant energies, but the more familiar you become with this process, and the more you work with plant energies, the more natural and intuitive it becomes.

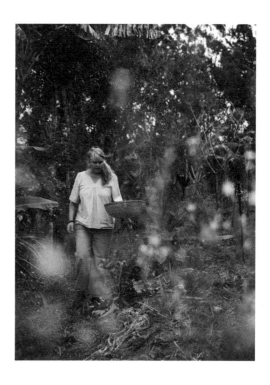

Making flower essences

For those who are drawn to them, making flower essences is very simple. They are very safe because they are 'vibrational' remedies, which means toxicity is not an issue. Vibrational remedies work by imprinting the energetic imprint of the plant onto water molecules. (For a beautiful visual understanding of this, you can explore Masaru Emoto's work with water.)

You can make an essence from any flower you are attracted to. However, it is important to approach the process with an intuitive understanding and awareness of nature and what you are doing.

Some plants want to share their essence and others do not. Before making an essence, spend time in a meditative state to communicate with the plant devas and ask for their guidance and permission on exactly what to do and which plant to use.

What you'll need

a small glass bowl
pure, fresh spring or mountain stream water, collected in a glass container if possible
muslin (cheesecloth) or a fine sieve for straining
brandy, vinegar (apple cider or Japanese plum vinegar are both good) or colloidal silver as a preservative; you can also use other alcohols, such as vodka, but brandy is traditional
a dark glass sterilised bottle (about 100 ml) to store your 'mother essence'
two (or more) 20–25 ml dropper bottles

Choosing your water

The water used in your flower essence is very significant. Ideally, you want water that has an energy field or charge to it. This makes clean stream or spring water the perfect source. Freshly caught rain water can also be used if it is from an unpolluted area. Ideally, catch fresh rain water in a glass bowl or jar and use it within a few days.

If you don't have access to clean spring or stream water, buy bottled spring water.

Do not use tap water, as it often comes from large dams where the water is chemically sterilised.

Choosing flowers for your essence

Before picking the flowers, use your intuition and ask for permission. You may 'hear' a word in your mind, see an image or get a 'gut feeling' or sense of the answer. Try to remain energetically neutral as you do this, and not to impart your own energy into the flowers. I find it helpful to stay in a state of gratitude for them; you can talk lovingly or sing to the flowers to help cultivate this. When you feel you have a connection, pick the flowers and place them in your glass bowl of spring water.

Harvesting the flowers

Some practitioners like to use scissors or leaves to pick the flowers, to avoid touching them as they drop into the bowl of water. Others feel fine to pick them with their hands.

This is not an infusion, so the flowers do not need to be immersed. You can cover the surface of the water with flowers, or just use as many as you have. For large flowers, you may use only one or two.

For a 'living' flower essence, fill your glass bowl with spring water and place the bowl among the still growing, unpicked flowers, with one or more of the flowers sitting in or just above the water.

The sun & sacred geometry

Leave your bowl and flowers in the sun for at least 2 hours, and up to 6 hours. You will get a stronger essence if you put the bowl and flowers in full sun for at least 2–4 hours.

I have also made storm and moon essences that felt very powerful.

If this is something you feel comfortable doing, you can stand in a labyrinth or spiral while making your flower essences. If you cannot create a labyrinth or spiral in your yard, print out a paper one and sit your bowl of flowers on that.

Making the flower essence 'mother'

When ready to strain, pour your flower water through a sieve lined with muslin (cheesecloth), into a sterilised jug.

Pour the water into your sterilised dark glass dropper bottle until it is half full. Fill the bottle to the top with your chosen preservative (brandy, vinegar or colloidal silver) and seal with the lid. The mixture in this dropper bottle is your 'mother essence'.

The mother essence is 50% flower essence water and 50% brandy or other preservative.

Flower essence stock bottles

The stock bottle is different from the dose bottle mentioned in the next paragraph. The stock bottle is the one a practitioner keeps in their clinic for making up flower essences. The stock bottle may sit in a dispensary for years, so the ratio of alcohol is higher to ensure a longer shelf life.

The dose bottle is the one the practitioner makes up for a patient who will use the drops over a period of weeks; it uses less alcohol so it tastes better, and because it doesn't need to last very long.

A stock bottle (used by the practitioner) uses two-thirds brandy. A dose bottle (given to the patient) uses one-third brandy or vinegar.

For a 25 ml stock bottle, you'd use roughly 8 ml water and 16 ml brandy (⅔ brandy, ⅓ water). To this you add either 4 or 7 drops of the 'mother essence'.

Flower essence dose bottles

To make a dose bottle to give to someone, fill a 25 ml bottle with two-thirds water (16 ml) and one-third (8 ml) brandy or vinegar. Add 4 or 7 drops from your stock bottle and your flower essence is now ready to use.

How to use a flower essence

Usually, drops of a flower essence are placed directly under the tongue or in a small glass of water to be sipped. You can also add them to your water bottle and drink throughout the day.

Some common dosages are:

- 7 drops morning and night, when you wake up and before bed
- 4 drops 3 times a day.

Remedies are most often used for 2–4 weeks. Some may be needed for months, or up to a year — or at regular intervals several times a year.

You can muscle test or use your intuition to guide you as to how many drops you use, based on whether the issue you are taking it for feels changed or resolved.

Plant spirit qualities

When making and using essences from the plants in this book, you can refer to the 'Plant Spirit Qualities' listed at the start of each chapter, but above all, always trust your own intuition and guidance, because a plant may have a use that is particular to you as an individual.

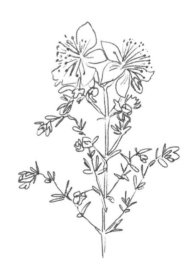

Equipment

You don't need lots of fancy gadgets to use wild plants in lots of different ways — whether as food or in herbal remedies. Here are some common kitchen items that will get the job done.

Cast-iron or stainless steel frying pan
A good-quality cast-iron frying pan is a great investment. As well as stovetop cooking and baking, they are amazing for campfire cooking (and even for cooking campfire cakes and breads). If properly cared for, they won't lose their surface or need to be replaced. As time goes on, they become seasoned and are less and less prone to sticking. Also, cooking in a cast-iron pan can bump up the iron content of your food, which is a good thing for most people — unless you have haemochromatosis (a condition caused by excess iron absorption).

If you don't want the extra iron, stainless steel is also a good choice and will become non-stick if used properly and seasoned. These pans do a great job of frying but are generally not as good for campfire baking.

Jug blender
When living with nature and eating natural foods, a blender is a godsend. There are now so many portable and rechargeable options that you can literally take one anywhere you go. They're great for making both food and herbal medicines — and a quick smoothie of fruit and 'weeds' is one of the simplest and most nutritious meals you can have!

Stick blender
I use my stick blender as much as my jug blender. Stick blenders are great for quick sauces that can be made in a Pyrex jug. They're also good for smaller quantities of plants, where you don't have enough to put in a jug blender.

Food processor
When making whole foods, a food processor is really handy for grinding nuts, seeds and wild plants, and for making nut-based pastry.

Hand-held mixer
An electric hand-held mixer is essential for making icing, and recipes such as vegan marshmallows (see page 220) that use aquafaba (the liquid from a tin of chickpeas).

Coffee grinder
I don't even drink coffee, but I use my coffee grinder constantly — to grind wild seeds into flour; dried herbs into powder for capsules, infused oils or for adding to smoothies; and grinding dried mugwort into powder for moxa.

Mortar and pestle
If you don't have a blender or coffee grinder, a mortar and pestle is the next best thing for grinding fresh and dried herbs and spices. Asian grocery shops usually supply them. Get a good granite one that can handle anything, and keep it on the bench.

Pyrex measuring jug
A Pyrex measuring jug (or one made from clear oven-safe glass) is a very versatile and useful piece of equipment. You will use it over and over for cooking meals and making herbal preparations, and using it as a bain marie for melting waxes for ointments and creams.

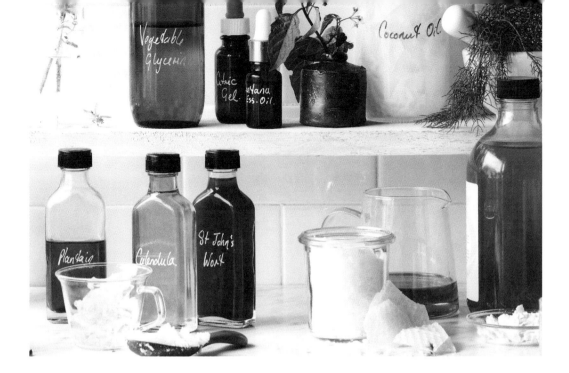

A good pot (or billy)

I'm assuming you have a good pot. Please tell me you have a good pot. A good pot is the cornerstone of human civilisation. You will need it to make soup, steam vegetables and weeds, melt waxes, brew herbal teas, and make steam for inhalations. A billy is a beloved campfire pot, and I know more than one person who has used the same billy for decades and wouldn't go anywhere without it.

Sieve

If you're making herbal medicines, or a good cup of tea, then a sieve is pretty vital. Many methods of herbal medicine-making require the extraction of the herbal constituents in a menstrum (liquid used to extract the herbs) that is then strained. This includes infused oils, glycetracts, teas and decoctions.

Muslin

You can use muslin (cheesecloth) to line your sieve to provide a finer grade of filtration, resulting in a cleaner and smoother medicine. It's also good for making vegan cheese and nut milks.

Recycled jars

A good variety of recycled jars can store your food and medicine for days, weeks or years. Keep a good supply of different sizes. Make sure to label them with what you put inside.

Amber bottles and jars

These are ideal for storing your finished herbal medicines because the darker glass protects them from light and heat, which causes them to oxidise and deteriorate more quickly. It's good to have a few different sizes. While amber bottles and jars are ideal, don't let not having one stop you from making herbal medicines. Clear glass can be stored in a cool, dark cupboard or in the fridge to get the same effect.

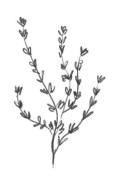

Ingredients & raw materials

For this book, I've tried to keep this ingredients list as simple as possible, and to reuse the same base ingredients in as many recipes as possible, so you don't have to keep sourcing new products. Many of these ingredients can be bought from the same supplier, to save on shipping.

Waxes

Waxes provide the structure and firmness of balms, salves and ointments. They also create a waterproof barrier on the skin, protecting it against infection and excess moisture. They are also long lasting and help preserve the herbs suspended in them.

Olivem 1000

A combination of fatty acids derived from olive oil, olivem 1000 is a 100% plant-based emulsifying wax that is similar in composition to the oils naturally found on the surface of our skin — and it also spreads well on the skin, with a nice, non-greasy moisturising effect. It is a good emulsifier that can be used in water and oil combinations such as creams and lotions, as well as balms and ointments.

Sunflower wax

Made from pure sunflower oil, sunflower wax is a vegan emollient — meaning it maintains moisture on the skin's surface. It helps provide texture and firmness to balms and ointments, without the need for preservatives. It is also GMO free, contains no trans fats, and can be sustainably produced.

Beeswax

Beeswax has a long history in medicine making for its texture, antimicrobial and preservative qualities, and its ability to act as a carrier for medicinal oils and resins. With bee populations around the world in danger from habitat loss, pesticides and disease, I have not used beeswax in this book, but if you have your own source of healthy bees, or are able to source beeswax ethically and locally, you can substitute it for other waxes.

Butters

Vegetable butters act as emollients that retain moisture and soften and protect the skin. As well as helping moisten the skin, they provide a nice smooth, creamy texture, and often a nice fragrance as well.

Cocoa butter

Cocoa butter is a firm yellow butter obtained from the cocoa seed. Its firmness makes it ideal for use in pessaries, suppositories and lip balms because it holds its shape. It is an excellent emollient, retains moisture, and softens and protects the skin. It is high in vitamin E and is a good carrier for herbs and oils.

Shea butter

Also known as karité, shea butter comes from the fat found in the kernels of seeds from the shea tree found in East and West Africa. Shea butter has long been used as a moisturiser to protect skin and hair from extreme heat or cold. Shea is an excellent emollient and is particularly useful for dry, ageing and damaged skin. It is the best lip balm I have ever used and the only thing that prevents me getting cold sores from wind, sun and snow. It looks beautiful and is an ingredient in many creams, balms and hair products, though it can be used on its own very effectively. It can be sourced organically and sustainably in a purified form.

Gels

Gels are useful when you want to cool the skin, for instance in cases of burns and inflammation. They dry matte and have a soothing, cooling quality. Many creams and ointments trap heat in the skin, aggravating 'hot' conditions like burns, inflamed eczema or rosacea. Gels are cooling and soothe inflammation.

Aloe vera gel

Rich in vitamins, minerals and amino acids, this soothing gel is extracted from the leaf of the *Aloe barbadensis* plant. The skin of the leaf is removed and the clear gel inside is extracted. The cooling and hydrating gel soothes and restores dry and damaged skin and is often used for sunburn, minor burns, windburn and shaving rashes. It is also good for bites, stings and pain or inflammation on the skin. It tones and heals acne-prone skin, and helps with eczema and psoriasis. You can use it directly from the plant, or buy an organic gel. However, most purchased gels contain preservatives to stop decomposition.

Laponite gel

Laponite gel is a man-made, clay-based gelling agent made from silica and minerals. It is a mixture of natural earth oxides that have been milled to fine particles that, when added to water, produce a stiff gel that holds its shape and dries smooth and matte when applied to the skin. It holds tinctures, plant juices, and essential and infused oils. It remains stable much longer than fresh aloe vera gel, and can be stored in the fridge for up to a year in some cases. It is ideal where there is heat and inflammation in the skin that can be exacerbated by oily substances. It is one of my favourite ways to apply plant juices directly to the skin.

Oils

Vegetable oils (like olive oil, rice bran oil, almond oil, and so on) have a wide range of benefits including softening the skin, improving circulation in the tissues below the skin, and protecting the skin from the damaging effects of environmental pollution and some of the effects of sun damage. Many also have healing properties and reduce scarring and inflammation. Vegetable oils act as a great carrier for herbal constituents, in particular essential oils and resins, which can be extracted by infusing herbs in oil to use as a base for balms, salves and ointments.

Castor oil

Castor oil is derived from the seeds of the castor bean plant (*Ricinus communis*, a.k.a. castor seed).

Castor oil improves lymphatic drainage, blood flow and thymus gland health, making it highly beneficial for the immune system. Its effect on the lymphatic system also improves overall circulation to major organs such as the heart and lungs.

Due to its anti-inflammatory, pain-relieving properties, castor oil is often used as a natural treatment for arthritis pain, joint swelling and inflammation, and can be applied directly to aching joints, muscles or tissues or used in a castor oil pack by putting a cloth and a hot water bottle over the area. It can also help with wounds and pressure ulcers, thanks to its moisturising and antimicrobial, antifungal and antibacterial properties.

Castor oil has long been used as a home remedy for constipation when taken internally. On the skin, castor oil can relieve dryness or irritation by preventing water loss. For acne, it penetrates deep into the skin, softening and hydrating the skin and fighting bacterial overgrowth that can clog pores. Clinical trials have confirmed that it is also effective against *Staphylococcus aureus*, which is linked to the development of acne.

It is also thought to improve hair growth by increasing blood circulation to hair follicles. Be sure to avoid getting it in your eyes.

Rice bran oil

Rice bran oil is rich in tocotrienols, the compounds in vitamin E involved in immune function and blood vessel health. It also contains oryzanol, which has been shown to suppress several enzymes that promote inflammation. Its plant sterols and poly- and mono-unsaturated fats (the 'good fats') have been studied for their health benefits in lowering cholesterol levels and reducing the risk of type 2 diabetes. These plant sterols help reduce the risk of heart disease, obesity and heart attack.

On the skin, its anti-ageing action and antioxidant properties combat the harmful effects of free radicals responsible for ageing. It moisturises skin cells, promotes blood circulation, protects against ultraviolet radiation and pollution, and reduces skin inflammation and scarring. Its non-greasy feel on the skin is pleasant. I like using rice bran oil as a base ingredient for infused oils because its clear colour and minimal scent makes it easy to assess how much herb has been extracted into the oil. When making large batches of an infused oil, its low cost is also helpful.

Olive oil

Extracted from the fruit of the olive tree (*Olea europaea*), olive oil is naturally high in healthy monounsaturated fatty acids (MUFAs). These fatty acids are linked to a variety of health benefits associated with a Mediterranean diet, including improved circulation and a lower incidence of atherosclerosis and cardiovascular disease, improved cholesterol and triglyceride levels. They are also associated with reduced risk of weight gain, obesity, insulin resistance and type 2 diabetes.

The polyphenols in extra virgin olive oil are considered anti-inflammatory and help to slow the effects of ageing in the heart and blood vessels, thereby reducing age-related cognitive decline and neurodegeneration.

The brain requires a high level of the fatty acids in olive oil for memory, focus, clear thinking and mood regulation. Extra virgin olive oil contains antioxidants called secoiridoids, which help

switch on genes that contribute to anti-ageing effects and reduce cellular stress.

On the skin, olive oil provides deep hydration, reduces inflammation and swelling, reduces the appearance of fine lines and wrinkles, and lessens the effects of sun damage, although it does not have a high enough SPF to use as a sunscreen on its own. It also reduces puffiness, and helps soothe dry or irritated skin, as well as balance oily skin.

Coconut oil

This edible oil is extracted from the meat of matured coconuts. While often touted as a 'healthy' fat, it is still a saturated fat, and has the capacity to increase blood cholesterol and triglycerides if over-consumed. A small amount is healthy as part of a balanced whole food diet.

This oil is rich in medium-chain fatty acids (MCFAs), in particular a type called lauric acid, which contributes to the oil's anti-inflammatory, antimicrobial and antifungal properties. Lauric acid reacts with saliva to form a soap-like substance that can help reduce cavities, dental plaque build-up and gum disease.

Being mildly antibacterial, it has been shown to reduce inflammation and help heal certain skin conditions, including fungal infections, eczema, psoriasis and dermatitis. It is an excellent emollient that helps retain moisture in the skin. On the hair, it helps repair damage from heat and chemical treatments.

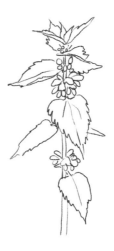

Solvents

Solvents such as glycerine, vinegar and alcohol are used to extract and preserve the active phytochemicals (plant compounds) found in medicinal plants, so they can be consumed as herbal preparations and stored for long periods.

Vegetable glycerine

Also known as glycerol or glycerin, vegetable glycerine is a clear liquid typically made from soy bean, coconut or palm oils. Glycerine can also be derived from animal products or petroleum, so check to make sure you have a sustainable, organic, plant-sourced product. Vegetable glycerine is odourless, and has a mild, sweet taste with a syrup-like consistency.

It has a variety of uses internally, including keeping athletes hydrated for longer, improving their endurance and performance. As a laxative, it helps counter constipation.

Vegetable glycerine also assists in the treatment of some types of glaucoma, taken orally as an osmotic agent, reducing build-up of pressure in the eyes by drawing fluid out of the tissue; it can also be used in a weak solution as eye drops to counter irritation and pain.

Glycerine is commonly used in skin care products for its excellent emollient, softening, smoothing and moisture-retaining properties. These properties are helpful in treating dry, rough, cracked and irritated skin, as well as eczema, psoriasis, oily skin, acne, minor skin infections, wrinkles, redness and fine lines. It also speeds the healing of bruises and inflamed tissues.

Vegetable glycerine is very safe and gentle because it's an inert, non-toxic, non-irritant and non-reactant solvent. Preparations can be made for the most sensitive areas of the body as an antiseptic or analgesic, including the mucous membranes of the vagina and nasal passages. It's also gentle enough to use on damaged tissue from burns or injury.

Chemically, glycerine is a sugar alcohol, primarily derived from animal and plant sources. Sugar alcohol does not contain the ethanol found in alcoholic beverages, so it can be used by

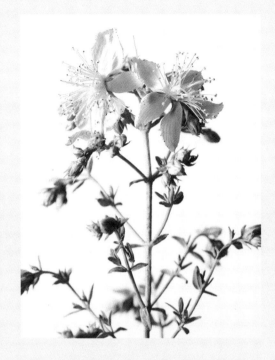

people who avoid alcohol. Also, despite the fact that it is called a 'sugar' alcohol, it is actually metabolised as a fat rather than a sugar, so it is generally safe for many diabetics.

Glycerine is ideal for extracting herbal constituents and preserving microorganisms that would otherwise be destroyed due to the sterilising and denaturing property of alcohol. This is particularly beneficial in the gut for maintaining a strong and diverse microbiome to assist with digestion and the assimilation of nutrients. Vegetable glycerine preserves aromatics, enzymes and polysaccharides, maintaining their taste and structural integrity.

It is also an effective solvent that can extract a wide range of herbal constituents (including most alkaloids, glycosides, volatile oils, waxes, resins, gums, balsam, polysaccharides, vitamins and minerals). Glycerine preserves herbal constituents for up to 1–2 years, so they can be used over longer periods than those obtained from fresh plants.

Apple cider vinegar

Made from fermented apples, apple cider vinegar is rich in acetic acid, B vitamins, polyphenols (plant-based antioxidants) and probiotics. It helps lower blood glucose levels and (along with dietary change and other supportive medicines) can be useful in managing insulin resistance and diabetes. In conjunction with a mildly calorie-restricted diet and an exercise plan, it helps reduce appetite and improve weight loss.

Apple cider vinegar is rich in minerals, in particular potassium, which is used in cellular transport, metabolism, respiration, blood health and nerve function. It is mildly antiseptic and may have a cooling effect where there is excess heat and inflammation on the skin.

For over 5000 years, apple cider vinegar has been used as a solvent to extract herbal medicines in the place of alcohol. It is only recently that the commercial benefits of preserving herbs in alcohol (such as stronger extraction of active constituents and greater shelf life) have led to widespread use of alcoholic tinctures.

For the home herbalist today, using apple cider vinegar as a solvent offers a cheaper and better-tasting alternative to commercial tinctures — one that is safe for all members of the community.

Apple cider vinegar is also better at extracting mucilage (which is poorly extracted in alcohol), which helps bring up mucus from the lungs, reduces coughing and improves breathing. It also assists the actions of stimulants, internally and externally, and supports the function of tonics and astringents.

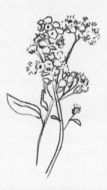

While pure alkaloids — highly active plant constituents with anti-inflammatory, analgesic, antimicrobial and antifungal properties — are not water soluble, alkaloid salts (formed when alkaloids bind with the acetic acid in vinegar) are soluble. Alcohol may produce a stronger alkaloid preparation, but in many cases, vinegar works sufficiently well as a solvent for healing a wide range of common ailments.

Preservatives

Preservatives have antimicrobial properties that stop herbal preparations becoming mouldy and rancid, prolonging their shelf life. Preservatives used by home herbalists include tincture of benzoin (benzoin is a resin collected from *Styrax benzoin* trees), citricidal (made from citrus seed extract), essential oils, glycerine, alcohol and honey. Preservatives are particularly important when making creams, as their water component makes them more susceptible to microbial contamination.

Citricidal

This potent antimicrobial is made from grapefruit seed extract and will help stop remedies spoiling due to microbial contamination.

If you find that citricidal isn't strong enough to prevent your creams spoiling, try adding an additional 5–10 drops of tincture of benzoin or essential oil per 100 g of cream.

Essential oils

Essential oils have many healing benefits, including being antimicrobial, anti-inflammatory, wound healing, improving circulation, and reducing scarring and pain. Many help calm the nervous system, reducing stress and anxiety. They also smell lovely and act as preservatives, improving the shelf life of herbal remedies.

Lavender *Lavandula angustifolia* (formerly *L. officinalis* or *L. vera*), *Lavandula latifolia*

Lavender oil is antiseptic and anti-inflammatory. It is wound healing, reduces scarring, soothes dry skin and is useful for minor burns and fungal or bacterial infections. It also relaxes the nervous system and reduces headaches, anxiety and insomnia.

Tea tree *Melaleuca alternifolia*

Tea tree oil, being antibacterial, antifungal and anti-inflammatory, is commonly used to treat acne, athlete's foot, lice, nail fungus and insect bites. It is generally useful for infections of the skin.

Lemon eucalyptus *Corymbia citriodora;* also known as *Eucalyptus citriodora*

Corymbia citriodora contains over 75% citronellal, a natural compound used in many mosquito repellents. This makes it a wonderful insect repellent. It is anti-inflammatory, antifungal, antiseptic, antibacterial and analgesic, and has calming properties that make it useful for meditation.

When used in an air diffuser, it can reduce exposure to airborne viruses by capturing them in the oil particles and deactivating them before they are inhaled.

When used as a surface disinfectant, it reduces bacterial infection and eliminates stale odours.

Frankincense *Boswellia serrata*; also known as olibanum

Frankincense has a long history of use in spiritual rituals and is still used today in various religious ceremonies. Its comforting and calming qualities make it ideal for reducing stress, stilling the mind and deepening meditation.

It strengthens the immune system against colds and flus, and inhalation can help relieve respiratory symptoms associated with bronchitis, congestion and asthma (along with other medication). When used topically for sprains, strains and minor inflammation, it is anti-inflammatory. It helps reduce skin blemishes, wrinkles, stretch marks, scars and minor wounds, and can balance oily or dry skin.

Rosemary *Rosmarinus officinalis*

Rosemary can increase blood circulation. It also improves blood supply to the brain, where it has the effect of improving memory and concentration.

As an anti-inflammatory it relieves pain in muscles and joints, and soothes headaches. It is also a natural insecticide.

In the respiratory system its antiseptic, antibacterial and antifungal properties help with colds, chest infections and allergies.

On the skin it prevents acne, and its antioxidant properties help reduce the appearance of wrinkles and age spots.

On the hair, its effect of increasing circulation in the scalp assists with hair growth and reduces dandruff, and the oil improves hair quality.

German chamomile *Matricaria chamomilla*

This deep blue oil is rich in a compound called bisabolol, which is known to have anti-irritant, anti-inflammatory, analgesic and antimicrobial properties. As such, it is highly effective for healing damaged skin, reducing the appearance of wrinkles, and as a treatment for acne due to its ability to reduce the number of bacteria on the skin. It helps reduces pain from muscle spasms, and can be used for burns, rashes and insect bites. For anxiety and restlessness, it is relaxing and calming and soothing.

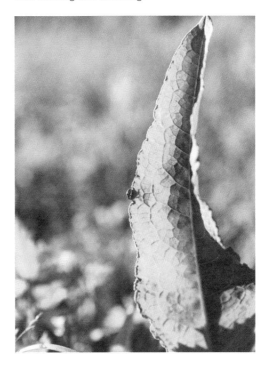

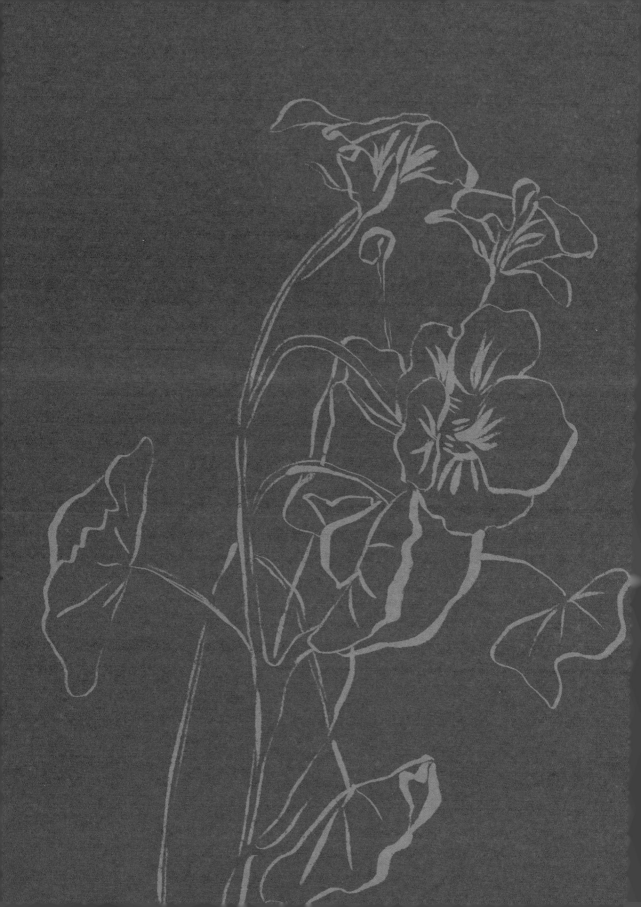

PART 3

Recipes

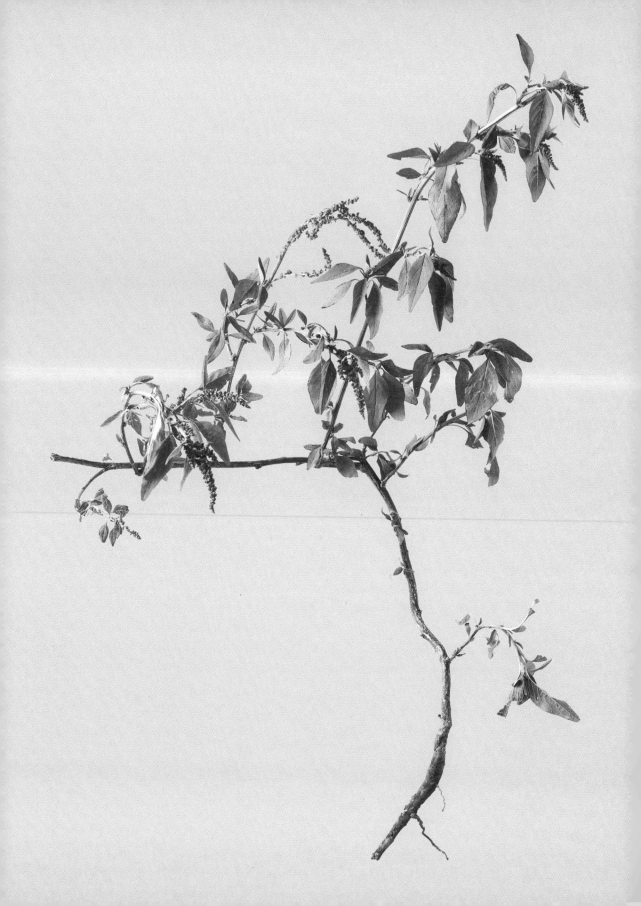

Amaranth

COMMON NAMES:

amaranth, pigweed

SPECIES:

There are over 60 *Amaranthus* species.
Common varieties include *A. blitum* (purple
and green), *A. viridis* (green and purple),
A. tricolor (domesticated purple flower,
multicoloured leaf) and *A. retroflexus*
(green leaf and flower, red root).

GENUS:

Amaranthus

FAMILY:

Amaranthaceae

DISTRIBUTION:

Native to North and South America.
Found in Europe, Asia, Africa, Australia
and New Zealand.

PLANT SPIRIT QUALITIES:

Amaranth is the plant of abundance, of all
needs being met. It helps you know you are
enough, you have enough, you do enough.
It will help you be more generous in giving
to yourself and others. Amaranth contains
all the essential amino acids — the building
blocks of protein that create new body cells.
Key word — abundance.

How to identify it

- The most characteristic feature of the amaranth plant is its flowering green or purple head, which has the distinctive slender, axillary to terminal paniculate spikes (a cluster of flowers with the youngest nearest to the top).

- Smaller spikes are located in the leaf axils below the spikes.

- The leaves grow in an alternate pattern and are ovate to lance-shaped, with distinct veins. They range from dull green to shiny or reddish green.

- The stems are erect, growing from 6–200 cm (2½ inches to 6 feet) tall.

- Stems are simple or branched, with a lower part that is thick and smooth, and an upper part that is usually rough with dense, short hair. They are greenish to slightly reddish, but usually red near the roots.

- The redroot amaranth (*Amaranthus retroflexus*) has a distinctive red root.

How to harvest

Seeds

Once the seed heads have turned from green or purple to brown, or once you can shake the flower head and seeds fall into your hand, the seeds are ready to harvest. If the flowering heads are really large, you can cut them and gently shake and massage them over a large bowl. There are often little insects; go gently so they are not damaged and can be placed back into the garden. You can also hang the seed head upside down with a bag wrapped around it for a few days.

Once you have collected all the seeds, you can winnow them by shaking the bowl gently and blowing off the husks and repeating until the husks are gone — or almost gone, depending on your level of patience.

If there is any moisture in the grains, it is good to spread them out in a dry place to dry for a day or two, or put them in a dehydrator overnight. Making sure they're completely dry before storing will reduce the risk of mould growing.

Once the grains are dry, store them in an airtight glass container. A recycled glass jar is perfect. Label it with the name of the grain and the date of harvesting.

Leaves

Amaranth leaves can be harvested all year. They are best collected in the morning when they are fresh and full of moisture.

You can use a sharp pair of scissors, or gently use your fingers to cut the leaves just above where the leaf meets the stem.

Generally, it's best to pick leaves from the bottom of the plant if you want to continue to harvest from the same plant.

Rinse the leaves in water to remove dirt or debris. Shake in a colander or pat with a towel to dry.

Use fresh, or freeze the leaves for later use.

Nutrients

Amaranth is one of the few plants containing high quantities of all the essential amino acids, making it a source of complete protein. It is one of the few grains to be high in lysine. It is also high in complex carbohydrates, minerals, vitamins (including several antioxidants) and fatty acids, making it a complete source of nutrition.

One cup (246 g) of cooked amaranth contains the following macronutrients: calories 251, protein 9.3 g, carbohydrate 46 g, fat 5.2 g. It also contains the minerals manganese, magnesium, phosphorus, iron, selenium and copper.

Culinary use

Amaranth has a large culinary use worldwide.

Native to Peru, it was a major food crop of the Aztecs, with some estimates suggesting it was domesticated between 6000 and 8000 years ago. The Aztecs used the grains as part of their religious ceremonies. When Hernán Cortés invaded the Aztecs' land in the 16th century, the Spanish outlawed amaranth on the grounds that it was being used in heathen ceremonies.

However, the plant prevailed and continued to be used in Africa, India and Nepal. Over the last twenty years, its use has spread to China, Russia, Thailand, Nigeria, Mexico, South America and the Western world, where it is sold in supermarkets and health food stores.

In Cambodia it is called *ptee*, and the leaf is used in cooking and to dip in a sauce called *tuk kroeung*. In India it has many names and is used in many dishes. It is eaten raw, cooked and in curries and bhajis. In Afghanistan and Pakistan it is called *ganhar*.

In Africa, in the Bantu-speaking regions of Uganda, it is known as *doodo*, and is commonly cooked with onions and tomatoes, or sometimes mixed with a peanut sauce.

It is called *mchicha* in Swahili.

In Kenya it is known as *terere* among the Kikuyu, Embu and Meru people, and *telele* by the Kamba people.

In Indonesia, it is known as *bayam*, in Thailand as *phak khom*, and in Suriname, *klaroen*.

In the West the seed is cooked and used as a cereal substitute in cakes and porridges.

Folk medicine

American herbalist Michael Moore recommends using the dried plant as an astringent, and the fresh plant as a cooling poultice. He suggests a tablespoon of chopped fresh leaves in a tea for the flu or gastroenteritis, and a douche made from a handful of fresh leaves in a pint of water for vaginal itching and inflammation.

The following species of amaranth are used in some countries for the following conditions.

Amaranthus blitum
The boiled leaves and roots are given as a laxative, and are also applied as an emollient poultice to abscesses, boils and burns. Root juice with sugar or molasses is traditionally given in dysentery.

Amaranthus viridis
The plant is cooling, antibiotic and laxative. It relieves stomach ache, stimulates the appetite and brings down fevers. It is used to soothe burning sensations, hallucination, leprosy, bronchitis, piles, leucorrhoea (white vaginal discharge) and constipation. The leaves are used as an emollient. The root is heating and an expectorant. It lessens the menstrual flow and excessive or discoloured vaginal discharge.

Amaranthus tricolor
The plant is cooling, antibiotic and laxative. It relieves constipation and stomach ache, stimulates the appetite and reduces fever. It is used to soothe burning sensations, hallucination, leprosy, bronchitis, piles and reduce excessive or discoloured vaginal discharge.

Research

Clinical trials on *Amaranthus* spp. have been done in the following areas: antibiotic,[1] anti-thrombotic,[2] anti-inflammatory, coronary heart disease and hypertension,[3] antioxidant[4] and diabetes.[5]

How to use it as a medicine

The root and leaves are used internally as a powder, infusion or decoction. Externally, the leaves and roots are used as a poultice.

CAUTIONS AND CONTRAINDICATIONS
Some species can cause allergies. More than a cup of raw fresh leaves eaten over several consecutive days can cause high levels of oxalates and nitrates to accumulate. Cooking leaves and grains makes them safe for regular long-term consumption.

Amaranth porridge

SERVES 2–4
30 MINUTES

GF

1 cup (200 g) amaranth grain

2 cups (500 ml) water or milk of your choice; if you soak the amaranth overnight you only need 1 cup (250 ml) liquid

Amaranth is a pseudo-grain rather than a cereal, making it gluten and grain free. It is also packed with protein, helping you power through your morning.

You can make this awesome super porridge as simple or as fancy as you please with the addition of your favourite toppings — any combination of milk, cream, yoghurt, your favourite fruits, sweeteners and spices such as cinnamon, ginger, cardamom or turmeric, or your favourite nuts and seeds.

I prefer to soak amaranth grain in cold water overnight to improve its digestibility. After soaking for 8–12 hours, simply drain and rinse and it's ready to cook.

Add the amaranth and half the milk to a saucepan. Bring to the boil, stirring frequently, then reduce the heat and simmer for 10–15 minutes, stirring now and then.

Once the milk is absorbed, pour in the remaining milk and continue to stir for another 10–15 minutes, until it has been absorbed again.

When cooked, the amaranth has a slightly grainy, gelatinous texture, and the grain can be firm on the outside and soft in the middle. It tastes a bit like the cob of sweet corn.

Serve with your favourite toppings.

Note

Because amaranth porridge takes a relatively long time to cook, I like to make one big batch for the week and store it in the fridge. That way it only needs to be reheated, or in summer can be eaten cold. It will last 3–5 days covered in the fridge.

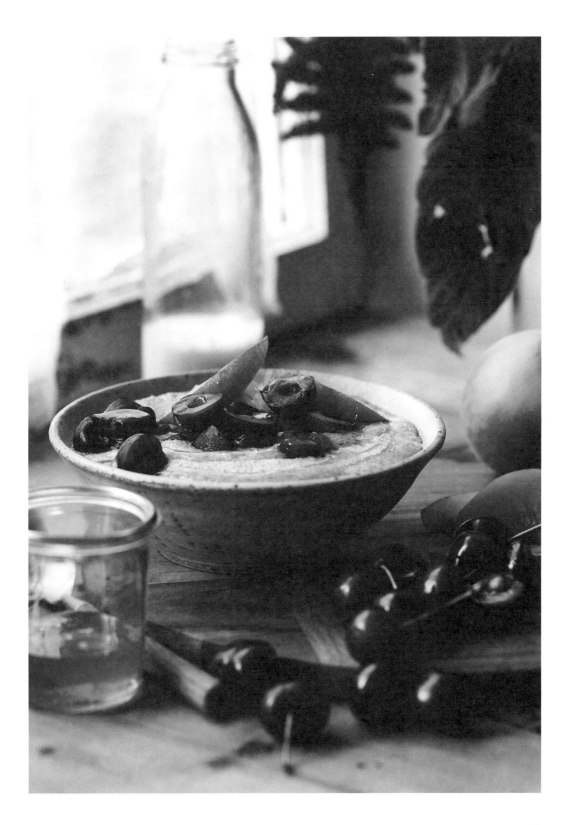

Amaranth-crusted tofu

SERVES 4
50 MINUTES

GF

1 cup (100 g) cooked amaranth grains
400 g (14 oz) firm tofu

GOCHUJANG SAUCE

2 tablespoons gochujang paste (Korean chilli paste)
2 tablespoons rice vinegar
1 tablespoon sesame oil
1 tablespoon maple syrup

LEMONY AMARANTH LEAVES

4 handfuls of fresh amaranth leaves
2 tablespoons lemon juice
1 teaspoon olive oil

This flavourful dish uses both the grain and leaves of the amaranth plant. It is packed with protein and minerals from the amaranth and tofu, and is a good one to make if you have any left-over amaranth porridge (page 58) in the fridge. I like to garnish the dish with sliced spring onion (scallion), shallot or red capsicum (pepper).

The lemony amaranth leaves are a delicious side dish for just about any meal. Enjoy them hot straight away, or let them marinate in the fridge for up to 3 days, to add to salad bowls for lunches.

Heat the oven to 180°C (350°F). Line a baking tray with baking paper.

Mix all the gochujang sauce ingredients together in a small bowl. Add the amaranth and mix well to coat the grains.

Cut the tofu into 6 slices, then coat all over with the saucy grains, smearing the mixture on thickly. Carefully transfer to the baking tray.

Bake for 25–30 minutes, until the coating looks slightly firmer; don't try to turn the tofu during baking, as the coating may fall off. It will still be a bit soft, but will look baked and crispy on the edges.

Just before serving, prepare the lemony amaranth leaves. In a pan, bring 2 cups (500 ml) water to the boil and blanch the amaranth leaves for 30–60 seconds. Drain in a colander, then return to the pan and mix the lemon juice and olive oil through. Season to taste.

Remove the tofu from the tray using a spatula. Serve on a bed of rice or salad greens, with a side of lemony amaranth leaves.

Wilted wild greens

SERVES 4 AS A SIDE DISH
15 MINUTES

GF

3 handfuls of roughly chopped wild greens
2 tablespoons lemon juice
2 teaspoons olive oil
2 lightly sautéed garlic cloves (optional)

You can use any wild greens growing around you — such as a mix of amaranth leaves, nettles, nasturtium, purslane, cobbler's pegs, nodding top, plantain, oxalis, chickweed, blackberry nightshade leaves, fat hen, cleavers, wild garlic and dandelion.

Great garnishes include pine nuts, toasted almond slivers and preserved lemon.

In a large saucepan, bring 4 cups (1 litre) water to a rolling boil. Add the leaves and blanch for 30 seconds.

Drain the leaves in a colander, tip them into a bowl and gently toss the remaining ingredients through. Season to taste and serve.

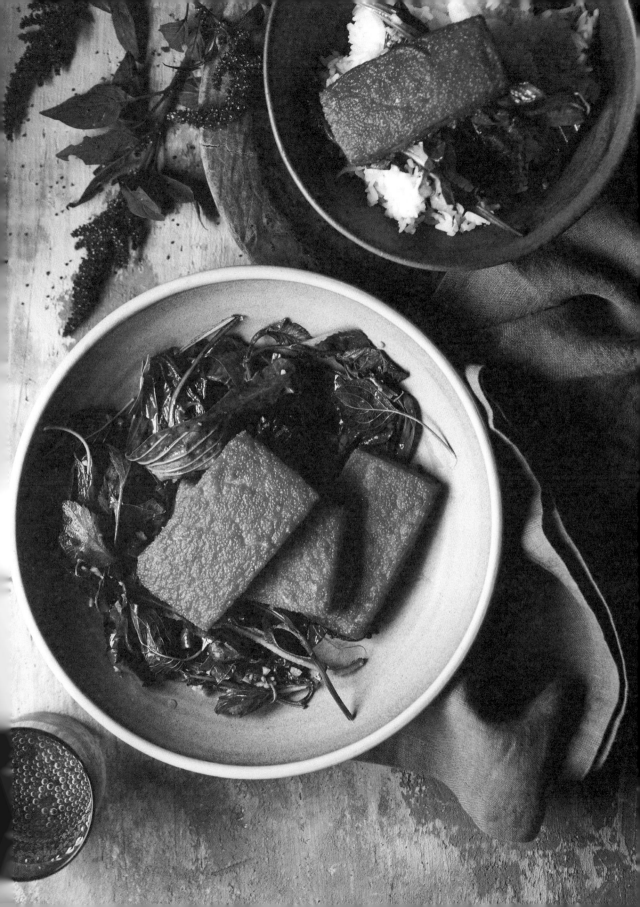

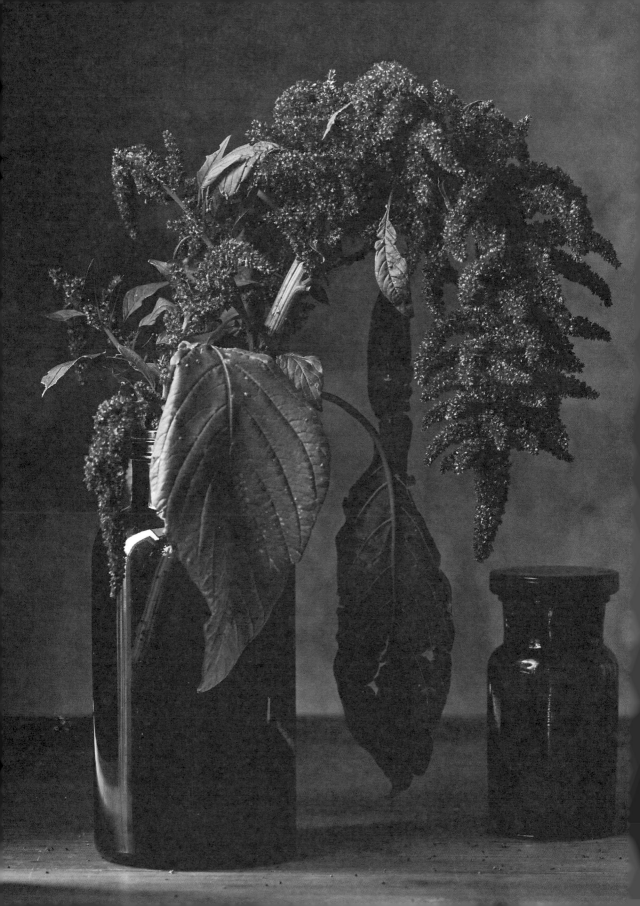

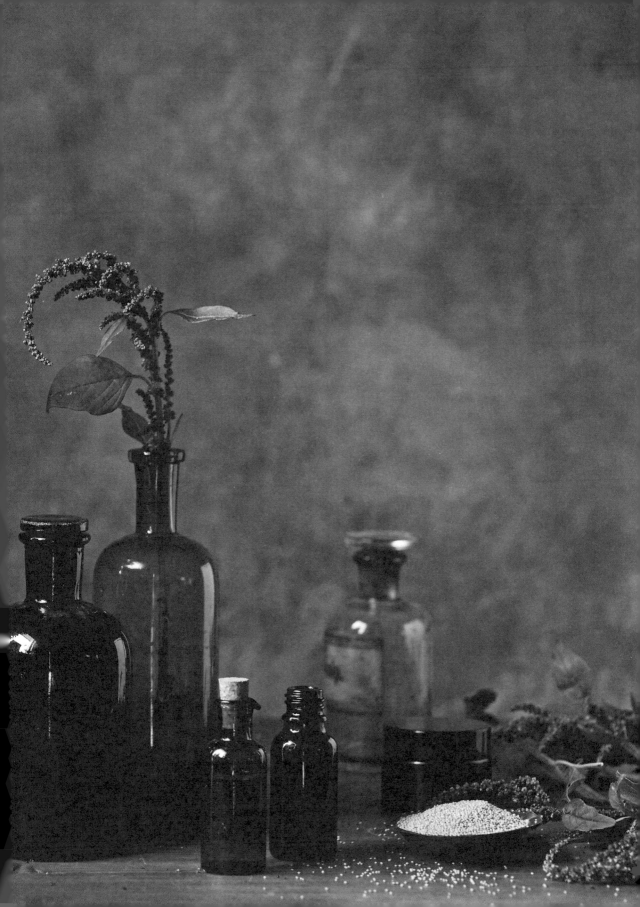

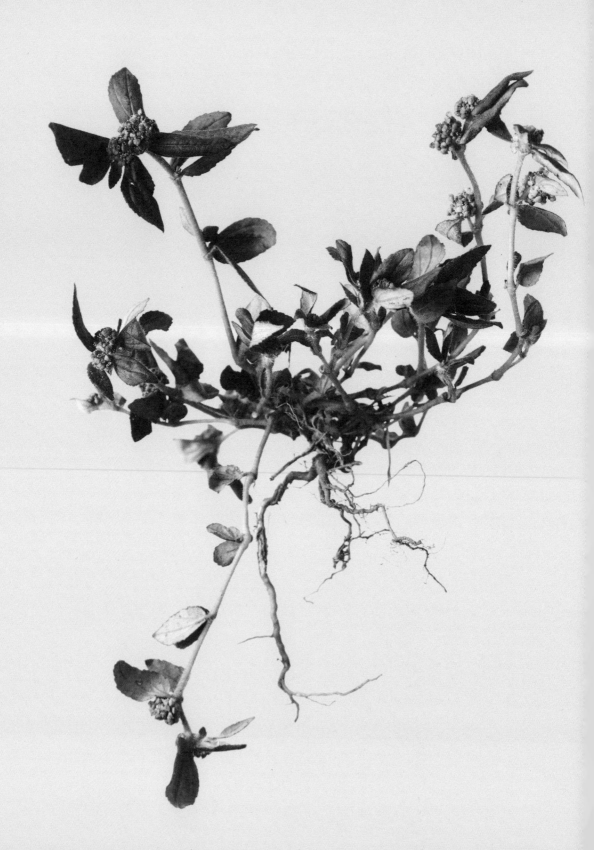

Asthma weed

COMMON NAMES:

asthma weed, euphorbia

Parietaria judaica (known as pellitory), is also called asthma weed, but is a different plant.

SPECIES:

Euphorbia hirta

GENUS:

Euphorbia

FAMILY:

Euphorbiaceae

DISTRIBUTION:

Originated in the southern US and Mexico. It is now pantropical, as it is so widely distributed throughout the tropical regions of the world.

PLANT SPIRIT QUALITIES:

Asthma weed helps us to 'let go' of emotional burdens such as guilt, fear and grief. Asthma weed is there to set us free — to guide us to a safe place where we no longer need to hold on to pain. You can use this as an essence if someone is having a panic attack, by rubbing it on their crown or heart. **Key words — letting go, reassurance, trust.**

How to identify it

- Asthma weed is an erect or prostrate annual herb that can grow up to 60 cm (2 feet) long.
- It has a solid, hairy stem that produces a white latex. Stems can be green or pink.
- There are stipules present (tiny leaves in pairs at the base of the leaf stalk).
- The leaves are simple, oval-shaped, hairy on both the upper and lower surfaces (but particularly on the veins underneath the leaf), with a finely dentate (serrated) margin.
- Leaves occur in opposite pairs on the stem, and can be dark green or a reddish/purple colour.
- The flowers are unisexual and are found in an inflorescence (a cluster at each leaf node). They look like little pompoms occurring at each leaf node.
- Flowers lack petals and are generally on a stalk.
- The fruit is a capsule with three valves, and produces tiny, oblong, four-sided red seeds.
- The plant has a white or brown taproot.

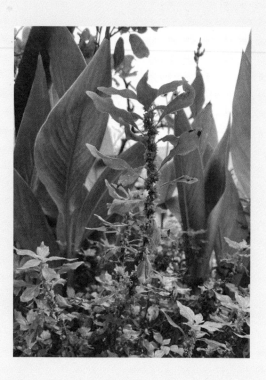

How to harvest

Asthma weed grows abundantly and is often found in disturbed areas such as roadsides, gardens and waste grounds. As these areas are often contaminated with pollution, herbicides, pesticides and dog faeces, make sure you have healthy plants that are not contaminated (see guidelines for safe wildcrafting on page 16).

For medicinal use and drying, the best time to harvest asthma weed is during its flowering stage, typically in late spring or early summer. At this stage, the plant's active constituents are most potent. For culinary and fresh plant use, the young leaves are best harvested in early spring.

It's a good idea to wear gloves and long sleeves while handling asthma weed, as its milky sap can cause skin irritation in some individuals.

Use secateurs or sharp scissors to cut the stems just above ground level. You can harvest the entire plant; however, the leaves, stems and flowers are the most potent parts for medicinal use.

Plants can be used fresh, or dried for later use.

Nutrients

Protein, beta-carotene, vitamin C, sodium, potassium, calcium, sulphur, phosphorus, iron, manganese, copper and zinc.

Culinary use

Fresh young leaves and stems can be cooked as a pot herb. They are best eaten in small amounts (about a handful) in chutneys or as a cooked vegetable. Don't eat daily for more than a couple of weeks as it may cause gastric irritation if used too often.

Parietaria judaica (pictured in the undergrowth) is also called 'asthma weed' (or 'pellitory'), but is a different plant to *Euphorbia hirta,* which also has medicinal properties.

Folk medicine

In Africa, *Euphorbia hirta* is used traditionally for female disorders and respiratory ailments, especially coughs, bronchitis and asthma. Based on the Doctrine of Signatures — a concept developed in the 15th century, which describes how herbs that look like a body part can heal that body part — the plant has been used to increase milk flow in lactating women because of its milky latex.

In Madagascar, people have used it as a diuretic, antidiarrhoeal, antispasmodic and anti-inflammatory. It is also used for coughs, chronic bronchitis and other respiratory disorders.

In Angola, it has been used against diarrhoea and dysentery, especially amoebic dysentery. The extract is also used as eardrops. Apart from respiratory conditions, it is also used for the treatment of boils, sores and in promoting wound healing.

In India, *E. hirta* has traditionally been used to treat worm infestations, and for dysentery, gonorrhoea, jaundice, pimples, digestive problems and tumours. The decoction of the root has been used to stop vomiting, in chronic diarrhoeas and fevers, and also for snakebite.

In Africa and Australia, the leaf extracts of *E. hirta* are also used to treat hypertension and oedema.

Research

Clinical trials have confirmed its use in the following areas: antioxidant,[1] anti-inflammatory,[2] asthma and allergies,[3] arthritis,[4] antiviral,[5] antibacterial and biofilm eradication,[6] antifertility activity, antifungal, anti-amoebic activity, antidiarrheal activity, diuretic, antimalarial, promoting breast development and breast milk production.[7]

How to use it as a medicine

Asthma weed is used as a powder, an infusion or a tincture.

CAUTIONS AND CONTRAINDICATIONS
Large doses cause gastrointestinal irritation, nausea and vomiting. The sap of the fresh plant can cause skin irritation. Best for short-term use (1–2 weeks).

Asthma weed can also be used in:
- Asthma weed glycetract
- Asthma weed tea

Fresh asthma weed chutney

SERVES 3 AS A CONDIMENT
40 MINUTES

GF

1 handful of washed and chopped fresh asthma weed leaves and stems

½ teaspoon salt

1 tablespoon olive oil

½ teaspoon mustard seeds

½ teaspoon cumin seeds

1 small onion, chopped

2–3 garlic cloves, chopped

1 small handful of chopped coriander (cilantro) leaves

¼ cup (20 g) grated coconut

1 tablespoon tamarind paste

2 tablespoons coconut sugar

2 small green chillies, chopped (adjust according to your spice preference)

1 tablespoon lemon juice

This recipe is based on an Indian-style vegetable chutney that can be enjoyed as a delicious and healthy condiment with various Indian or vegetable dishes. It works best with fresh young asthma weed leaves and stems, harvested in early spring, as the new growth is less bitter — but do use gloves when harvesting, as the sap can irritate the skin. This chutney has a long history of use as an antiparasitic and for gastrointestinal disorders.

It's very important to follow the boiling, soaking, draining and rinsing instructions below, to neutralise the toxicity in the sap.

Place the asthma weed in a saucepan with the salt and 2 cups (500 ml) water. Bring to the boil, then reduce the heat and simmer for 10 minutes. Turn off the heat and leave to soak in the cooking water for 15 minutes. Strain off and discard the cooking water.

Rinse the asthma weed in fresh water, then squeeze out the excess water through a colander or a piece of muslin (cheesecloth). This process is important to neutralise the toxicity of the irritating sap.

The asthma weed is now ready to use. If it is in a hard clump, gently loosen it with your hands. Set aside.

Heat the olive oil in a frying pan over medium heat. Add the mustard seeds and cumin seeds, listening for the crack and crackle as they pop, then add the onion and garlic and sauté for 5 minutes, until they start to look slightly translucent.

Add the cooked asthma weed and chopped coriander and cook for 2 minutes.

Stir in the grated coconut, tamarind paste, coconut sugar and chilli, mixing well, then cook for another minute. Take off the heat and allow to cool.

Once cooled, transfer the mixture to a blender or food processor. Add the lemon juice and blend to a paste; if needed, you can add a little water to adjust the consistency.

Taste the chutney and season with a little more salt and lemon juice if necessary.

Your chutney is now ready to serve. It will keep in an airtight container for a week in the fridge, or in the freezer for 3 months.

Serve in a small dish, with dal or curry, and pappadams or roti.

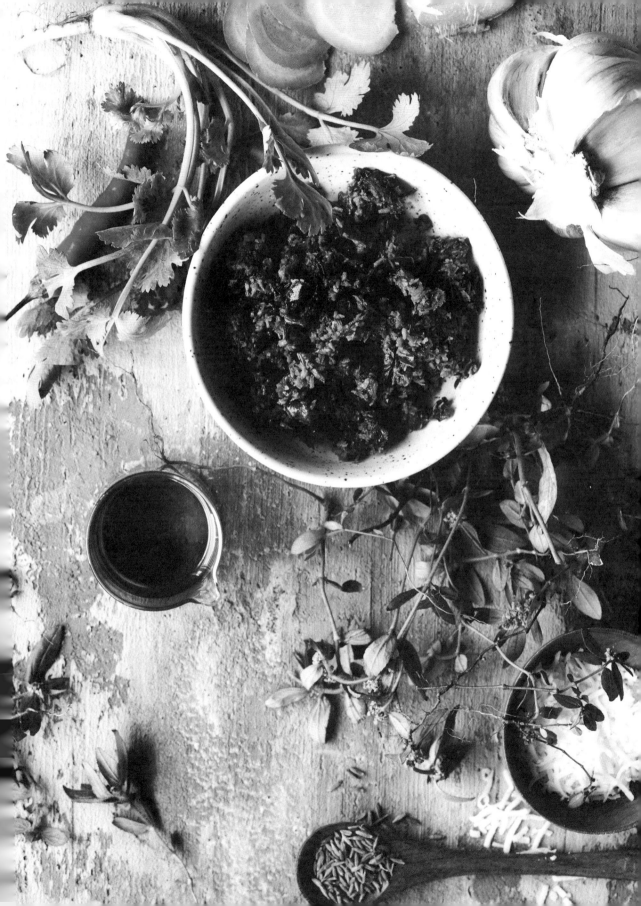

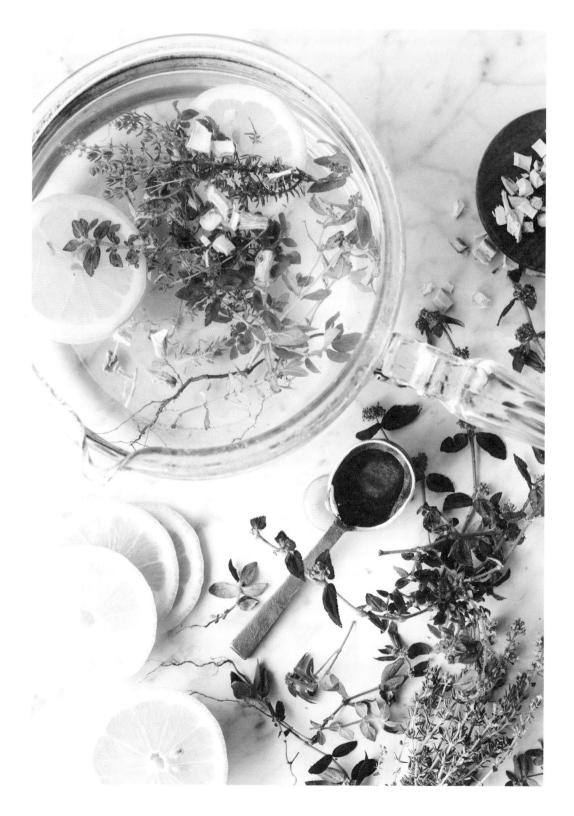

Asthma weed cough syrup

This syrup is an excellent remedy for respiratory ailments such as dry spasmodic coughs and bronchitis, where it helps relax the bronchioles, and reduces the cough reflex. Its anti-inflammatory and anti-allergic effects also make it useful for hay fever and mild asthma. (If you are on asthma medication, consult your prescribing doctor and a trained herbalist before using this remedy.)

**MAKES ABOUT 200 ML
(7 FL OZ)
30 MINUTES**

GF

20 g (¾ oz) dried asthma weed leaves and stems

20 g (¾ oz) dried marshmallow root

10 g (¼ oz) dried thyme leaves

½ cup (110 g) raw or golden cane sugar or ½ cup (125 ml) honey (optional)

1 tablespoon lemon juice

Sterilise a 200–300 ml (7–10½ fl oz) glass jar (an amber bottle is ideal) in the dishwasher, or in a pot of boiling water for 10 minutes (see page 23).

Add the dried herbs to a saucepan with 2 cups (500 ml) water. Bring to the boil, then boil gently over medium heat for 20 minutes, or until the liquid has reduced to 1 cup (250 ml).

Line a sieve with muslin (cheesecloth) and place over a bowl. Strain and compost the herbs, then pour the strained liquid back into the pan.

If using sugar, add it now and stir until dissolved, then boil for about 5 minutes.

If using honey, take the pan off the heat, then mix the honey through to incorporate.

Pour the syrup into your sterilised jar or bottle. Seal with the lid, then label it 'Asthma weed cough syrup', add the ingredients to the label (with the Latin names for the variety you've used) and with the date made.

Store the cough syrup in the fridge, where it will last up to 3 months. If the cough has passed, you can store the syrup in the freezer, where it will last up to 12 months.

Note
Soaking the marshmallow root in cold water overnight before boiling will extract more marshmallow mucilage (slimy goo) that has the healing properties.

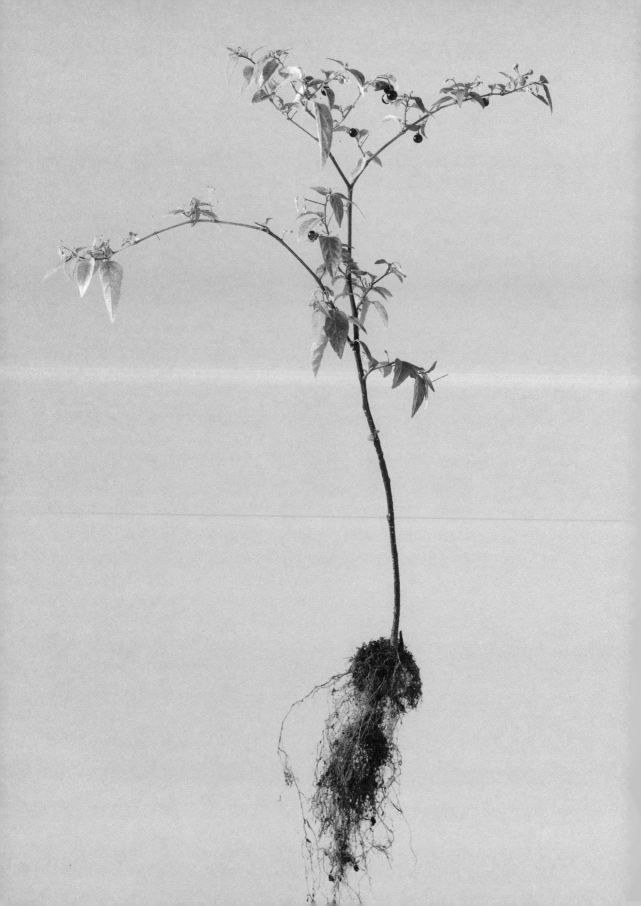

Blackberry nightshade

COMMON NAMES:

blackberry nightshade, black nightshade

SPECIES:

Solanum nigrum

GENUS:

Solanum

FAMILY:

Solanaceae

DISTRIBUTION:

Originated in Europe and Asia. Naturalised in North and South America, Australia, New Zealand and South Africa.

PLANT SPIRIT QUALITIES:

Blackberry nightshade helps balance the right and left hemispheres of the brain, which can be useful for nervous system integration, and switching between creative and analytical work. It can help with meditation and clairvoyance; like a power cord you can plug into the universal wall socket, it will make the energies of the universe available to you. **Key words — integration, communication.**

How to identify it

- Blackberry nightshade has upright branching stems, which are sparsely hairy (or occasionally hairless) and rough in texture.
- The leaves are green (or purplish-green when young). Oval, elongated or egg-shaped, they taper to a point at the tip, and are alternately arranged on stalks.
- The small, star-shaped flowers are borne in several-flowered clusters in the leaf forks near the tips of the branches.
- The flower clusters have a main stalk that is 1–2 cm (½–¾ inch) long, and each flower also has its own stalk. The flowers have five white petals that are fused at the base. They have a yellow centre, five small greenish sepals, five yellow stamens, and an ovary topped with a style and stigma.
- Flowering occurs throughout the year.
- The round fruit (berries) turn from green to black or purplish-black. The berries generally point downwards, with sepals that generally point outwards.
- The berries contain numerous small seeds.

Note

Some people think this plant is toxic because they confuse it with deadly nightshade (*Atropa belladonna*), which has a dark purple flower and is poisonous. My rule of thumb is only eat the berries if you can see the flowers.

Green blackberry nightshade berries can be toxic in much the same way as green potatoes. They are both from the Solanaceae family and contain high levels of solanine, which can be toxic if ingested. The berries are safe to eat once they have turned dark black and easily drop off the plant.

How to harvest

Berries
Harvest the berries when they have turned black. They will start green, then turn purple, before turning shiny black. When they are ripe, they fall easily into your hand.

You can rinse the berries and remove any stems or twigs.

They can be eaten fresh, or frozen for later use.

Leaves
The leaves can be harvested all year. The best time to harvest the leaves is in the morning when they are fresh and full of moisture.

You can use a sharp pair of scissors or gently use your fingers to cut the leaves just above where the leaf meets the stem.

Generally, it's best to pick leaves from the bottom of the plant if you want to continue to harvest from the same plant.

Rinse the leaves in water to remove dirt or debris. Shake in a colander or pat with a towel to dry.

Use fresh, or freeze the leaves for later use.

Nutrients

Protein, fat, carbohydrate, fibre, calcium, phosphorus, iron, vitamin A, thiamine (B1), riboflavin (B2), niacin (B3), vitamin C.

Culinary use

The fully ripe blackberries have a mildly sweet tomato-like flavour, and can be used like any berry in jams, pies, chutneys, salads, smoothies or, best of all, fresh off the plant. The leaves can be eaten as a pot herb.

Folk medicine

In Nepal, *Solanum nigrum* has traditionally been used to treat pain, inflammation and fever. In Africa, it is used for a diverse range of conditions, from ringworm to warts, bedwetting, erysipelas (acute streptococcus bacterial infection), snakebite and venomous animal stings, burns, conjunctivitis, glaucoma, trachoma, cataracts and skin disorders. In India, it is used for stomach ache, stomach ulcer, rabies, wound healing, cough, liver tonic, indigestion, to increase fertility in women, asthma and whooping cough.

Australian herbalist Pat Collins makes a balm that she uses to treat cold sores, herpes and neuralgia.

Research

Clinical trials have confirmed its use in the following areas: antiviral, including against hepatitis C, and potentially in Covid-19 and post-Covid symptoms,[1] reduces pain,[2] anti-inflammatory and antioxidant,[3] anticonvulsant/antiseizure,[4] hepatoprotective,[5] antitumour, antibacterial and neuroprotective.[6]

How to use it as a medicine

The berries, leaves, roots and stems are all used in medicines. Most commonly the leaves, roots and stems are made into an infusion, powder or tincture.

CAUTIONS AND CONTRAINDICATIONS
Green fruit has been associated with nausea, vomiting, diarrhoea, headache, dizziness, loss of speech, fever, sweating, rapid heart beat and pupil dilation. Ripe fruit and cooked leaves are considered safe. Plants of the Solanaceae family have been associated with increased joint pain in people with arthritis. Avoid if allergic to the Solanaceae family.

Blackberry nightshade can also be used in:
- Wild wilted greens
- Blackberry nightshade tea

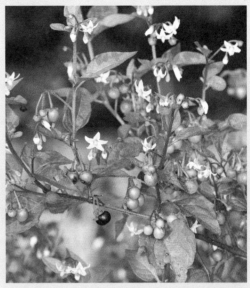

^ Blackberry nightshade (*Solanum nigrum*)

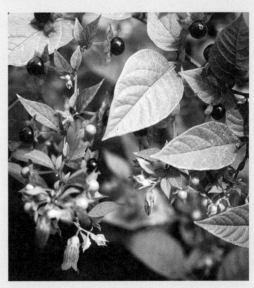

^ Deadly nightshade (*Atropa belladonna*). This plant is toxic, and potentially lethal. If you can see purple flowers, don't ingest this plant. Never eat nightshade berries unless you can see the flowers! Blackberry nightshade (top) has white flowers; deadly nightshade (above) has purple flowers.

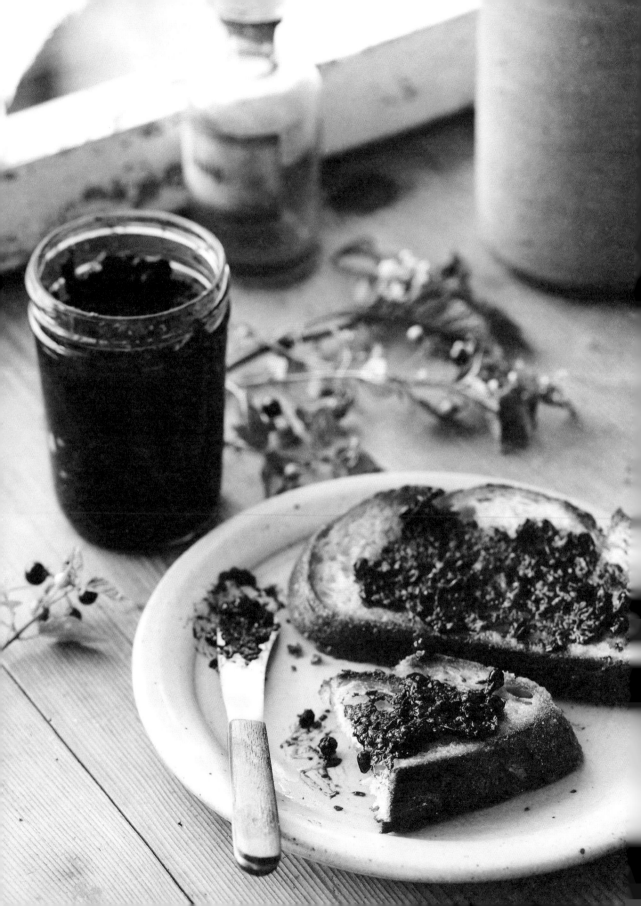

Blackberry nightshade jam

MAKES ¾–½ CUP JAM
20 MINUTES

GF

1 cup (160 g) fully ripe fresh blackberry nightshade berries

2 tablespoons raw sugar

1 teaspoon lemon juice

The bright purple colour of this jam is pure magic. Smear it on your favourite sourdough for a deliciously fun wild food breakfast or snack, or swirl it through muesli, smoothies and yoghurt.

For this jam, use only fully ripe blackberry nightshade berries. They are ripe when they are pure black and fall off easily in your hand; don't use any that are still light purple or green. Because the plant always has both ripe and unripe berries, you can collect the black ones as they ripen and freeze them, until you have enough for this jam. If you have lots of ripe berries from your blackberry nightshade harvest, you can easily double the recipe.

Sterilise a glass jar in the dishwasher, or in a pot of boiling water for 10 minutes (see page 23).

Put the berries in a saucepan and lightly mash them with a fork to release some of the juice. Stir in the sugar and lemon juice.

Bring to the boil, then reduce the heat and simmer for about 10–15 minutes; the more berries, the longer it will take to reach setting point. Keep stirring so the jam doesn't stick to the bottom.

To check if it's ready, dip a cold spoon into the mixture, wait a few seconds for it to cool, then wipe your finger across the spoon. When the jam is the right consistency, your finger will leave a jam-free streak on the spoon.

When it's ready, pour the mixture into your sterilised jam jar. Seal with the lid, then label the jar with the ingredients and date made.

Unopened, the jam will keep in a dark cupboard for 12 months. Once opened, it will keep in the fridge for 3–6 months.

Blackberry nightshade, nodding top & artichoke spelt pizza

MAKES 4
1¼ HOURS

As well as being delicious together on this wholesome, home-made vegan pizza, the addition of wild edibles, with all their nutritional and medicinal compounds, also helps make pizza night a little healthier. Artichokes, blackberry nightshade and nodding top leaves, for instance, all have a degree of liver protective effects.

Feel free to adapt the toppings. If you don't have nodding top leaves, you can use baby spinach, fresh basil or other wild greens instead. Some vegan cheeses are amazing and quite nutritious, while some are disgusting and bizarre, both nutritionally and in terms of taste, so it pays to shop around.

PIZZA BASES
(MAKES 4 SMALL BASES)

1 teaspoon instant dried yeast

1 teaspoon sugar

⅔ cup (170 ml) lukewarm water

2 cups (280 g) plain (all-purpose) spelt flour (white spelt is softer and less dry, but brown is more nutritious … your call!)

½ teaspoon salt

¼ teaspoon garlic powder (optional)

1 tablespoon olive oil

TOPPINGS (PER BASE)

1 tablespoon olive oil

2 garlic cloves, crushed (or use roasted garlic)

1 teaspoon dried Italian herbs

1 tablespoon toasted pine nuts or almond pieces

1 small handful of fresh blackberry nightshade leaves

1 small handful of fresh nodding top leaves

¼ cup (40 g) pitted green olives

½ cup (110 g) artichoke hearts

75 g (2½ oz) vegan cheese

Start by making the pizza bases. Combine the yeast, sugar and water in a small bowl and leave for 5–10 minutes, until bubbles start to form.

In another bowl, mix together the flour, salt and garlic powder. Make a well in the centre, then add the yeast mixture and olive oil. Mix together with your hands or a spoon to form a ball of dough.

Turn the dough out onto a floured surface and knead by hand for 5–10 minutes, until it's stretchy and not sticky; you may need to add more flour or water to get the right consistency.

When it feels good, put it in a clean bowl, cover with a tea towel and let it rise for an hour or so. It should double in size.

Preheat the oven to 250°C (480°F), or as high as your oven will go. Turn the dough out of the bowl and cut into four even pieces. Roll each piece on a floured surface into a pizza round. If you don't need all the pizza bases, you can layer baking paper between the ones you're not using and freeze them.

Transfer your rolled pizza base to a pizza tray. Spread or drizzle the olive oil over the pizza dough, then sprinkle with the garlic, herbs and nuts. Arrange the other topping ingredients on top.

Bake for 12–15 minutes, or until the pizza base is golden brown. Serve immediately.

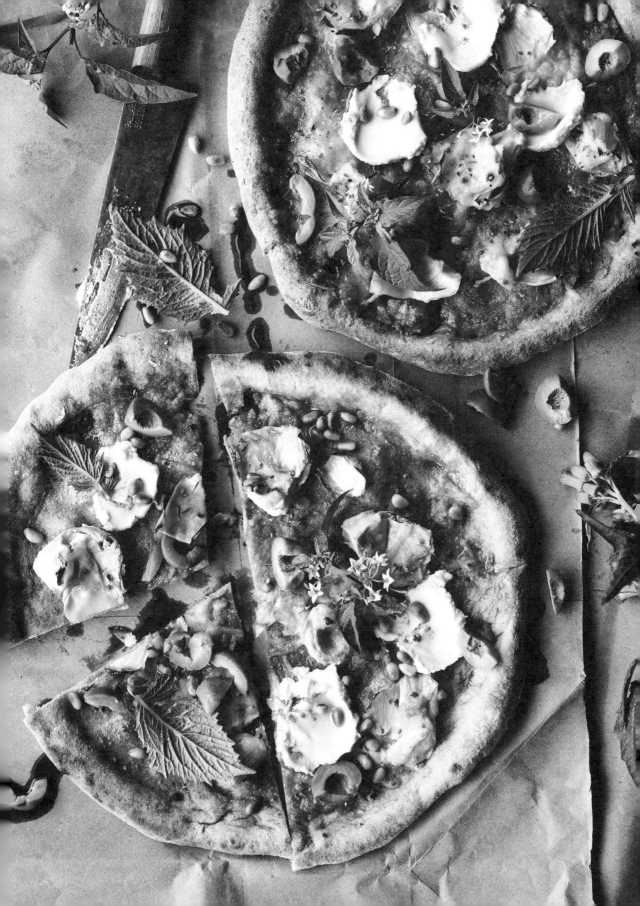

Blackberry nightshade cold sore balm

MAKES 30 G (1 OZ)
20 MINUTES

2 teaspoons infused blackberry nightshade oil (see notes)

2 teaspoons infused St John's wort oil and/or infused lemon balm oil (see notes)

1 teaspoon castor oil

1 teaspoon sunflower wax

5 drops of peppermint or tea tree essential oil, or 2 drops of each

This nerve pain ointment is good where there is any nerve-related pain, including cold sores, herpes, shingles, nerve pain in the face and jaw, or any nerve pain with a sharp, shooting sensation. Always seek medical attention for nerve pain.

This balm was inspired by Pat Collins' wonderful book on wild foraged plants, *In Touch with the Earth: Pat's herbal recipes.*

In a Pyrex or other heatproof glass jug, combine the blackberry nightshade oil, St John's wort oil, castor oil and sunflower wax. Place the jug in a saucepan, then pour about 5 cm (2 inches) water into the pan to make a water bath.

Bring the water to a slow boil, then reduce the heat to a simmer. Stir the mixture in the jug until the wax has melted, about 8–10 minutes.

Take off the heat and stir in your chosen essential oil.

Pour into a sterilised amber glass jar (see page 23), or recycled lip balm pot, and allow to set.

Seal with the lid, then label with the ingredients, date made, and an expiry date of 12 months. If making multiple batches, add a batch number.

Best stored in a dark, cool cupboard or drawer.

HOW TO USE THIS BALM

Apply to the affected area as often as possible throughout the day. Be sure to wash your hands thoroughly with soap and water before and after use, or apply the ointment with an ear bud so as not to spread infection.

Notes

Make an infused blackberry nightshade oil using fresh leaves, stems, and black berries, using the fast method for fresh herb-infused oils on page 31.

Fresh lemon balm leaves and fresh St John's wort flowers can be added when making your blackberry nightshade oil. However, I prefer to make St John's wort oil using fresh flowers, and the slow method for infused oils on page 30, which takes 2 weeks.

If you don't have St John's wort or lemon balm, just use 4 teaspoons blackberry nightshade oil in this ointment.

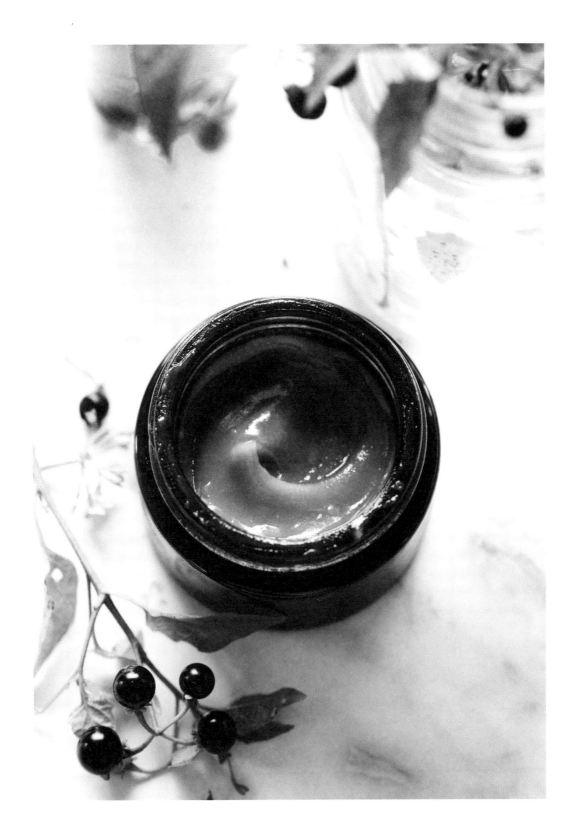

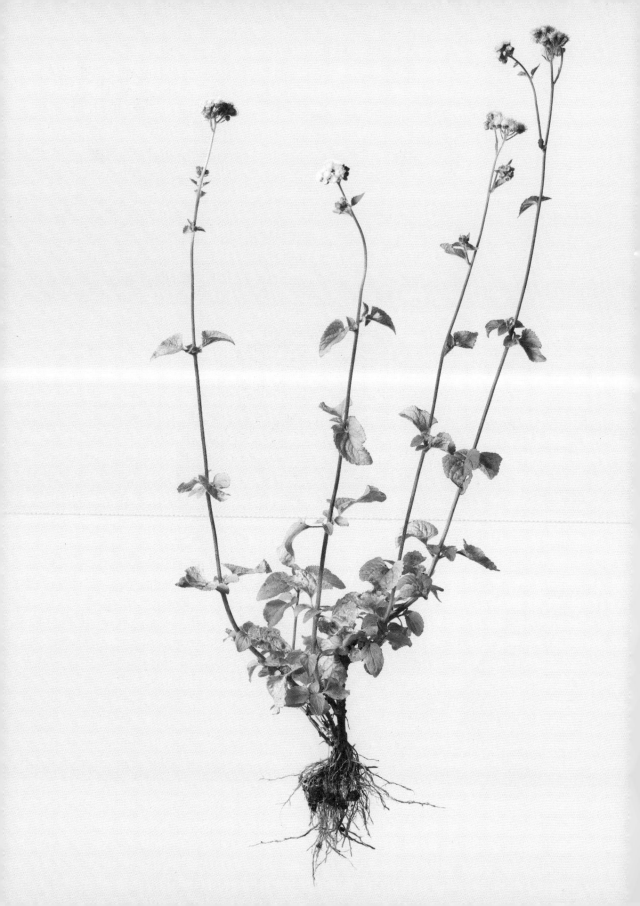

Blue top

COMMON NAMES:

blue top, billy goat weed, blue billy goat weed, floss flower, blue mink

SPECIES:

Ageratum conyzoides (blue top, billy goat weed) and *Ageratum houstonianum* (blue billy goat weed, floss flower, blue mink)

GENUS:

Ageratum

FAMILY:

Asteraceae

DISTRIBUTION:

Originated in Central and South America and the West Indies. Now naturalised in Asia, Africa, Brazil and Australia.

PLANT SPIRIT QUALITIES:

Blue top helps you clear emotional pain by helping you express it, so that it can be released and healed. When we don't give 'voice' to our pain it remains trapped and unheard in our body, causing physical and emotional problems. Blue top is a powerful remedy for any sort of emotional healing or release work. **Key words — healing, emotions, expression.**

How to identify it

- The flat-topped flowering heads are one of the main features of blue top (*A. conyzoides*). Composite flowers of cream to pale blue to lilac are arranged in dense clusters at the tips of the branches.
- The entire plant is covered in fine white hairs, which make it soft and furry.
- It has ovate leaves with tapering points and serrated margins. The leaves are variable in size and shape, and are strongly scented.
- The fruit is a dry seed head (achene), which is about 2 mm (1/16 inch) long, brown to black in colour, and topped with a tuft of hair (a pappus).

Note

Blue top (*A. conyzoides*) is often confused with **blue billy goat weed (*A. houstonianum*)**.

A. conyzoides leaves tend to be more ovate or lance-shaped, with more serrated edges, while *A. houstonianum* has more heart-shaped leaves without serrations (see photos opposite).

A. conyzoides has a more compact flower head; *A. houstonianum* has longer, fluffier flower heads.

A. conyzoides has only a few hairs on the bracts surrounding its flower heads. *A. houstonianum* has numerous sticky hairs on the bracts around the flower heads, and the hairs tend to be longer.

These are subtle differences, and the similarity of the common names can make them difficult to distinguish. There is so much confusion between the two that information from non-scientific sources is also difficult to distinguish.

The uses of the two plants tend to be very similar, with both being used for wound healing, insecticidal activity, diabetes and inflammation.

How to harvest

This plant usually grows beside roadsides, in paddocks, in rural farming areas or areas of housing development. Make sure pollutants such as herbicide sprays, animal faeces or industrial and building chemicals have not contaminated the plants. (See Safe Wildcrafting on page 16.)

Plants should be harvested when they are about 20 cm (8 inches) tall.

Cut the plants from the stem about 5 cm (2 inches) above the ground, so the plant can regrow.

You can rinse the plants and dry them in a colander, or pat dry with a towel.

Plants can be used fresh, frozen for future use, or dried and used as tea.

Nutrients

Vitamin C, B vitamins, vitamin E, zinc and iron.

Culinary use

There is mention of blue top's usefulness as an edible plant, but it seems to be used more commonly as a medicinal plant.

Folk medicine

Blue top is used for fevers, and tick and insect bites. Crushing the leaves and rubbing on the bite helps rapidly reduce pain and swelling.

In Central Africa, it is used to treat pneumonia, wounds and burns.

In India, it is traditionally used mainly as an antibacterial, but also in dysentery and kidney stones.

In Asia, South America and Africa, an aqueous extract of this plant is used as an antibacterial. In Cameroon and Congo, the traditional use is for fever, rheumatism, headache and colic. In Brazil, aqueous extracts of leaves or whole plants have been used to treat colic, colds, fevers, diarrhoea, rheumatism, spasms and burn wounds. It is recommended as an antirheumatic.

In Bangladesh, *A. conyzoides* is called *oochunt*, and a macerated form of the whole plant is taken twice a day for diabetes.

How to use it as a medicine

Ageratum spp. is used as an infusion, a macerate and a tincture. It is also used as a poultice, and the fresh plant is applied directly to the skin.

Research

Clinical trials have confirmed its use in the following areas: antimicrobial,[1] antifungal,[2] analgesic and anti-inflammatory,[3] benign prostatic hypertrophy,[4] polycystic ovarian syndrome,[5] wound healing,[6] antioxidant,[7] antidiabetic,[8] reducing muscle spasm, radioprotective, reducing the effects of gamma radiation, antimalarial activity.[9]

CAUTIONS + CONTRAINDICATIONS

Due to the presence of pyrrolizidine alkaloids, it should not be used by those with liver disease or pregnant women.

Blue top can also be used in:

- Blue top tea
- Blue top glycetract
- Anti-inflammatory gel
- Wild weed powder

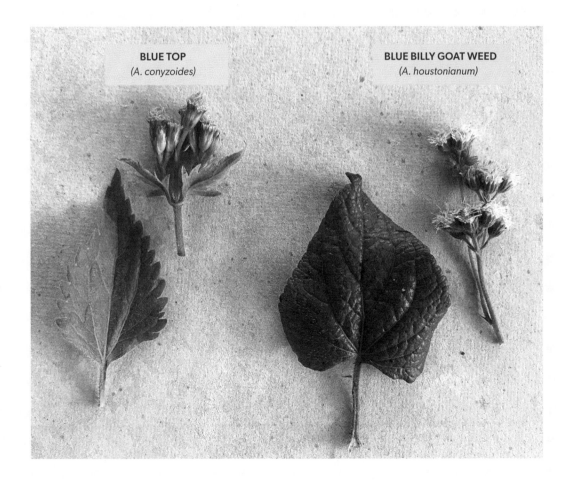

BLUE TOP
(A. conyzoides)

BLUE BILLY GOAT WEED
(A. houstonianum)

Blue top eczema & psoriasis cream

MAKES ½ CUP (125 ML)
20 MINUTES INFUSING
+ 40 MINUTES

2 tablespoons dried blue top leaves, stems and flowers

2 tablespoons blue top infused oil (see note)

1½ tablespoons olivem 1000

1½ teaspoons vegetable glycerine

12 drops of citricidal (citrus seed extract)

5–10 drops of lavender and/or German chamomile essential oil (optional)

½ teaspoon blue butterfly pea powder (optional, for colouring; the cream will be pale green without it)

Note

Make your infused blue top oil either by the slow method (2 weeks) on page 30, or the fast method (1–2 days) on page 31.

If you have very dry eczema or psoriasis, this cream can add moisture and soften the skin. Being anti-inflammatory, it also helps reduce pain and itching.

Many people find creams trap too much heat for their eczema, so they may be better off using a cooling gel, such as the anti-inflammatory gel on page 90.

I find the blue top in this remedy really effective, but if it doesn't grow nearby, you can use broadleaf plantain (see page 92) instead.

Infuse the dried blue top in ½ cup (125 ml) hot boiled water for at least 15–20 minutes, or overnight for a strong infusion.

Pop some ice cubes in a large bowl half filled with water, to have an ice bath ready for when you are mixing your cream. (You can leave the ice bath in the fridge or freezer until needed.)

Strain and compost the herbs. Pour the infusion into a small saucepan, but leave it off the heat.

In a Pyrex or other heatproof glass jug, combine the blue top infused oil, olivem 1000 and glycerine. Place the jug in another saucepan, then pour about 5 cm (2 inches) water into the pan to make a water bath. Bring the water to a slow boil, then reduce the heat to a simmer. Frequently stir the mixture in the jug until melted.

Add the citricidal to your blue top infusion in the other pan. Heat the infusion until close to boiling point — but take it off the heat as soon as bubbles form.

The oil mixture and the infusion need to be as close as possible to the same temperature to incorporate smoothly and avoid a gritty cream, so as soon as the wax has melted and the infusion is near boiling, pour the melted oil mixture into the infusion, place the saucepan in the ice bath (this will help the mixture thicken much more quickly) and start mixing with a fork or whisk.

When the cream has cooled for a minute or two, add the essential oil and butterfly pea powder, if using. Stop mixing when the mixture has thickened to the consistency of whipped cream — you don't want to overmix your cream as it may separate. It can take around 10–15 minutes for the cream to cool and thicken.

Spoon into a sterilised glass jar (see page 23). (If the jar isn't sterile, the cream will go mouldy within a couple of weeks.) Seal with the lid, then label with the ingredients, date made, and an expiry date of 3 months. If making multiple batches, add a batch number.

Best stored in the fridge.

HOW TO USE THIS CREAM

Apply to the skin 2–3 times daily for eczema, psoriasis, dry flaky skin, bites and itches.

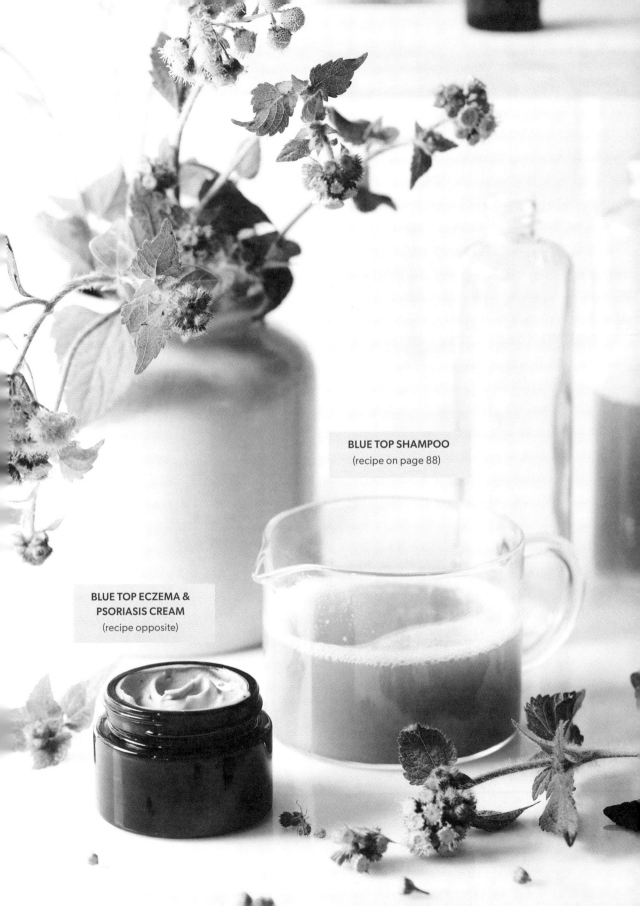

BLUE TOP SHAMPOO
(recipe on page 88)

**BLUE TOP ECZEMA &
PSORIASIS CREAM**
(recipe opposite)

Blue top shampoo

MAKES 1 CUP (250 ML)

**OVERNIGHT INFUSING
+ 15 MINUTES**

¼ cup (3 g) dried blue top leaves, stems and flowers

½ cup (125 ml) castile soap

20 drops of citricidal (citrus seed extract)

10 drops of peppermint essential oil (optional)

½ teaspoon coconut oil or argan oil

This shampoo is such a great home-made alternative to shop-bought anti-dandruff shampoo. It feels cooling and soothing to a dry, itchy, scaly or irritated scalp. The peppermint oil helps bring blood flow to the scalp and provides a cooling, soothing sensation. However, be careful of getting it in your eyes and mouth. If you are sensitive to peppermint you may want to leave it out.

Infuse the dried blue top in ½ cup (125 ml) hot boiled water overnight to make a strong infusion, or for at least 30 minutes.

Strain the liquid into a bowl and compost the herbs. Add the remaining ingredients to the liquid and stir slowly, incorporating them all, but not making it too bubbly.

Pour into a recycled container and put the lid on. Using a waterproof pen, label and date the bottle with an expiry date of 1 month. (The shampoo has a short expiry date, so it's best made in small batches.)

Leave the shampoo in your shower, ready to use. If it makes your hair feel a bit dry, use a conditioner afterwards, or rinse with apple cider vinegar, which is also good for relieving dandruff.

Blue top poultice

MAKES 2–3 DRESSINGS

20 MINUTES

2 large handfuls of coarsely chopped fresh blue top leaves, soft stems and flowers; discard any woody stems, as they won't blend easily

¼ cup (60 ml) water

Blue top is a great first aid remedy for itchy, irritated skin from bites and stings from ticks and insects, and from prickly plants such as stinging nettle. It's also helpful for arthritic pain and inflammation.

Use the fresh plant when you are outdoors to soothe a bite or sting. Remove the insect, then simply gather a small handful of blue top leaves, stem and flowers, about the size of a large marble, chew it a bit to get the juice out, then rub it directly onto the bite or sting.

If the irritation persists, gather a few big handfuls of blue top and make this poultice.

Put the herbs in a blender with the water and blend to make a paste.

TO USE THE POULTICE

Apply the paste to the irritated area, cover with a gauze bandage or dressing, then leave it on for a few hours or overnight. Change the dressing every 12 hours and apply a fresh poultice if needed. Drinking blue top tea may also be helpful (see teas on pages 22–23). Any left-over paste will keep in a sterilised glass jar (see page 23) in the fridge for up to 3 days, or in the freezer for up to 3 months.

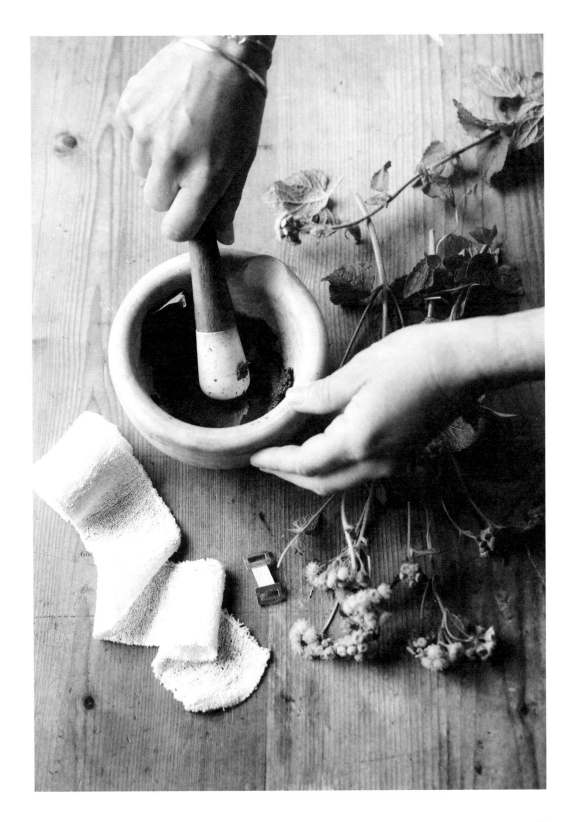

Anti-inflammatory gel

MAKES 60 G (2 OZ)
20 MINUTES

This gel dries matt, has a cool, smooth texture, and works amazingly well for bites, burns, pain, inflammation, sore muscles and arthritis. It contains laponite (see page 38), which has its own cooling and soothing properties that can be enhanced by adding anti-inflammatory herbs, such as those below.

- **Blue top (*Ageratum conyzoides*)** — has shown some analgesic activity in animal studies, and has anti-inflammatory effects. Leaf extracts have been shown to improve movement in people with arthritis.

- **Comfrey (*Symphytum officinale*)** — has been used traditionally for its pain-relieving and anti-inflammatory properties, and can reduce swelling and pain associated with sprains, strains, bruising and arthritis.

- **Sow thistle (*Sonchus oleraceus*)** — some studies have shown sow thistle can reduce painful stimuli and modulate pain.

- **Chickweed (*Stellaria media*)** — traditionally, fresh chickweed leaves have been employed as a poultice for inflamed skin.

- **Tropical chickweed (*Drymaria cordata*)** — clinical studies have demonstrated analgesic properties superior to indomethacin (an anti-inflammatory drug), and fever-reducing properties comparable to aspirin.

- **Citricidal** — a potent antimicrobial made from citrus seed extract that helps prevent remedies from spoiling due to contamination by microorganisms.

2 large handfuls of coarsely chopped fresh anti-inflammatory herbs (see above)

3 heaped tablespoons laponite gel (or aloe vera gel)

6 drops of citricidal (citrus seed extract)

5–10 drops of peppermint essential oil

Collect fresh anti-inflammatory herbs from the list above. (They often grow together, which makes collecting at two or three of them easy.)

Juice the plants in a juicer, or whiz them in a blender and strain them through muslin (cheesecloth). Keep juicing until you have at least 10–20 ml (¼–¾ fl oz) of juice. (Sometimes it takes nearly a full cup of herbs before any juice starts to come out.)

Put your laponite gel in a bowl and slowly stir in the green juice, keeping a nice thick consistency with a dark, rich, brilliant green colour. You may not need all the juice; any left-over juice can be frozen in an ice cube tray for 3 months, to make another batch.

When you are happy with the gel's consistency, gradually mix in the citricidal and peppermint oil until well incorporated. When adding essential oils, start with half the number of recommended drops, then do a skin patch test to feel the strength of the oil before adding more. The essential oil can also be left out if you are sensitive to it.

Place the gel in a small sterilised glass jar (see page 23), then seal with the lid and label it with the ingredients and date made. Store your gel in the fridge, where it will keep for 1 month.

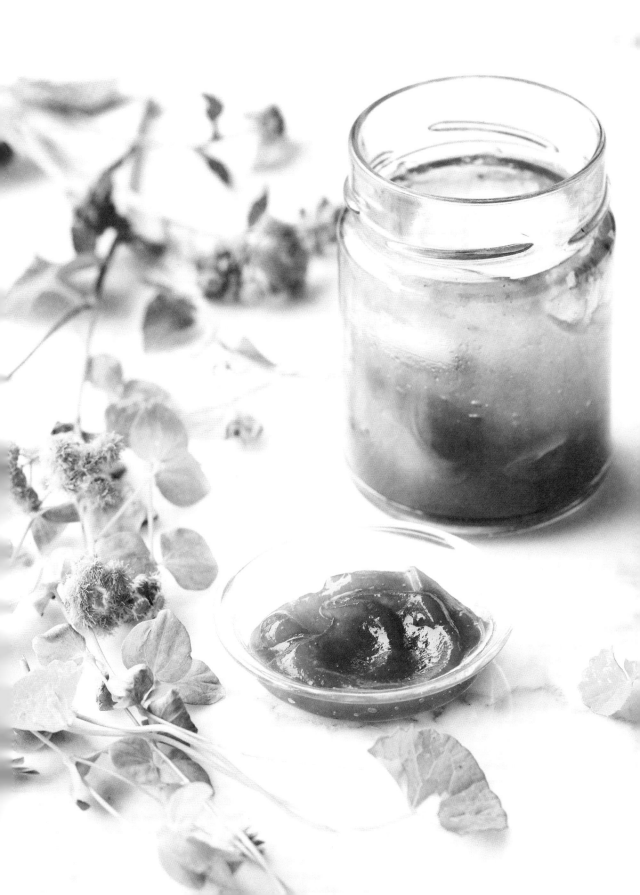

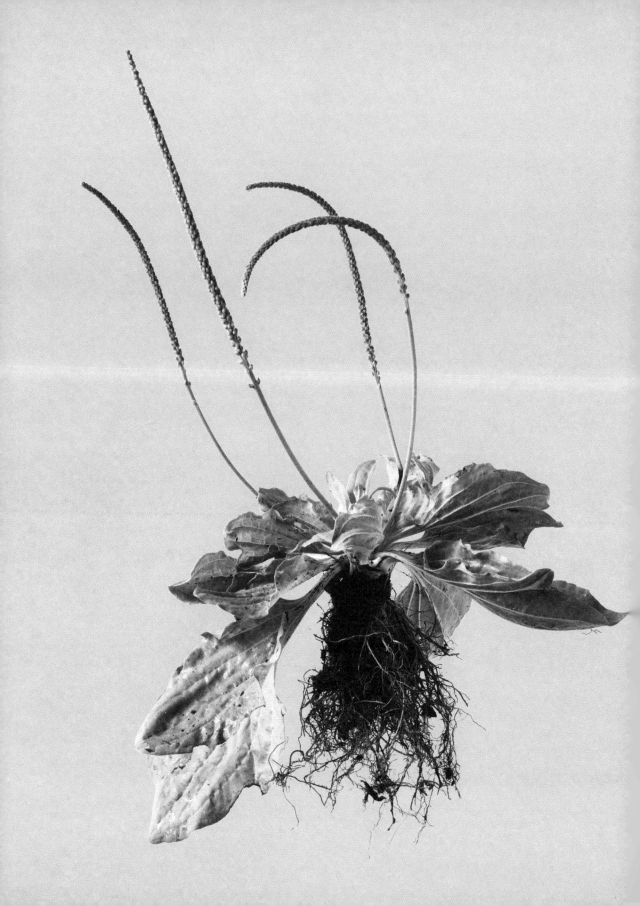

Broadleaf plantain

COMMON NAMES:

broadleaf plantain, greater plantain, bartang seeds

SPECIES:

Plantago major

GENUS:

Plantago

FAMILY:

Plantaginaceae

DISTRIBUTION:

Native to Europe, and Northern and Central Asia, but has widely naturalised throughout the world.

PLANT SPIRIT QUALITIES:

Plantain helps give us internal discipline and fortitude, so we can stay on track and focus our effort. It also helps us deal with 'authority issues' or anger in more mature and constructive ways, rather than just lashing out. The role of benevolent discipline is to set things right without harming anyone. **Key words — discipline, focus.**

How to identify it

- This perennial plant forms a basal rosette, with large oval leaves that have a smooth margin.
- The leaves have 5–9 large, distinct parallel veins that diverge in the wider part of the leaf.
- The leaves attach directly to the base without a stalk, but do have a narrow part at the base of the leaf.
- It has long, upright flower stems, which can be 5–40 cm (2–16 inches) long, and end with an inflorescence of dense flowers.
- The flowers are small and greenish-brown, with purple stamens.
- Flowers are wind pollinated.

How to harvest

Seeds

Broadleaf plantain will go to seed in mid to late summer. Look for the tall stalks with brown or black seeds.

Cut the seed stalks at the base.

Put the seed stalk heads in a paper bag and give it a shake to collect the seeds — or shake the stalks over a large bowl. You can leave the bag or bowl under the stalk for a day or two to catch more seeds.

When you have the seeds, remove any debris by gently rubbing the seeds through your hands and blowing away the debris and chaff.

Store the seeds in a cool, dry dark place, such as a paper bag or a glass jar in a dark cupboard.

Label the bag or jar with the name of the plant and the date harvested.

Make sure you leave some plants unharvested, so the colony of plants can reproduce.

Leaves

The leaves can be harvested all year. The best time to harvest the leaves is in the morning, when they are fresh and full of moisture.

You can use a sharp pair of scissors or gently use your fingers to cut the leaves just above the base of the plant.

Generally, it's best to pick leaves from the bottom of the plant if you want to continue to harvest from the same plant.

Rinse the leaves in water to remove dirt or debris, then shake in a colander or pat with a towel to dry.

Use fresh, or freeze or dry the leaves for later use.

Nutrients

Protein, carbohydrate, fatty acids, potassium, copper, manganese, iron, sulphur, calcium, vitamins C and K.

Culinary use

Plantain leaves are best eaten young, before they become too tough. They can be eaten cooked or raw, finely chopped and added to salads or soups. The seeds have a nutty flavour and are high in protein. If you can get enough of them, they can be dried and ground into a flour to make bread. The seeds can also be cooked like sago or porridge.

Folk medicine

A range of biological activities have been found from plant extracts, including wound-healing activity, anti-inflammatory, analgesic, antioxidant, weak antibiotic, immunomodulating and anti-ulcer activity. Some of these effects may account for the use of this plant in folk medicine for a range of diseases related to the skin, respiratory organs, digestive organs, reproduction, the circulation, for pain relief and against infections.

In Ireland, *Plantago major* has been used to treat wounds and bruises. It has accompanied European colonisation around the world, which has given rise to the name 'Englishman's foot', as it seems to spring up in the wake of white settlers. Plantain is one of the plants that is mentioned in the Saxons' 'nine herbs charm'. The Anglo–Saxons used it to treat smallpox. It is referred to in literature by both Chaucer and Shakespeare. An old remedy to stop vomiting consisted of a cake made from plantain seeds, egg yolk and flour. When mixed with rose oil, plantain juice rubbed on the temples and forehead was said to have 'helped lunatic persons very much'. The healer and midwife Trotula of Salerno used plantain for uterine haemorrhages, claiming it could restore the very essence of a woman. The British Pharmacopoeia recommends it for cystitis with blood loss and bleeding haemorrhoids.

Plantain has a long history of use as a topical application for slow-healing wounds, and can be used for ulceration anywhere in the body, both internally and externally.

Author and educator Katrina Blair recommends it for drawing out venom from bites and stings, as well as drawing out infection from a wound, and improving healing time. She also uses it to reduce the risk of infection from contaminated water due to its ability to inhibit the growth of *Escherichia coli* and *Streptoccus pneumoniae*, and to purify the water.

How to use it as a medicine

Plantain is used as an infusion, a tincture or glycetract, and commonly as a poultice.

Research

Clinical trials have examined its use in the following areas: wound healing,[1] antioxidant, immunomodulating,[2] antibacterial and antiviral effects,[3] liver protective[4] and anti-asthmatic.[5]

Broadleaf plantain can also be used in:
- Wild wilted greens
- Wild weed pesto
- Wild greens powder
- Plantain tea
- Plantain glycetract

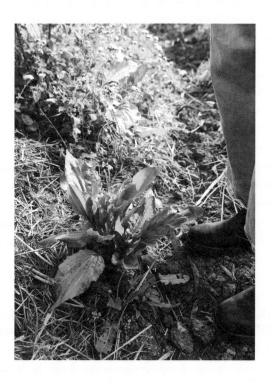

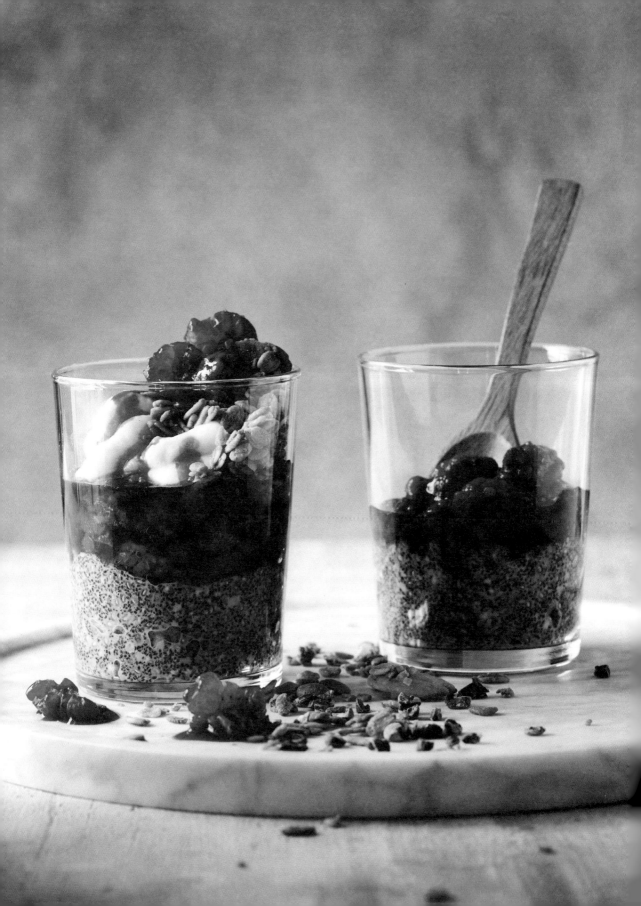

Plantain seed pudding

MAKES 2

**OVERNIGHT SOAKING
+ 15 MINUTES**

GF

¼ cup (65 g) plantain seeds

1 tablespoon chia seeds

1 tablespoon hemp seeds

2 tablespoons finely chopped
walnuts

1 tablespoon dried cranberries
or sultanas

¾ cup (185 ml) milk of your
choice

1 tablespoon maple syrup

1 teaspoon pure vanilla extract

½ teaspoon ground spices,
such as cinnamon, cardamom,
ginger or turmeric (optional)

1 cup (125 g) frozen or fresh
raspberries

1 tablespoon orange juice
(optional)

TOPPING OPTIONS

coconut, cacao nibs, muesli,
fresh berries, your favourite
yoghurt

As well as being grain and gluten free, this pudding is a protein and mineral powerhouse, and can be enjoyed like a chia pudding. If you don't have small intestinal bacterial overgrowth (SIBO), it is healing and soothing to the digestive tract and makes a great food for gastric irritation or mild constipation. In India, plantain seeds are called *bartang bee*j or *bhurtang beej*, and are mixed with water and given to babies to improve digestion.

Plantain seeds can be harvested from your plants or purchased online by searching 'plantago, bartang beej'. Though you can use the seeds on their own, they have quite a strong flavour and I find them nicer in a mix of other seeds.

Lightly crush the plantain, chia and hemp seeds using a mortar and pestle. Tip the seeds into a bowl. Add the walnuts, cranberries, milk, maple syrup, vanilla and spices, if using. Mix together, then cover and leave to soak on the kitchen bench overnight.

The next morning, if the pudding is too hard and dry, stir in a bit more milk to get a nice consistency.

If using frozen raspberries, you can quickly thaw them in a small pan over low heat until soft; I like to add a splash of orange juice to give them a nice citrus tang.

Spoon the pudding into two serving glasses, and either layer the raspberries through or place on top. Serve with the yoghurt and your favourite toppings.

Plantain & charcoal drawing ointment

This ointment can be used like the traditional Amish charcoal salve, or the classic medicine cabinet remedy called Magnoplasm, which are both used for drawing out everything from splinters to pimples to big pus-filled boils and carbuncles (a cluster of boils).

Any small foreign body or pus-filled sore can be drawn out of the skin with this awesome remedy. Change any dressings daily.

MAKES ¼ CUP (60 ML)
20 MINUTES

2 tablespoons plantain infused glycerine (see note)

1 teaspoon sunflower wax

1 teaspoon olivem 1000

1 teaspoon castor oil

1 teaspoon epsom salts (magnesium sulphate)

1 teaspoon activated charcoal powder

1 teaspoon bentonite clay

10 drops of tea tree oil

Place all the ingredients, except the tea tree oil, in a Pyrex or other heatproof glass jug. Place the jug in a saucepan, then pour about 5 cm (2 inches) water into the pan to make a water bath.

Bring the water to a slow boil, then reduce the heat to a simmer. Stir the mixture in the jug occasionally while you wait for all the ingredients to melt — about 15–20 minutes.

Remove from the heat, then stir in the tea tree oil.

Pour the mixture into a sterilised glass jar (see page 23). Seal with the lid, then label with the ingredients, date made, and an expiry date of 12 months. If making multiple batches, add a batch number.

Best stored in a dark, cool cupboard or drawer.

TO USE FOR SPLINTERS, BOILS AND PUS REMOVAL

Cover the affected area with the ointment, then cover with a dressing. Change the dressing every 12–24 hours.

Note

To make the plantain infused glycerine, infuse ½ cup (2.5 g) dried plantain leaves in ½ cup (125 ml) pure vegetable glycerine and ¼ cup (60 ml) distilled water for 2 weeks.

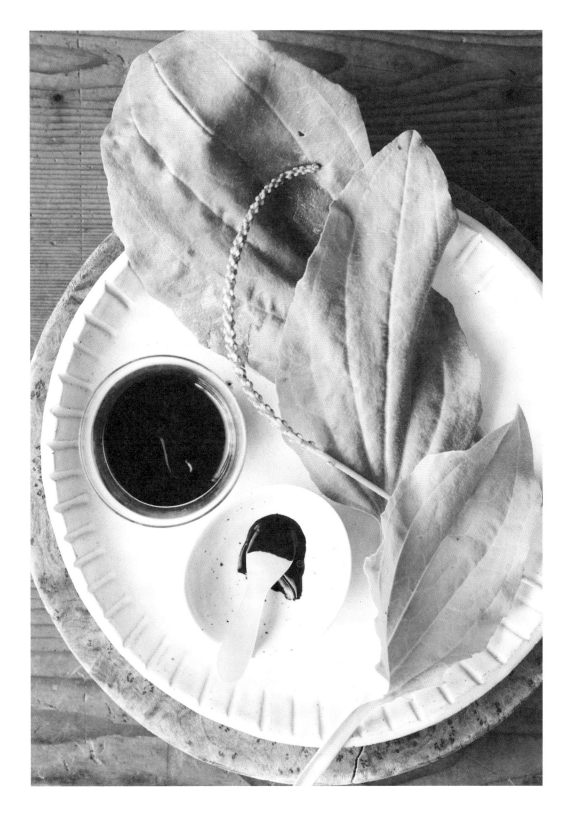

Plantain ointment

MAKES 50 ML (1¾ FL OZ)
20 MINUTES

Plantain can reduce inflammation and swelling. Its antimicrobial properties inhibit the growth of a wide range of bacterial and fungal infections, and it can assist with blood clotting to reduce bleeding time. This plant has a moisturising effect on the skin, which helps promote faster wound healing by reducing scar formation and improving the formation of new tissue and blood vessels.

50 ml (1¾ fl oz) plantain infused oil (see note)

5 g (⅛ oz) shea butter

5 g (⅛ oz) sunflower wax

Note
Make your infused plantain oil either by the slow method 2 weeks) on page 30, or the fast method (1–2 days) on page 31.

Add all the ingredients to a Pyrex or other heatproof glass jug. Place the jug in a saucepan, then pour about 5 cm (2 inches) water into the pan to make a water bath.

Bring the water to a slow boil, then reduce the heat to a simmer. Stir the mixture in the jug frequently until the wax has melted, about 8–10 minutes.

Pour the mixture into a sterilised amber glass jar (see page 23) and allow to set.

Seal with the lid, then label with the ingredients, date made, and an expiry date of 12 months. If making multiple batches, add a batch number.

Best stored in a dark, cool cupboard or drawer.

Plantain poultice for wounds & ulcers

MAKES 2–3 DRESSINGS
10 MINUTES

Plantain leaves can go directly on the skin (the laying on of leaves). It is important not to get dirt into the wound, so wash the leaves in salt water first. Air-dry the leaves, then place the clean, dry leaves directly over the wound. To hold the poultice on, wrap a bandage around the leaves, and change the dressing daily.

If any red streaks are coming from the wound, it means an infection has entered the bloodstream and needs medical care. Deep, serious or infected wounds need topical and/or internal antibiotics and require immediate medical attention.

2–3 large, whole, clean fresh plantain leaves, washed in salty water

1 small bandage

Place the fresh leaves over the wound or ulcer and bandage it. Leave it on overnight. Change the dressing every 12 hours using fresh leaves. It's a good idea to drink some plantain tea as well. (See the section on teas on pages 22–23.)

Keep checking for any signs of infection — including redness, swelling, or any pus or watery fluid coming from the wound. If you notice any infection, seek immediate medical treatment.

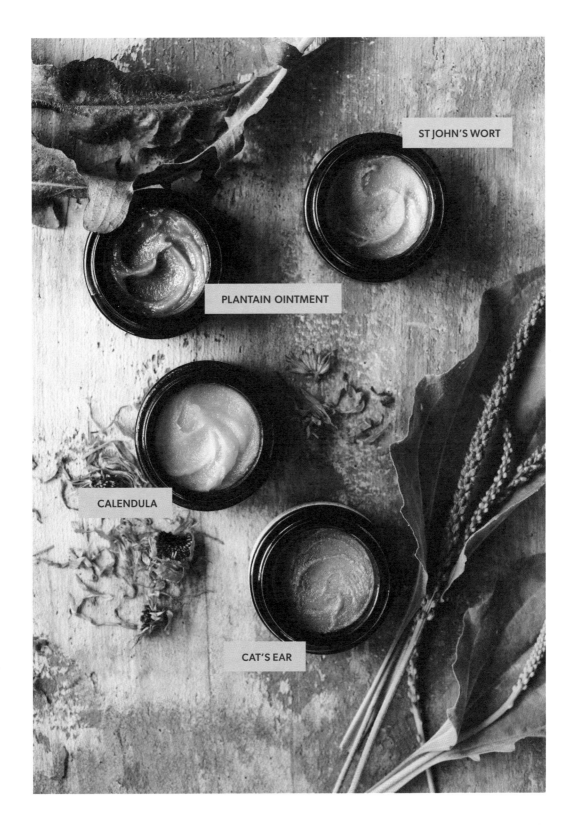

ST JOHN'S WORT

PLANTAIN OINTMENT

CALENDULA

CAT'S EAR

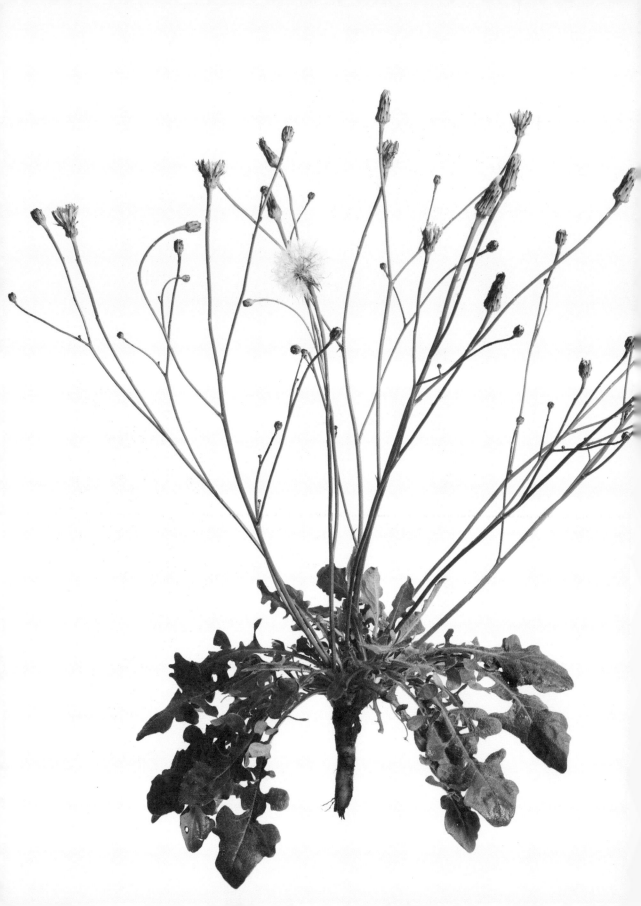

Cat's ear

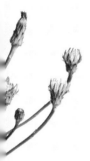

COMMON NAMES:

cat's ear, flatweed

SPECIES:

Hypochaeris radicata

GENUS:

Hypochaeris

FAMILY:

Asteraceae

DISTRIBUTION:

Native to Europe, and found in North and South America, Japan, Australia and New Zealand.

PLANT SPIRIT QUALITIES:

Cat's ear helps open your mind to new possibilities and perspectives, to have a broader view of life and see things in a fresh way. It gives you the courage to break out of a rut, and to release old habits and addictions, to inspire a sense of adventure and new beginnings. **Key words — open mind, greater perspective, possibility.**

How to identify it

- Cat's ear has a basal rosette and looks similar to dandelion (see photo opposite).
- The leaves are toothed, but are more asymmetrical than dandelion leaves, and with more rounded margins.
- Unlike dandelion, the leaves have hairs on the top and underneath.
- The stem is solid with multiple branches, while dandelion has a straight, hollow stem with no branches.
- Cat's ear can have many flowers on the ends of its branching stems, while dandelion has a single flower.
- The flower heads are solitary on branched stems, and are up to 5–15 mm (¼–½ inch) in diameter, with bracts 2.5 cm (1 inch) long.
- The flowers are made of yellow ray florets.
- The achene (seed head) is orange-brown, 4–7 mm (¼–⅜ inch) long, and carries two rows of pappus (hairs) that are 8–14 mm (⅜–½ inch) long.

How to harvest

Leaves

The best time to harvest cat's ear is spring or early summer before flowering, when leaves are at their most tender. You can use a sharp pair of scissors or gently use your fingers to cut the leaves from the base of the rosette.

Generally, it's best to pick leaves from the bottom of the plant if you want to continue to harvest from the same plant.

Rinse the leaves in water to remove dirt or debris. Shake in a colander or pat with a towel to dry.

Use fresh, or freeze leaves for later use.

Leaves can also be dried in a dehydrator, laid out in a well-ventilated cardboard box in a sunny spot, or hung in a dry, well-ventilated spot until dry.

When dry, store in a glass jar or paper bag out of the light.

Label with the name of the plant and date collected.

Roots

Harvest in spring or early summer before flowering, when most nutrients are found in the roots.

When harvesting the root, use a spade to dig deeply around it, then gently excavate the dirt around the root with your fingers to try to get the root out without it breaking.

Rinse the roots in water to remove dirt. Shake in a colander or pat with a towel to dry.

Roots can be dried in a dehydrator, laid out in a well-ventilated cardboard box in a sunny spot, or hung in a dry, well-ventilated spot.

Nutrients

Vitamin A, beta-carotene, protein, calcium, phosphorus and copper.

Culinary use

Cat's ear leaves can be used raw in salads, or boiled, steamed or sautéed. The roots can be roasted and used to make a coffee, in the same way as dandelion roots.

Folk medicine

Hypochaeris radicata has been used in traditional medicine for its anti-inflammatory, diuretic and liver protective activity, and also for treating kidney problems. It has been used for the treatment of wound healing and skin diseases caused by pathogens, and for jaundice, rheumatism, dyspepsia, constipation, hypoglycaemia and kidney disease in traditional medicinal practice in Tamil Nadu, India.

How to use it as a medicine

Cat's ear can be used as an infusion (leaf), decoction (root), tincture (both root and leaf) or powder.

Research

Clinical trials have confirmed its use in the following areas: antioxidant,[1] antibacterial,[2] antifungal.[3]

CAUTIONS + CONTRAINDICATIONS

Use with caution if allergic to the Asteraceae family. The leaves are high in oxalates, so are best eaten cooked.

Cat's ear can also be used in:

- Wild wilted greens
- Cat's ear infused oil
- Cat's ear tea
- Cat's ear glycetract

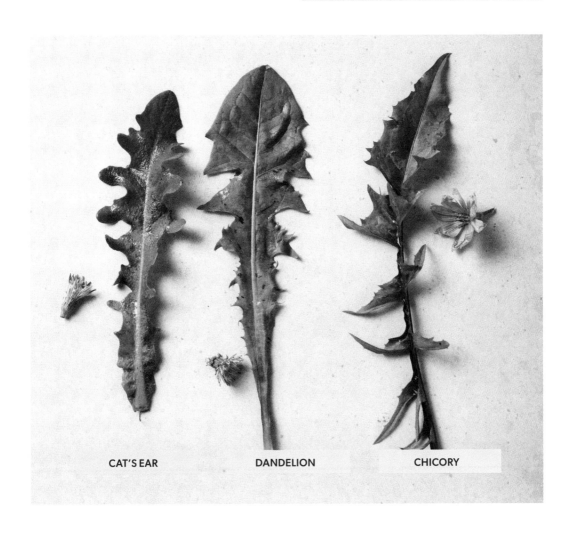

CAT'S EAR | DANDELION | CHICORY

Cat's ear savoury pancakes

MAKES 4
30 MINUTES

Cat's ear is high in vitamin A and minerals, and has antioxidant, antibacterial and antifungal properties. It is often called 'false dandelion' because it looks similar to dandelion (especially the eye-catching yellow flower), and can be eaten in a similar way. I find it's best eaten cooked to reduce oxalates (a compound found in many fruits and vegetables) and because the leaves are furry (which feels bleh on the tongue).

My favourite way to consume furry leaves such as cat's ear, comfrey, borage and cleavers is to make them into a pancake. These green pancakes look great, are bursting with green goodness and feel so wholesome.

1 cup (140 g) plain (all-purpose) spelt flour

1½ cups (375 ml) milk of your choice

1 handful finely chopped fresh cat's ear leaves

1 cup (50 g) baby spinach leaves

1 teaspoon salt

1 tablespoon olive or walnut oil, for pan-frying

Sift the flour to remove any lumps, then place it in a blender jug. Add the milk, cat's ear, spinach and salt and blend for 2 minutes, until you have a smooth green batter.

Heat a frying pan over medium heat and add the oil.

Add one-quarter of the batter to the frying pan, swirling the pan straight away to form the batter into a circle. Cook for 1–2 minutes, until the top is dry and has changed colour to darker green.

Flip the pancake over and cook the other side for 1–2 minutes. Once cooked, you can keep the pancake warm in the oven on the lowest setting until the rest are cooked, to politely feed the hungry horde, or gobble yours immediately with your favourite toppings.

Topping ideas: cashew cheese (see page 178), vegan feta, avocado, sautéed mushrooms, olives, capers, pickles, sauerkraut, fresh greens, sprouts, edible flowers and nut butters.

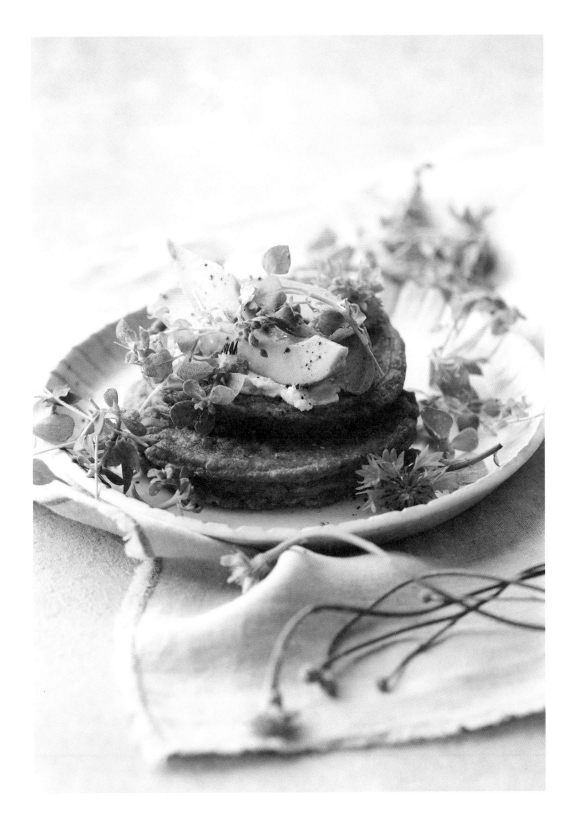

Cat's ear root coffee

Cat's ear roots make a delicious caffeine-free coffee substitute, with a mild, nutty, slightly sweet taste. These roots are rich in minerals and antibacterial and antifungal compounds, and are a good source of fibre and prebiotics. Follow the instructions for harvesting cat's ear roots on page 104. You can use them either fresh or dried.

SERVES 1; MAKES 1 CUP

15–30 MINUTES ROASTING + 5 MINUTES

GF

1 tablespoon roasted cat's ear roots or powder (see note)

milk of your choice (optional)

sweetener of your choice (optional)

If using roasted roots, place in a saucepan with 1 cup (250 ml) water. Bring to the boil, simmer for 5 minutes, then strain into your cup.

If using powdered root, place it in a plunger or teapot, pour in 1 cup (250 ml) boiling water and let it sit for 3–5 minutes, depending on how strong you like it. Strain into your cup.

Enjoy your coffee either black, or with milk and/or sweetener.

Note

To roast cat's ear roots, use the method given on page 160 for roasting dandelion roots for making dandelion coffee. You can then cut the roasted roots into chunks and steep as directed above, or grind them into a powder using a coffee grinder.

Cat's ear antifungal ointment

This ointment is ideal for fungal infections of the skin, including ring worm and tinea.

MAKES 50 G (1¾ OZ)
20 MINUTES

50 ml (1¾ fl oz) cat's ear root infused oil (see note)

5 g (⅛ oz) shea butter

5 g (⅛ oz) sunflower wax

5–10 drops tea tree essential oil

In a Pyrex or heatproof glass jug, combine the cat's ear infused oil, shea butter and sunflower wax. Place the jug in a saucepan, then pour about 5 cm (2 inches) water into the pan to make a water bath.

Bring the water to a slow boil, then reduce to a simmer. Stir the mixture in the jug for 8–10 minutes, until all the ingredients have melted.

Take off the heat. Stir in half the tea tree essential oil until incorporated. Test the strength by carefully dabbing a tiny bit of ointment on your inner wrist (it will still be hot). Stir in more essential oil if desired.

Pour into a sterilised amber glass jar (see page 23) and allow to set. Seal with the lid, then label with the ingredients, date made, and an expiry date of 12 months. If making multiple batches, add a batch number. Best stored in a dark, cool cupboard or drawer.

Note

Make an oil infused with cat's ear roots either by the slow method (2 weeks) on page 30, or the fast method (1–2 days) on page 31.

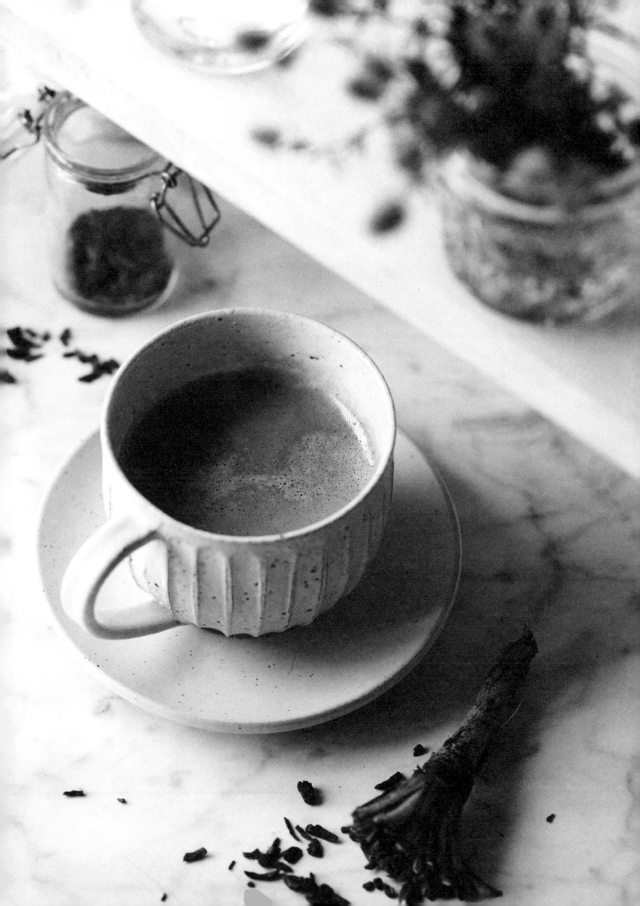

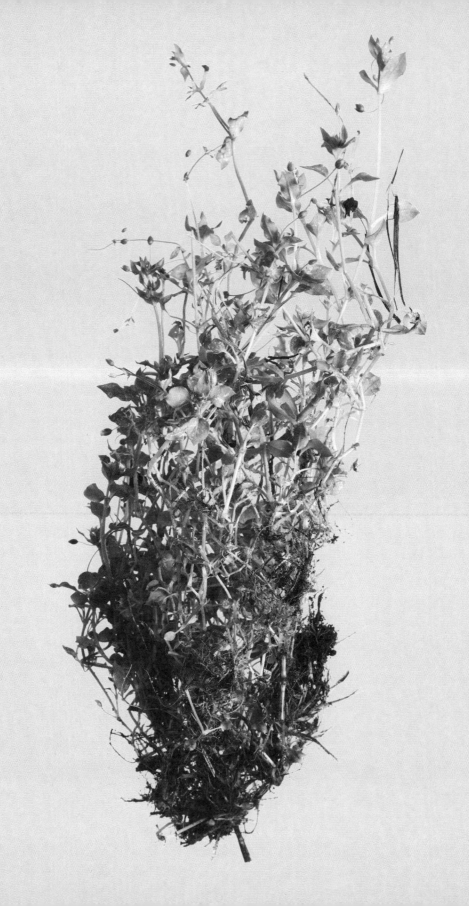

Chickweed

COMMON NAMES:

chickweed

SPECIES:

Stellaria media

GENUS:

Stellaria

FAMILY:

Caryophyllaceae

DISTRIBUTION:

Origins are uncertain. Distributed throughout North Africa, the Americas and Southern Europe, through the Middle East and the Indian subcontinent, to Malaysia and Australasia.

PLANT SPIRIT QUALITIES:

Chickweed clears stagnant energy or a heavy pain body caused by repetitive negative thoughts and emotions. It is good for shifting depression, guilt or shame, emotional release work, and even weight loss where overeating is caused by suppressed emotions. It is like starlight that shines into the darkness trapped in your energy body, dissipating it and allowing you to feel light and positive once again. **Key word — lightness.**

How to identify it

- Chickweed is a sprawling, light-green groundcover with weak, slender stems reaching up to 40 cm (16 inches).
- It has a line of fine tiny hairs running down the side of the stem. Often you will need to hold it up into the light to see the hairs.
- The leaves are oval and opposite, the lower ones with stalks.
- It has tiny white, star-shaped flowers with five very deeply lobed petals. The stamens are usually three, and the styles three.
- The flowers are followed quickly by the seed pods. It flowers and goes to seed at the same time.
- It has no visible sap. If you find what you think is this plant and it has a milky white latex sap, it is most likely petty spurge, which will cause sores on the skin.

How to harvest

Chickweed is a cool season annual that grows in autumn, sometimes throughout winter, depending on location, and into spring. Chickweed dies back in warm weather and will usually regrow the following season if conditions remain similar in the ground.

It is very easy to harvest with scissors, or gently pull up sections only, leaving enough for the patch to regenerate.

The whole plant — but mainly leaves, stems and flowers — can be eaten and used medicinally.

Nutrients

Rich in protein, vitamin A (carotenoids), vitamin B, vitamin C, minerals, iron, copper.

Culinary use

Used around the world as a pot herb and salad vegetable.

Folk medicine

Chickweed has a wide range of applications anywhere there is inflammation or ulceration. It is used frequently for inflammation of the gastrointestinal tract, and for arthritic and rheumatic pain.

It is also considered to be very cleansing and strengthening for the systems of elimination, such as the liver, kidneys and lymph.

It can also be used as a soothing poultice for hot, red and itchy or inflamed skin conditions, such as eczema and psoriasis.

A decoction of the whole plant has traditionally been taken after childbirth to promote breastmilk production, bring on menstruation and improve circulation.

How to use it as a medicine

Chickweed can be used as a tincture, an infusion, a poultice, a powder and a fresh juice (succus).

Research

Clinical trials have confirmed its use in the following areas: weight management,[1] antiviral,[2] antifungal,[3] liver protective.[4]

CAUTIONS + CONTRAINDICATIONS
None known.

Chickweed can also be used in:
- Wild weed pesto
- Wild wilted greens
- Wild greens powder
- Chickweed tea
- Chickweed glycetract
- Chickweed infused oil

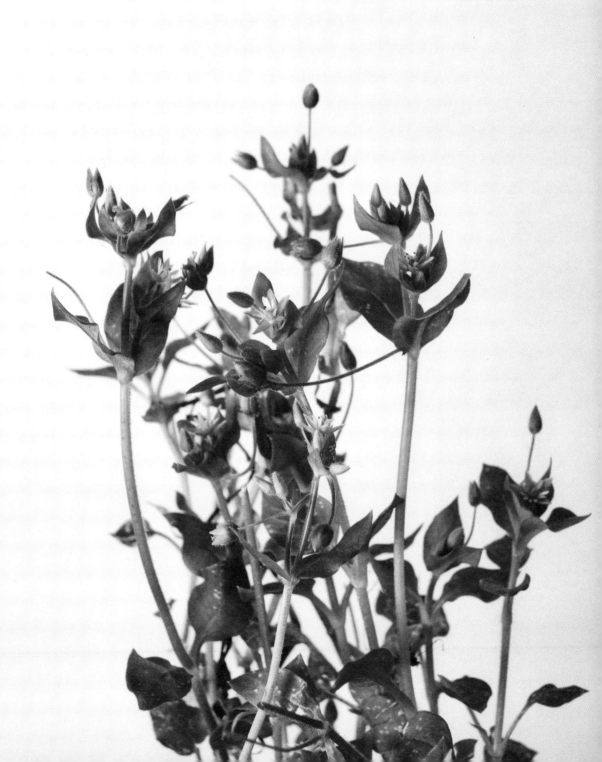

Spring salad

SERVES 2–4
20 MINUTES

GF

This salad is what I imagine fairies eat. It is so pretty and delicate in looks and taste, and so cleansing and purifying.

Chickweed is an excellent source of vitamin C, and is rich in compounds called saponins, which act like dishwashing detergent on a greasy pan, and help break down fats in the body. The edible herbs and flowers are also bursting with fibre, vitamins and minerals.

The fennel is calming to the gut and helps improve digestion. Pears also soothe the digestion, assist bowel movements and also have a low glycaemic index, helping blood sugar regulation.

Edible flowers can be bought in some health food shops, or collected from your garden or local area. Common edible garden flowers are nasturtium, viola, violet, pansy, calendula, rose, hibiscus, chamomile, lavender, cornflower and dandelion flowers.

This salad should definitely be eaten wearing a tiara and fairy wings — or at the very least a dab of glitter or a sparkly bindi.

1 handful of fresh chickweed leaves and stems

1 handful of salad leaves (lots of wild edibles such as dandelion, nasturtium, gotu kola, purslane, nodding top, cobbler's pegs, oxalis, fennel, herb robert and mallow)

¼ fennel bulb

1 pear

1 small handful of edible flowers (see above)

MAPLE CITRUS DRESSING

juice of 1 orange

juice of 1 lemon

1 tablespoon maple syrup

1 tablespoon olive oil or cold-pressed seed oil

¼ teaspoon salt

Wash and drain the chickweed and salad leaves and shake out the water, or pat dry. Place the leaves in a salad bowl.

Slice the fennel and pear into delicately thin strips. Add to the leaves and gently toss the salad.

Mix together the dressing ingredients and either serve on the side and let people add their own, or gently toss through the salad.

Scatter or delicately arrange the flowers over the top, so they don't go soggy, and serve straight away, for maximum freshness and prettiness.

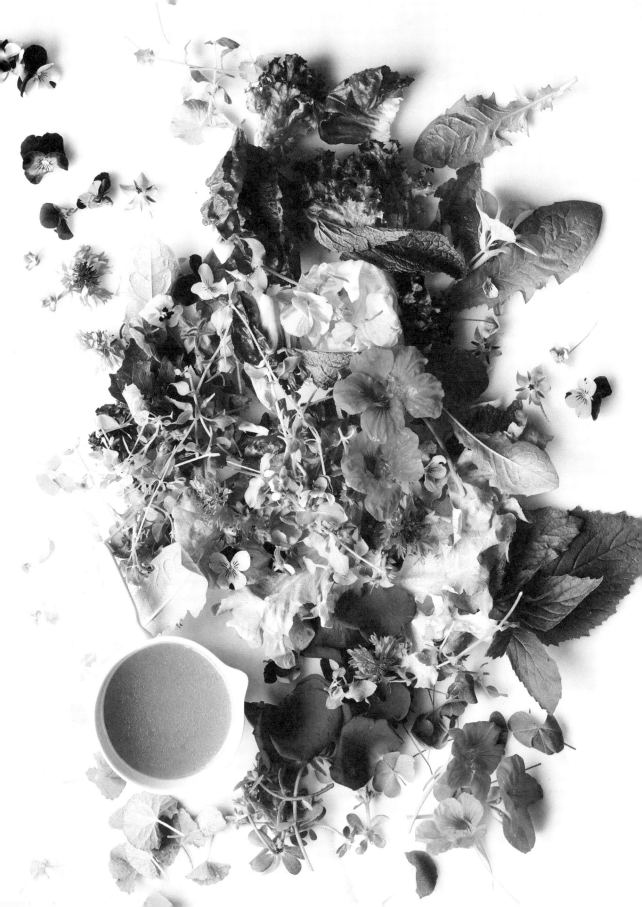

Chickweed, cashew & caper toasts

Chickweed can be eaten as a tasty salad vegetable in wraps, or on sandwiches or crackers. It's so handy having some in the garden, so you can duck out and grab a handful to pump up the fibre, vitamin C and health benefits of your lunch. This is one of my favourite ways to use it as a topping.

MAKES 2
10 MINUTES

2 slices of sourdough bread

1 tablespoon vegan butter
or olive oil

2 tablespoons cashew cheese
(page 178)

¼ red onion, thinly sliced

1 teaspoon regular capers, or
nasturtium capers (page 229)

1 small handful of fresh
chickweed leaves and stems

½ lemon

Toast the sourdough bread slices, then spread with the butter or olive oil and cashew cheese.

Arrange the onion and capers on top, then garnish each slice generously with chickweed.

Squeeze the lemon juice over the top, season with a pinch of salt and pepper and enjoy straight away.

Chickweed, cucumber & apple juice

This cleansing juice helps to support the lymphatic system, regulate blood sugar, support weight control, cool inflammation and detoxify the body.

SERVES 1; MAKES ABOUT
1 CUP (250 ML)

15 MINUTES

2 green apples

1 cucumber

3 handfuls of fresh chickweed
leaves and stems

1 sprig of mint

ice cubes (optional)

Chop the apples and cucumber and place them in a juicer. Add the chickweed and mint and blitz into a juice.

If you don't have a juicer, you can blend the ingredients using a blender, then either strain the juice, or drink it with all the fibre (for extra gut health).

Add water to taste, and some ice cubes if you like cold drinks.

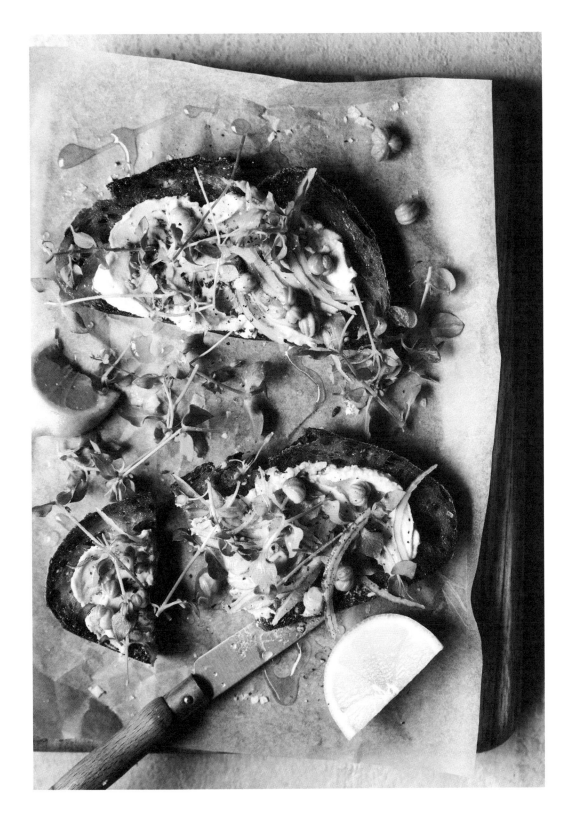

Chickweed skin cream

MAKES ½ CUP (125 ML)

30 MINUTES OR OVERNIGHT INFUSING + 40 MINUTES

2 tablespoons dried chickweed, or 1 handful of fresh chickweed leaves and stems

3 tablespoons chickweed infused oil (see note)

1½ tablespoons olivem 1000

1 teaspoon vegetable glycerine

12 drops of citricidal (citrus seed extract)

Note

Make your infused chickweed oil either by the slow method (2 weeks) on page 30, or the fast method (1–2 days) on page 31.

Chickweed cream is traditionally used to alleviate hot, red, itchy or inflamed skin conditions such as dermatitis, eczema, psoriasis, hives, allergic rashes, bites and chronic itching. It is cooling and soothing, helping reduce redness, swelling and itching.

Before starting this recipe, read the section on making creams on page 34. This recipe uses two saucepans — one for your water infusion, and the other for your waxes and oils.

Infuse the dried or fresh chickweed in ½ cup (125 ml) hot boiled water overnight, or for a minimum of 30 minutes.

Strain and compost the herbs, then pour the infusion into a small saucepan, but leave it off the heat.

Pop some ice cubes in a large bowl half filled with water, to have an ice bath ready for when you are mixing your cream. (You can leave the ice bath in the fridge or freezer until needed.)

In a Pyrex or other heatproof glass jug, combine the chickweed infused oil, olivem 1000 and glycerine. Place the jug in another saucepan, then pour about 5 cm (2 inches) water into the pan to make a water bath. Bring the water to the boil, then reduce the heat to a slow boil. Stir the ingredients in the jug frequently until the wax has melted, about 8–10 minutes.

Add the citricidal to your chickweed infusion in the other pan. Heat the infusion until close to boiling point — but take it off the heat as soon as bubbles form.

The oil mixture and the infusion need to be as close as possible to the same temperature to incorporate smoothly and avoid a gritty cream, so as soon as the wax has melted and the infusion is near boiling, pour the melted oil mixture into the infusion, place the saucepan in the ice bath (this will help the mixture thicken much more quickly) and start mixing with a fork or whisk. (If making a large batch, a stick blender will be much faster.)

Stop mixing when the mixture forms nice stiff peaks like whipped cream; this can take 8–10 minutes.

Spoon into a sterilised amber glass jar (see page 23). Seal with the lid, then label with the ingredients, date made, and an expiry date of 3 months.

This cream is best stored in the fridge.

Chickweed anti-inflammatory gel

Like the fresh juice or ice below, this gel can be used for anything that is red hot and itchy on the skin — including conditions such as hives, eczema, psoriasis, chickenpox, bites and heat rashes. Try a small area first to make sure there is no reaction, before applying it to areas of affected skin.

MAKES 30 ML (1 FL OZ)
15 MINUTES

2 tablespoons laponite gel (or aloe vera gel)

1 handful of fresh chickweed leaves and stems

6 drops of citricidal (citrus seed extract)

Place the gel in a small bowl.

Juice the chickweed to give 1 teaspoon of fresh juice, or pound using a mortar and pestle and squeeze the mixture through some muslin (cheesecloth).

Pour the juice into the gel and stir to blend into a beautiful green mixture. Stir in the citricidal, which acts as an antibacterial agent that will make the gel last longer.

Place in a sterilised glass jar (see page 23), then seal with the lid. Label with the ingredients and date made and store in the fridge.

A gel made with aloe vera will last 3–4 days in the fridge. If you used laponite, your gel will last up to 3 months in the fridge.

Chickweed ice

MAKES 4–6 ICE CUBES
10 MINUTES

4 handfuls of fresh chickweed leaves and stems (or as much as you can sustainably harvest)

Chickweed is great for soothing red, itchy and inflamed skin. I like to use the juice directly on the skin, but it can also be added to drinks for a cooling, cleansing drink.

Because chickweed is abundant for only half the year, I freeze the juice in ice cube trays so I can thaw as needed.

Juice the chickweed in a juicer. If you don't have a juicer, blitz it in a blender with a little water, then strain through muslin (cheesecloth).

Pour the juice into ice cube trays and freeze. Your chickweed ice will last in the freezer for up to a year.

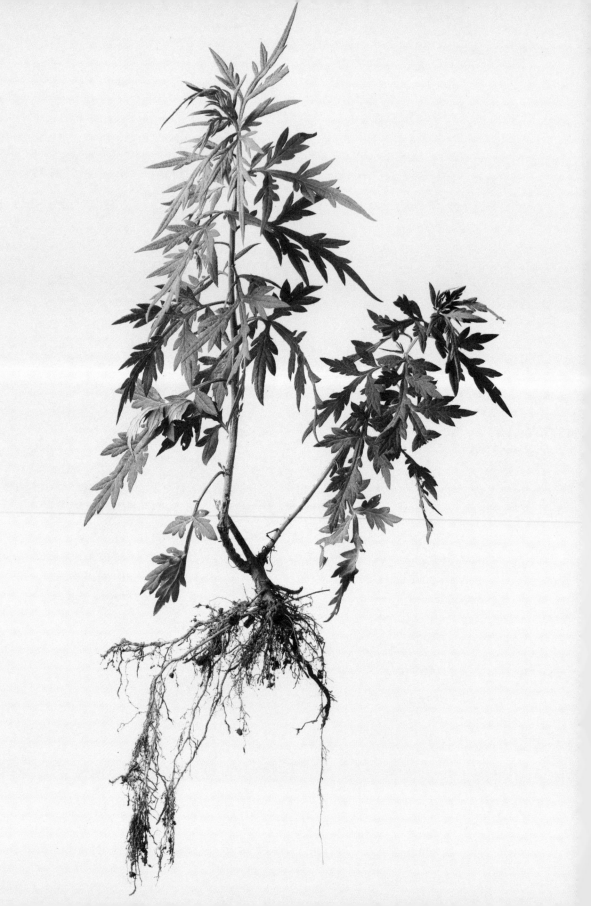

Chinese mugwort

COMMON NAMES:

Chinese mugwort, tree mugwort, verlot's mugwort, mugwort

In Chinese, it is known as *ai ye*. Mugwort is the common name for at least 10 species in the genus *Artemisia*. In Europe, mugwort most often refers to the species *Artemisia vulgaris*, known as common mugwort.

SPECIES:

Artemisia verlotiorum

GENUS:

Artemisia

FAMILY:

Asteraceae

DISTRIBUTION:

Native to eastern Asia, in particular south-western China and northern Japan. It is naturalised in Great Britain, Europe, North Africa and Australia.

PLANT SPIRIT QUALITIES:

Mugwort opens doors. It can be useful for meditation or shamanic journeys. If a birth or death is being drawn out due to fear, uncertainty or holding on, mugwort can help the soul make the transition by acting as a guide between the worlds. It helps you accept the light and the darkness within yourself without judgement, to see your shadow self and know yourself more fully. Chinese mugwort is wise, and will keep you safe. **Key words — seeing, multidimensional communication, acceptance.**

How to identify it

- Chinese mugwort grows 1–3 metres (3–9 feet) high and 1.5 metres (5 feet) wide.
- It has multiple tall green stems that are generally unbranched.
- The leaves are dark to greyish green, with a whitish underside.
- The lance-shaped leaves are 5–10 cm (2–4 inches) long and 3–8 cm (1¼–3¼ inches) wide. They are lighter than the stem colour and are deeply lobed.
- It has reddish flowers that are very small and found on elongated, branching terminal spikes. It flowers in late summer and autumn.
- The root is a branching fibrous rhizome.

Note

Artemisia verlotiorum can be distinguished from *Artemisia vulgaris* by its height, and by its long, thin, lance-shaped leaves. *A. vulgaris* is generally much smaller, with a fatter, rounder leaf. It also has darker green leaves. A new hybrid, *Artemisia x wurzellii*, has been identified as a cross between *A. vulgaris* and *A. verlotiorum*.

How to harvest

Leaves and stems can be harvested in late spring or early summer before flowering. The stems can be thick and woody, so use secateurs to snip branches below the leaf nodes. The plant often grows back even more vigorously after pruning.

Nutrients

Not identified.

Culinary use

Not a common culinary food.

Folk medicine

Not a lot is written about this species of mugwort, but it may have been used in a similar fashion to similar species of mugwort.

It is used as moxa in traditional Chinese medicine, and for its relaxant effects in the respiratory, circulatory, digestive and nervous system.

It is used in the folk medicine of Tuscany, Italy, as a remedy for hypertension.

It can be used as an insect repellent or placed in cupboards to keep moths away.

How to use it as a medicine

I use this species mainly for making smudge sticks or moxa, which can be used for energetic clearing, or held near the skin to ease inflammation. It is useful for healing inflammation.

It can also be made into an infused oil that can be used externally and massaged into the chakra points for over-excitability and to help with sleep, dreaming and visioning, or as an antifungal for fungal skin infections.

It can be drunk as a tea for hypertension and inflammation.

Due to its high thujone content, it should only be used short term (1–3 days) and in moderation (1–2 cups of tea per day).

Research

Clinical trials have confirmed its use in the following areas: anti-inflammatory,[1] anti-convulsant and pain relieving,[2] blood pressure lowering[3] and antifungal.[4]

CAUTIONS + CONTRAINDICATIONS

This plant can cause uterine contraction, so should be avoided in all stages of pregnancy. Large amounts can be toxic due to the high thujone content. It can also cause a rash and hay fever in sensitive individuals. Large amounts have been associated with tumours in animals with excess consumption.

Chinese mugwort can also be used in:

• Chinese mugwort tea

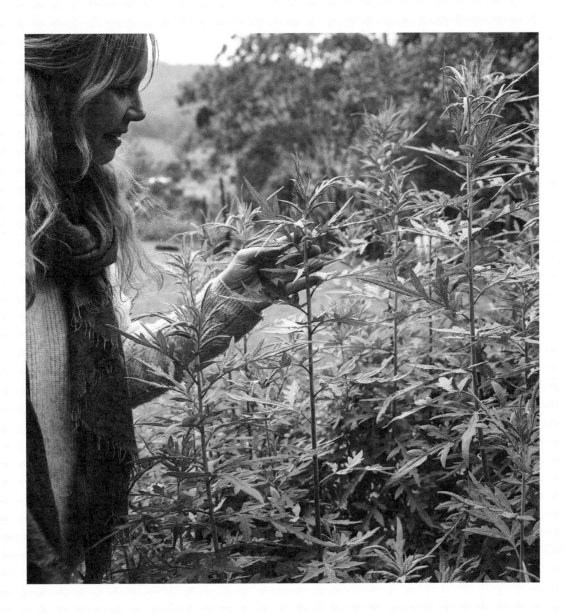

Chinese mugwort smudge stick

MAKES 1 SMUDGE STICK

30 MINUTES OR OVERNIGHT INFUSING + 40 MINUTES

1 metre (3 feet) of embroidery thread or twine

1 bunch 10–20 cm (4–8 inch) long stems of dried Chinese mugwort

Note

The easiest way to dry a bunch of freshly harvested Chinese mugwort stems is to leave them in a dehydrator for 12–24 hours. You can also dry them in the oven at the lowest heat with the door ajar for 4 hours, or in a cardboard box in the car for 1–2 days, turning the plants two or three times a day.

Throughout human history, Indigenous cultures have used the smoke from burning herbs in cleansing and purification rituals. The practice of 'smudging' often incorporates symbolic elements of all four elements: Water, Earth, Fire and Air. Aspects of cultural appropriation can easily creep into these rituals, so please always be mindful to explore them with sensitivity, humility and some research. However, it is human nature to evolve these rituals into new ones that reflect our own unique circumstances and personal histories.

Start by establishing an intention of gratitude to the Chinese mugwort plant. Energetically, you can use Chinese mugwort to access multidimensional states and see the multifaceted parts of yourself. It also helps you discern what qualities and relationships to cultivate in yourself and with others you encounter in this and other realms. Chinese mugwort is wise, and will keep you safe.

HOW TO MAKE A MUGWORT SMUDGE STICK

Cut the embroidery thread or twine into three 10 cm (4 inch) pieces, and one 70 cm (26 inch) piece.

Bind the dried stems and leaves in a bunch by tying the 10 cm (4 inch) threads around the bottom, middle and top. Now wrap the long piece of thread tightly around the base, then loosely work your way up, then back down the stem, in a criss-cross pattern. Tie into a knot at the bottom and trim off any excess thread or twine.

TO USE THE SMUDGE STICK

Make sure you have a glass jar with a lid or some sand to extinguish the smudge stick when you are finished. Light the dried herb bundle with a lighter, then blow gently so it starts smoking.

To smudge a person, blow the smoke up and down their body — including the arms and legs and front and back. Some people like to use a feather or a small leafy branch to move the smoke across the body.

To smudge a room, blow the smoke into the room — especially in the corners, windows and doorways, and any areas of concern. Again, a feather or leafy branch can be helpful to move the smoke around the space. Extinguish the stick in a jar of rice, or by placing it in a glass jar with a lid so it can't get any more oxygen.

Do not use if pregnant.

Chinese mugwort anti-inflammatory balm

This balm can be used to help alleviate pain and inflammation, arthritis, sore joints, headaches, period pain and heavy menstrual bleeding, and is useful in treating fungal infections of the skin, as well as tinea, ringworm and candida. **Do not use if pregnant.**

MAKES 30 ML (1 FL OZ)
20 MINUTES

1 tablespoon infused mugwort oil (see note)

1 teaspoon castor oil

1 teaspoon sunflower wax

Combine all the ingredients in a Pyrex or other heatproof glass jug. Place the jug in a saucepan, then pour about 5 cm (2 inches) water into the pan to make a water bath.

Bring the water to a slow boil, then reduce the heat to a simmer. Stir the mixture in the jug until the wax has melted.

Pour into a small sterilised glass jar (see page 23) and allow to set.

Seal with the lid, then label with the ingredients, date made, and an expiry date of 12 months. If making multiple batches, add a batch number.

Rub the ointment into the affected area 2–3 times a day, or as often as needed.

Best stored in a dark, cool cupboard or drawer.

Note
Make your infused mugwort oil either by the slow method (2 weeks) on page 30, or the fast method (1–2 days) on page 31.

Moxa sticks

**MAKES 2 MOXA STICKS
40 MINUTES**

Traditional Chinese medicine (TCM) practitioners use moxibustion ('moxa' for short) with mugwort to help clients move stagnation of Qi and blood, and dry damp heat or cold, and believe it can help relieve swelling, bruising, pain, inflammation, arthritis, sore joints, musculoskeletal issues, headaches, period pain, heavy menstrual bleeding, as well as immune and respiratory conditions.

You can use moxa on your own, or under the guidance of a TCM practitioner. Avoid in infectious diseases, fevers and haemorrhages. **Do not use if pregnant.**

4 cups (30 g) dried
Chinese mugwort

YOU WILL ALSO NEED

coffee grinder (or mortar and pestle)

a 20 x 20 cm (8 x 8 inch) sheet of mulberry paper or rice paper, or similar thin but strong paper (you can buy these cheaply online on sites such as Etsy)

a utensil with a handle that is 1–2 cm (½–¾ inch) wide and about 20 cm (8 inches) long

glue (see note)

a small clean paintbrush

a chopstick (optional)

good ventilation

a lighter, or small candle

a glass with rice in it, or a jar with a lid that fits the moxa stick inside

Note

Make your own glue by mixing together 1 teaspoon of xanthan gum and 6 teaspoons of warm water and stirring for 5–10 minutes until the gum has fully dissolved and is lump free. (This is the glue used by cigar makers.) Or, you can simply make a paste using equal parts flour and water.

In batches, grind the mugwort into a fluffy powder using a coffee grinder. (You can use a mortar and pestle, but it'll take a long time.)

Lightly roll the paper once around your chosen utensil handle, like you're rolling up sushi. Brush a line of glue all the way down the paper on the handle, then roll the rest of the paper around the handle. (Don't roll the paper too tight, or you won't be able to get it off the handle.) When you get to the end, seal the other long paper edge down with glue, to make a long cylinder. Slide the paper about 5 mm (¼ inch) off the end of the handle, fold the overhanging paper edges over and seal with glue, to enclose it.

Now slide the whole paper cylinder off the handle. Put small pinches of mugwort into the cylinder and tamp the herb down with your utensil handle, or a chopstick. It can take 10–15 minutes to fill the moxa stick, so relax into it. Make sure the mugwort is tightly packed.

Seal the top end with paste. Let it dry and it's ready to use. (I like to tie some twine around one end, so I remember to light the other end.)

HOW TO USE THE MOXA STICK

Make sure you have good airflow in the room so it doesn't get too smoky. Burn the end of your moxa stick with a lighter or candle. It can take a while to light properly.

Hold the stick 2–3 cm (1 inch) away from the back of your hand to see if you can feel the heat. Do not check by touching the end! Moxa will burn you, so keep it away from the skin at all times.

Hold the stick like a paintbrush. When you can feel the heat, you can use the stick on yourself or another person by holding it 2–3 cm (1 inch) away from the area or acupressure point. It should feel warm and pleasant. If it starts to feel too hot, move the stick slightly further away, or to another point. You can hold it over each spot for about 2–3 minutes using a spiral, back-and-forth or pointing motion. If ash builds up on the end of the stick, roll it off into your jar.

When the treatment is finished, extinguish the moxa by stubbing it out in a jar with rice in it, or putting it in a jar and screwing the lid on so no air gets in. Don't put it out with water, as you will ruin the stick for its next use. Seal in a jar and use within 12 months.

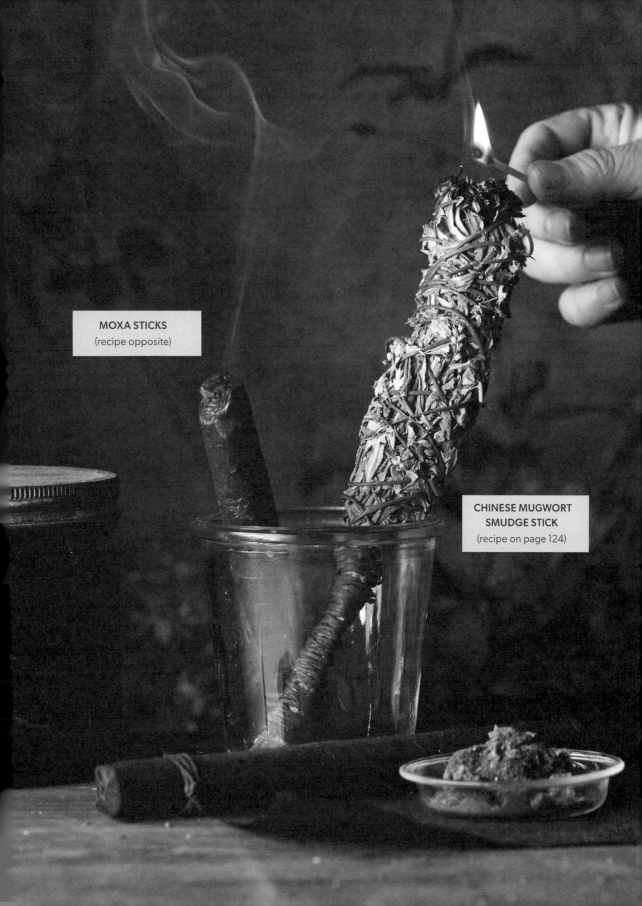

MOXA STICKS
(recipe opposite)

**CHINESE MUGWORT
SMUDGE STICK**
(recipe on page 124)

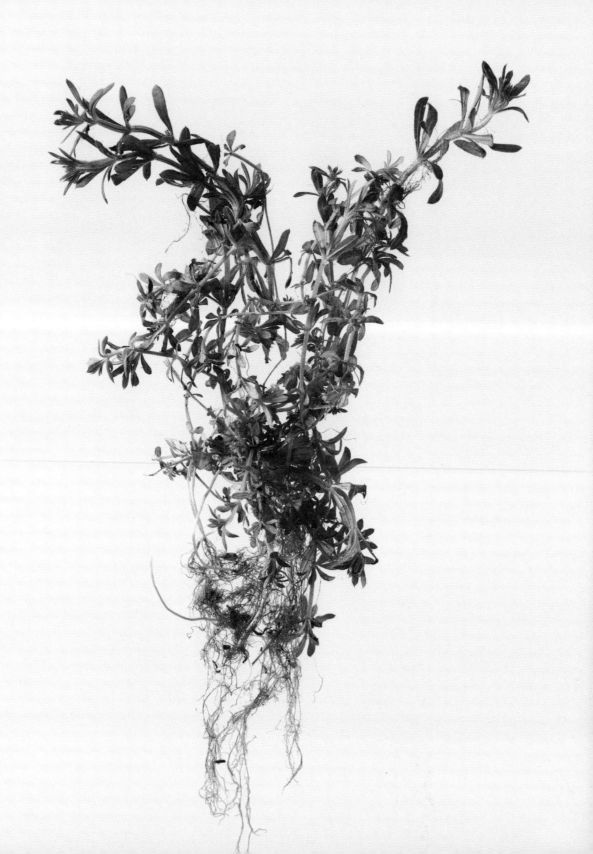

Cleavers

COMMON NAMES:

cleavers, clivers, sticky weed, goose grass

SPECIES:

Galium aparine

GENUS:

Galium

FAMILY:

Rubiaceae

DISTRIBUTION:

Native to Europe, Africa and Asia, from Britain and the Canary Islands to Japan. Naturalised in North, South and Central America, Canada, Australia, New Zealand and some Oceanic islands.

PLANT SPIRIT QUALITIES:

Ironically, given how this plant 'holds on' so tightly when it sticks to you, cleavers is about letting go of things that are keeping you stuck, or that no longer serve you, but you may be holding on to, afraid to let go — jobs, relationships and identities that you have outgrown, but are afraid to let go. In the body it helps move toxins through the lymphatics so you can eliminate them. In your life, it can move things that are keeping you stuck, to create a new path and identity for yourself. **Key words — letting go, identity.**

How to identify it

- The most distinguishing feature of cleavers are the small, velcro-like hooked hairs that grow out of the leaves, stems and fruit, which attach themselves to anything that comes in contact with them.
- It is a creeping groundcover with stems that branch out, sometimes growing to knee height.
- The flowers are very small (1 mm long and 1–2 mm across) and are white with four petals, fused together at their base, and with four tiny yellow stamens.
- Flowers are arranged in small, spreading clusters (1–9 flowers) on short side branches.
- It flowers mostly in late spring and early summer.
- The leaves are narrow or lance-shaped, 1–8 cm (½–3¼ inches) long and 2–10 mm (¹⁄₁₆ –½ inch) wide, with pointed tips and tiny backward-pointing prickles along their margins.
- The whorled leaves radiate from a single point and wrap around the stem. They are stalkless, and are found in groups of 6–9 at each of the stem joints.
- It has two-lobed, kidney-shaped fruit, which easily break into two one-seeded parts when mature.
- The small fruit (2–6 mm/¹⁄₁₆–¼ inch across) are densely covered with hooked hairs. They are green or purplish-green in colour when young, turning grey, greyish-brown or brown as they mature.
- The tiny round seeds are 2–3 mm.
- The root system is branching, fibrous and shallow.
- The plant is very effective at spreading by reseeding itself.

How to harvest

Cleavers is a cool season annual that grows in spring through summer, and sometimes all year in temperate climates.

Leaves
The plant is very easy to harvest as it pulls out of the soil with little effort. In order to not pull up the roots accidentally, you may want to harvest with scissors, or else gently pull up sections only, leaving enough for the patch to regenerate.

The whole plant, but mainly the leaves and stems, can all be eaten and used medicinally.

Seeds
When seeds are visible and have turned greyish brown, you can harvest the plant by cutting the stems and putting them upside down in a paper bag or over a large bowl to dry. Once dry, gently massage the leaves so the seeds fall into the bag or bowl.

Nutrients

Cleavers is rich in silica, minerals and vitamin C.

Culinary use

The leaves and stems can be used as a vegetable. It is unpleasant raw in salad, as it is too prickly, but can be juiced if you want to use it fresh. When cooked, the hairs soften, making it a good pot herb. It can also be used in stir-fries.

If you have the patience for it, the little round green fruits of cleavers can be collected, dried and roasted as a coffee substitute.

Leaves and stems can be used for tea.

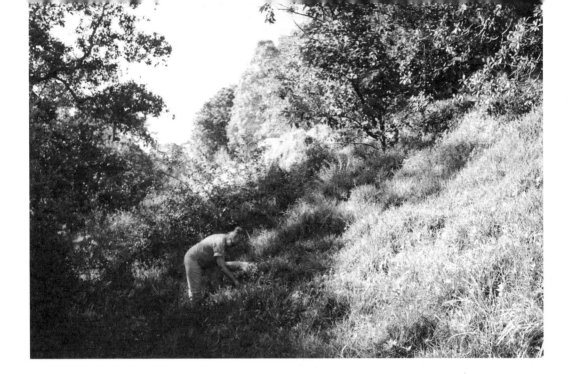

Folk medicine

Traditionally, cleavers has been used to great effect as a diuretic to treat the kidneys, urinary system and lymphatics. It also has a history of external use for ulcers, wounds, burns, bites and stings. It has been used to break up urinary gravel, to soften hardened lymph nodes and break down fibrosis.

The American herbalist Matthew Wood uses it for the nervous system, where he finds it effective for oversensitive nerve endings, tightened tendons (Dupuytren's contracture and Morton's neuroma), and ticklish or itchy skin.

Research

Clinical trials have confirmed its use in the following areas: immune modulation,[1] antibiotic,[2] antioxidant[3] and healing ulcers.[5]

How to use it as a medicine

Cleavers can be used as a tea, a tincture, a cream, a poultice or a fresh juice (succus).

CAUTIONS + CONTRAINDICATIONS
Avoid if taking blood-thinning medication. Caution with aspirin and in pregnancy. Cleavers can be a common allergen, so use a small amount first to check for allergic reactions.

Cleavers can also be used in:
- Cat's ear savoury pancakes
- Wild wilted greens
- Cleavers glycetract
- Cleavers tea

Cleavers, potato & quinoa balls with cleavers dipping sauce

MAKES 18 BALLS
1½ HOURS

GF

½ cup (125 ml) mayonnaise

½ cup (125 ml) light-flavoured oil (such as rice bran), for frying

CLEAVERS DIPPING SAUCE

½ cup (125 ml) vegan plain yoghurt, or ¼ cup (65 g) tahini plus ¼ cup (60 ml) water

2 garlic cloves, crushed

juice of 1 lemon

½ teaspoon salt

½ cup cleavers

CRISPY QUINOA COATING

⅔ cup (135 g) raw quinoa

1 teaspoon smoked paprika

1 teaspoon onion salt

1 teaspoon dried Italian herbs

POTATO BALLS

4 medium Dutch cream or other waxy/boiling potatoes that will hold their shape

2 handfuls of fresh cleavers, washed and finely chopped

2 garlic cloves, crushed (optional)

Cleavers are rich in minerals, especially silica, which strengthens the hair, skin and nails. Here's a great way to get the mineral-rich cleavers into your food — without them cleaving to your tongue, which they do if you eat them raw. Using the crispy quinoa coating instead of traditional breadcrumbs also makes these gluten-free.

These balls make nice finger food at a party, or can be served with a big salad as a light meal or lunch. The creamy dipping sauce adds a lemony garlic flavour and another dose of minerals to the dish.

Put all the dipping sauce ingredients in a blender and whiz until smooth. Taste and adjust any flavours as desired. Pour into a small serving bowl, then cover and leave in the fridge until needed.

Preheat the oven to 200°C (400°F).

To make the crispy quinoa coating, put the quinoa in a saucepan with 1⅓ cups (330 ml) cold water. Bring to the boil, then boil over medium heat for 10–15 minutes, until light and fluffy. (Quinoa also cooks well in a rice cooker.)

Mix the paprika, salt and herbs through the cooked quinoa, then thinly spread the quinoa over a large baking tray (or over two smaller ones if needed). You want the grains to go dry and crispy.

Bake for 10 minutes. Remove from the oven and use a spatula to turn the grains, mixing the browner ones into the less cooked ones. Bake for another 10 minutes, until all the grains are crispy and golden.

Meanwhile, start making the potato balls. Peel the potatoes and cut into 2 cm (¾ inch) cubes. Place in a saucepan with 2 cups (500 ml) water and bring to the boil. Reduce the heat and simmer for about 20 minutes, until the potatoes are soft enough to mash. Strain the potatoes, then mash until smooth.

In another small saucepan of boiling water, blanch the cleavers for 10–15 seconds, then strain and press the water out of them.

Add the cleavers to the mashed potatoes, with salt and pepper to taste, and the garlic, if using (you might like to lightly fry it first). Mix them through, then roll into balls the size of golf balls.

To coat the potato balls, have your tray of crispy quinoa handy, and the mayonnaise in a bowl. Working one at a time, roll the balls in the mayonnaise, then in the quinoa coating. Bake for another 5 minutes on a tray lined with greaseproof paper.

Serve hot or cold, with the cleavers dipping sauce.

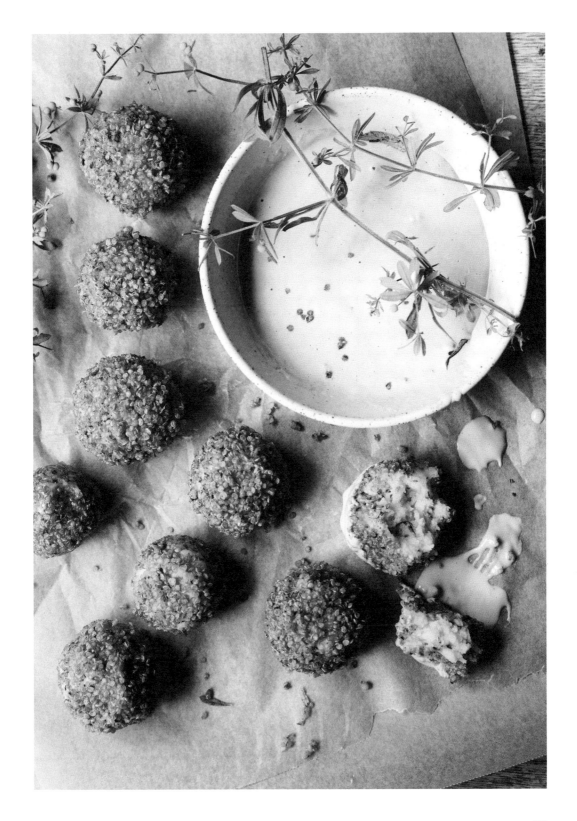

Cleavers coffee

SERVES 1; MAKES 1 CUP
15 MINUTES

1 tablespoon dried toasted
cleavers seed powder
(see note)

milk of your choice (optional)

sweetener of choice (optional)

Note

Follow the instructions on page 130 for harvesting and drying cleavers seeds. Once the seeds are dry, toast them in a frying pan for 5 minutes over medium heat until golden brown. Tip them into a bowl and let them cool completely, then grind the seeds to a powder using a coffee grinder. Any left-over powder will keep in a clean glass jar in the pantry for up to 12 months.

Cleavers seeds make a delicious coffee substitute, similar to regular coffee, with a mildly bitter, nutty and slightly sweet taste. These seeds are rich in minerals and have traditionally been used to help treat swollen lymph glands, oedema (swelling) of the face, arms, legs and ankles, as well as urinary tract infections. This coffee is ideal for anyone wanting to reduce their caffeine consumption.

Place the dried seed powder and 1 cup (250 ml) water in a saucepan and boil for 15 minutes.

Strain and drink either black, or with milk and/or sweetener.

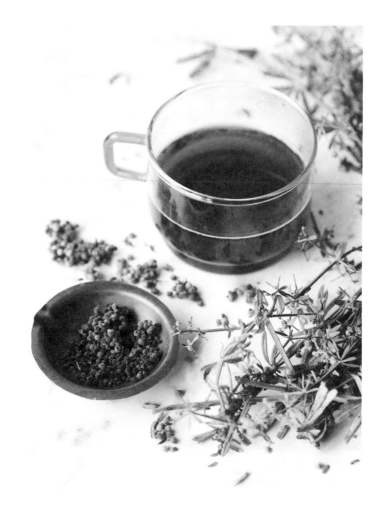

Cleavers lymph cream

MAKES ½ CUP (125 ML)
40 MINUTES

2 tablespoons dried cleavers, or 1 handful of fresh cleavers

3 tablespoons cleavers infused oil (see note)

1½ tablespoons olivem 1000

1 teaspoon vegetable glycerine

12 drops of citricidal (citrus seed extract)

5–10 drops of chamomile or lavender essential oil (optional)

Note

Make cleavers infused oil either by the slow method (2 weeks) on page 30, or the fast method (1–2 days) on page 31.

Herbalists have long used cleavers for its effects on the glands and lymphatic system. This moisturising cream helps firm the skin and reduce puffiness, and can be used for conditions such as acne, eczema, psoriasis, abscesses and boils, and for swollen lymph glands or fluid retention in the face, legs or ankles.

Before starting this recipe, read the section on making creams on page 34.

Infuse the dried or fresh cleavers in ½ cup (125 ml) hot boiled water for at least 30 minutes, or overnight for a strong infusion.

Strain and compost the herbs, then pour the infusion into a small saucepan, but leave it off the heat.

Pop some ice cubes in a large bowl half filled with water, to have an ice bath ready for when you are mixing your cream. (You can leave the ice bath in the fridge or freezer until needed.)

In a Pyrex or other heatproof glass jug, combine the infused oil, olivem 1000 and glycerine. Place the jug in another saucepan, then pour about 5 cm (2 inches) water into the pan to make a water bath.

Bring the water to the boil, then reduce the heat to a slow boil. Stir the mixture in the jug until the wax has melted, about 8–10 minutes.

Add the citricidal to your cleavers infusion in the other pan. Heat the infusion until close to boiling point — but take it off the heat as soon as bubbles form.

The oil mixture and the infusion need to be as close as possible to the same temperature to incorporate smoothly and avoid a gritty cream, so as soon as the wax has melted and the infusion is near boiling, pour the melted oil mixture into the infusion, place the saucepan in the ice bath (this will help the mixture thicken much more quickly) and start mixing with a fork or whisk. (If making a large batch, a stick blender will be much faster.)

Once it has cooled a bit, add the essential oil, if using. (Add 5 drops, then test some on your skin to see if you want to add more essential oil or not.)

Stop mixing when the mixture forms nice stiff peaks like whipped cream; this can take 8–10 minutes.

Spoon into sterilised glass jars (see page 23). Seal with the lid, then label with the ingredients, date made, and an expiry date of 3 months.

This cream is best stored in the fridge.

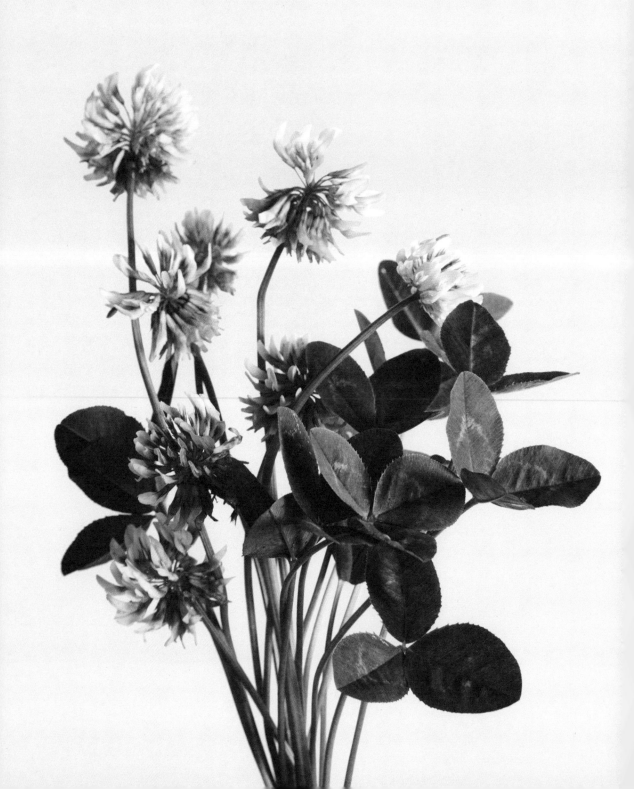

Clover, white

COMMON NAMES:

clover, white clover

SPECIES:

Trifolium spp. There are over 300 *Trifolium* species. *Trifolium repens* (white clover) is the most common one found in gardens.

GENUS:

Trifolium

FAMILY:

Fabaceae

DISTRIBUTION:

Native to Europe and Central Asia. It has been widely introduced worldwide as a yard crop, and is now also common in most grassy areas of North America, Australia and New Zealand.

PLANT SPIRIT QUALITIES:

Clover gives you the ultimate 'makeover' of your heart and psyche, helping to overcome poor self-esteem and poor body image, so you can see your true beauty for yourself. **Key words — beauty, self-esteem.**

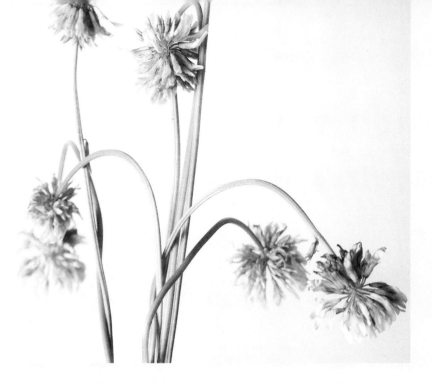

How to identify it

- White clover has creeping, hairless stems.
- Leaflets are hairless, and usually have white V-shaped bands across them.
- Unlike oxalis, to which it looks similar, it has a bland taste, with no sourness.
- It has many white to pinkish flowers in heads on long peduncles.
- The seed pod is usually 3–4 seeded.
- The root has below-ground rhizomes and above-ground stolons.

How to harvest

Flowers

Mainly it's the flowers that are used. Flowers are best cut off directly under the flower to get as little stem as possible.

Leaves

Use scissors to cut the stems near the ground. Do this gently to avoid uprooting the plant so that it can regrow. The leaves have the highest nutritional content before flowering. They mainly just taste like grass, but can be added to a salad along with other more delicious greens to boost nutrition.

Seeds

The flowering seed heads can be cut from the stems and put into a paper bag to dry and collect the seeds.

Make sure to harvest sustainably, and leave enough flowering plants to regrow.

Nutrients

Protein, sodium, potassium, calcium, magnesium.

Culinary use

Leaves and flowers are edible, either raw or cooked. Leaves can be used in salads and soups. Young flowers are nice in salads. Tea is often made from the flowers.

The root can be cooked and eaten as a vegetable.

Folk medicine

Traditionally, the flowers have been used in infusions for skin disease and as a blood cleanser. They have been used particularly for wounds, sores and boils.

Infusions have also been used for coughs, colds, fevers, leucorrhoea and gout.

They are also considered pain relieving, antiseptic, sedative, and expectorant.

In India *T. repens* is used for the treating intestinal worms. In Pakistan it is used for fever, meningitis, pneumonia, sore throats, abdominal pain, joint disorders, coughs, colds, fever and as an eye wash.

How to use it as a medicine

It is mainly used as an infusion.

Research

Studies have shown *T. repens* to be effective as an antioxidant[1] and in the treatment of diabetes.[2]

CAUTIONS + CONTRAINDICATIONS

White clover (*T. repens*) has little data, but appears to be safe in moderate doses as a food or tea. White clover releases a small amount of toxic cyanogenic glycosides (similar to those found in apple seeds) when its leaf tissues are damaged. Although many people eat it raw in small amounts (e.g. a small handful), if you're concerned, cooking can neutralise this toxin. The levels are non-toxic in flowers.

Clover can also be used in:

- Clover tea

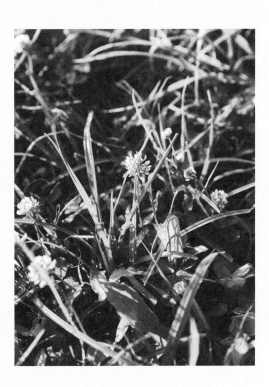

Clover syrup

This wonderfully simple syrup is like a vegan honey that has been scented with a patch of sweet-smelling fresh clover flowers. It can be used like honey on any kind of bread, in drinks and drizzled over breakfasts, yoghurt, pancakes or desserts.

MAKES ½ CUP (125 ML)
15 MINUTES

1 handful of freshly picked white clover flowers (use straight away)

½ cup (125 ml) water

1 cup (185 g) raw caster (superfine) sugar

1½ teaspoons lemon juice

Combine the clover flowers, water and sugar in a saucepan and gently bring to the boil. Reduce the heat and simmer for 10 minutes, until the syrup thickens.

Remove from the heat, pour the syrup through a sieve to strain out the flowers, and stir in the lemon juice.

Pour into a sterilised glass jar (see page 23) and store in the fridge, where it will keep for up to 6 months.

Mahalabia with clover syrup

This delicious Middle Eastern chilled dessert is light and fragrant, and spiced with cardamom, which goes beautifully with the subtle flavour of clover syrup. Perfect for summer evenings after a big meal, it can be made well ahead of time and left to chill in the fridge for special gatherings.

SERVES 2
30 MINUTES

2 tablespoons cornflour (cornstarch) or rice flour

1¼ cups (310 ml) milk of your choice

1 tablespoon raw caster (superfine) sugar

1 small handful of freshly picked white clover flowers, finely chopped, plus extra to garnish

½ teaspoon ground cardamom

2 tablespoons clover syrup (see above)

2 tablespoons chopped pistachios

In a cup, mix the cornflour with ¼ cup (60 ml) of the milk to make a smooth paste. Set aside.

Pour the remaining milk into a saucepan. Add the sugar, clover flowers and cardamom and warm over low heat for 3–5 minutes.

Add the cornflour paste and, stirring constantly, increase the heat to medium–high. Keep stirring for another 5 minutes or so, until the mixture thickens.

Pour into two serving cups or bowls and leave to cool slightly, then cover and chill in the fridge for at least 30 minutes, or until ready to serve.

Just before serving, drizzle a tablespoon of clover syrup over each pudding and garnish with pistachios and extra clover flowers.

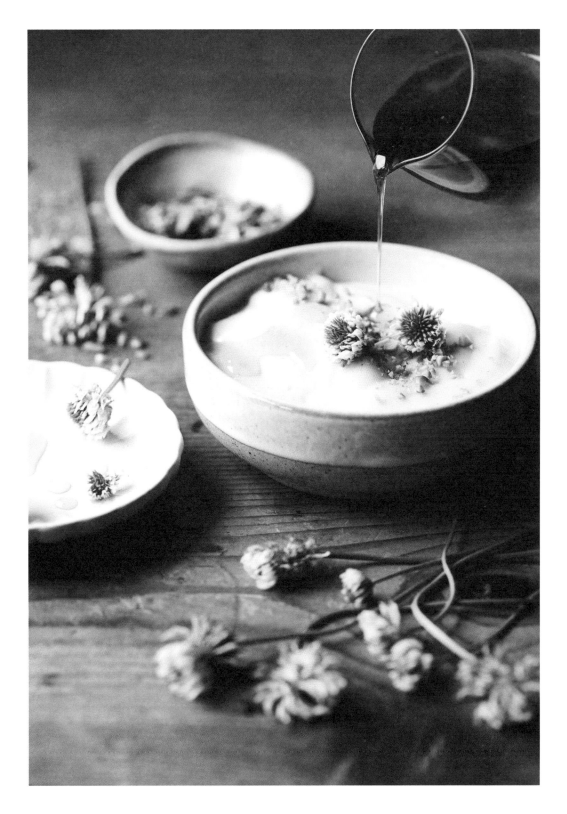

Clover cupcakes with orange cashew icing

These delicate little beauties are a delightful way to use white clover to boost the variety of plants in your diet for added fibre and nutrition. They are perfect for garden parties or fairy-themed birthday parties.

You'll need to plan on making the icing ahead, as the cashews need to be soaked for 2 hours before using.

MAKES 8 LARGE MUFFINS OR 10 SMALL MUFFINS

30 MINUTES

¾ cup (185 ml) milk of your choice

1 tablespoon orange juice

1½ cups (225 g) self-raising flour

½ cup (110 g) caster (superfine) sugar

¼ cup (60 ml) rice bran or sunflower oil

2 teaspoons pure vanilla extract

1 small handful of freshly picked white clover blossoms, finely chopped, plus extra flowers to garnish

ORANGE CASHEW ICING

1 cup (155 g) raw cashews

¾ cup (185 ml) orange juice

⅓ cup (80 ml) maple syrup

1½ tablespoons lecithin

1 teaspoon pure vanilla extract

a pinch of salt

½ cup (100 g) coconut oil, melted

3 teaspoons milk of your choice

To make the icing, soak the cashews in a bowl of water for 2 hours. Drain, then place in a blender with the orange juice, maple syrup, lecithin, vanilla and salt. Blend for 3 minutes, then add the melted coconut oil and blend for another 2 minutes. Transfer to a shallow bowl, then cover and chill in the fridge for at least 2 hours, or overnight.

Preheat the oven to 160°C (315°F). Line an 8-hole or 10-hole muffin tin with paper cases.

Pour the milk into a jug, add the orange juice and set aside to curdle and thicken, like a buttermilk.

Sift the flour and sugar into a bowl.

Add the oil and vanilla to your buttermilk jug and whisk gently to combine. Pour into the flour bowl and mix with a wooden spoon until the lumps are gone — but don't over mix, as air is needed to make the cupcakes light and fluffy.

Gently fold the clover blossoms through the batter. Pour the batter into the muffin tin, filling each hole only halfway, to give the mixture room to rise.

Bake for 10–15 minutes for small muffins, or up to 20 minutes for large muffins; a skewer should come out clean when poked in the centre. Allow to cool in the tin, then remove to a wire rack.

Take your icing out of the fridge and mix using an electric hand mixer or stand mixer You can add the milk teaspoon by teaspoon to get a smoother, softer consistency. You may not need the whole amount, so check the consistency before adding more. You want the icing to be soft, but still hold its shape in peaks and waves. It should not fall out of the mixing bowl when tipped upside down.

Spread the icing on the cupcakes and garnish each one with an extra clover flower.

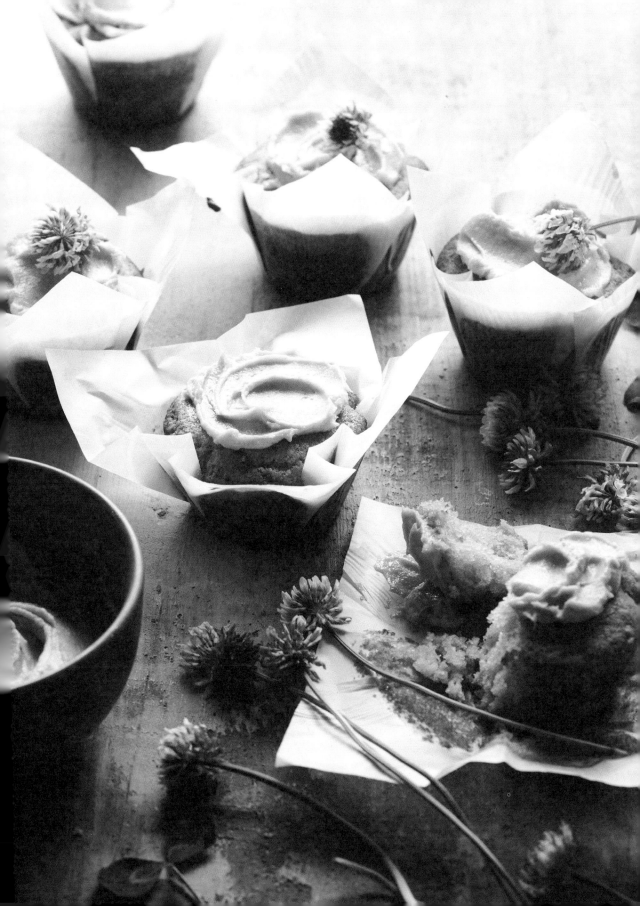

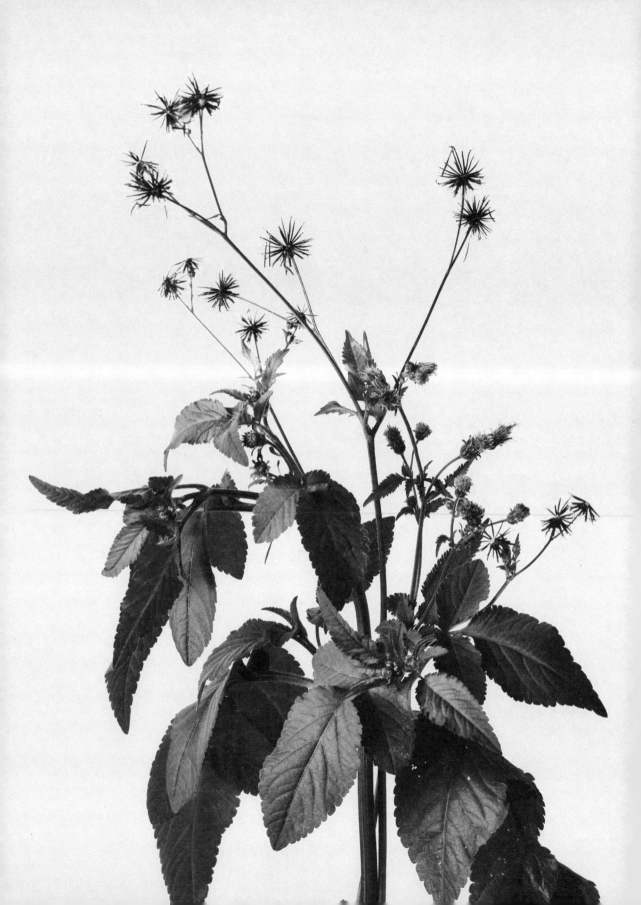

Cobbler's pegs

COMMON NAMES:

cobbler's pegs, farmer's friends, beggar's ticks, black jack, sticky beaks

SPECIES:

Bidens pilosa

GENUS:

Bidens

FAMILY:

Asteraceae

DISTRIBUTION:

Native to the Americas. Introduced throughout Europe, Asia, Africa, Australia and the Pacific Islands.

PLANT SPIRIT QUALITIES:

When you feel like giving up, cobbler's pegs helps you persevere. It inspires you to try from all different angles until you find what works. When you become frustrated, because it feels too hard or it's taking too long, cobbler's pegs brings grace to your struggle and helps you accept the timing of things while continuing to work towards them. **Key word — tenacity.**

How to identify it

- Cobbler's pegs are most easily identified by their black spiky seed heads, which stick to everything they touch.
- The plant has small, white daisy-like flowers, with 5–7 delicate white petals and a yellow centre.
- The leaves are oval or lance-shaped, with serrated edges. Each stem ends with a group of three leaves.
- The stems can be light green, dark green or reddish in colour.
- It has a fibrous root system.

How to harvest

Leaves

Cobbler's pegs are an annual that will die back in winter and regrow in spring. Leaves, stems and flowers are best harvested before the black seed heads appear in late summer to early autumn.

The young leaves and stems can be harvested throughout the growing cycle by cutting near the base with a pair of scissors. Leaving the roots intact will ensure the following year's growth.

Seeds

Seeds can be harvested in late summer to early autumn by gently pulling the burr-shaped heads off the plants, or by cutting the stems and letting them dry, then shaking the seeds into a paper bag.

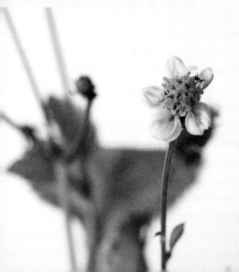

Nutrients

Protein, vitamin C, calcium, iron, potassium and magnesium.

Culinary use

Cobbler's pegs are an unpopular weed in Australia, but worldwide they are a common wild food. The plant is an incredibly high source of plant protein. The leaves, stems and flowers can be used raw in salads, cooked as a green vegetable, dried and stored for future use, or made into a tea. The seeds can be ground into a powder and applied as a local anaesthetic for cuts or toothache, or used as a fibre to improve digestion.

Folk medicine

Folkloric use has been documented in Australia, America, Africa and Asia, including the following conditions.

Gastrointestinal

Stomach ache, colic, constipation, diarrhoea, dysentery, appendicitis, enteritis, gastritis, intestinal worms, haemorrhoids, stomach ulcers, bacterial infections in the gastrointestinal tract.

Respiratory

Asthma, sore throats, colds, flu, tuberculosis, cough, earaches.

Infections

Acute infectious hepatitis, conjunctivitis, renal infections, yellow fever, malaria.

Female reproductive

Menstrual irregularities, period pain, morning sickness, heavy bleeding.

Systemic

Diabetes, metabolic syndrome, inflammation, arthritis, hypertension.

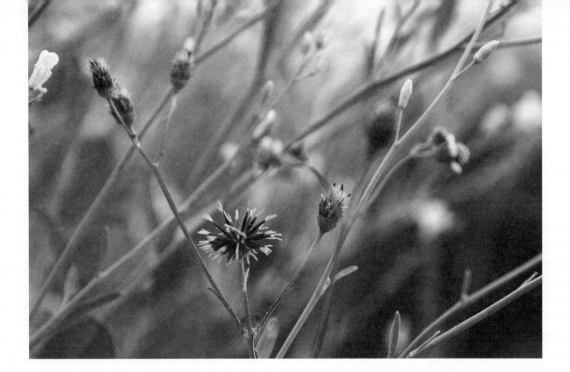

Externally
Cuts, burns, wounds, snakebite, nose bleeds.

Research

Clinical trials have confirmed its use in the following areas: anti-inflammatory,[1] antidiabetic and anti-hypoglycaemic,[2] anti-allergenic,[3] immune-modulating,[4] antioxidant,[5] antimalarial,[6] antibacterial,[7] antifungal,[8] antihypertensive, vasodilatory,[9] wound healing,[10] anti-ulcerative.[11]

How to use it as a medicine

All parts of the plant have traditionally been used as ingredients in folk medicine, including the leaves, flowers, stems, roots and seeds. It is usually prepared as a dry powder or tincture for external use, and as a powder, maceration, infusion or decoction to use internally. The fresh juice is a potent antibacterial.

CAUTIONS + CONTRAINDICATIONS
In areas that have soils high in silica and cadmium, *Bidens pilosa* can accumulate these compounds.

Cobbler's pegs can also be used in:
- Cobbler's pegs glycetract
- Cobbler's pegs tea
- Wild wilted greens
- Wild greens powder

Cobbler's pegs, lentil & tomato curry

SERVES 4

30 MINUTES + OVERNIGHT SOAKING (OPTIONAL)

1 cup (215 g) dried green lentils, or a 425 g (15 oz) tin of lentils

2 tablespoons olive or coconut oil

1 large onion, finely diced

2 small celery sticks, diced

1 thumb-sized piece of fresh ginger, peeled and grated (or 2 teaspoons ginger paste)

5 garlic cloves, crushed (or 2 teaspoons garlic paste)

1 fresh chilli, or ½ teaspoon chilli flakes or chilli powder

2 teaspoons ground coriander

1 teaspoon ground cumin

2 teaspoons garam masala

3 tablespoons tomato paste (concentrated purée)

3 fresh tomatoes, chopped

2 teaspoons salt

2 teaspoons rapadura or coconut sugar

3 handfuls of coarsely chopped fresh cobbler's pegs leaves

Packed with minerals, this delicious curry is also super high in protein, with cobbler's pegs having the highest protein content of all the wild plants I know — offering a whopping 24 grams of protein per 100 grams of fresh leaves. Cooked lentils also contain about 9 grams of protein per 100 grams, so this nutritious curry is perfect to enjoy on repeat.

It's wonderful served with steamed rice, lemon wedges, coconut yoghurt, and fresh cobblers pegs, parsley or coriander (cilantro). For a creamy dal version of this dish, stir in 200 ml (7 fl oz) coconut cream towards the end of cooking.

If using dried lentils, soak them in a bowl with plenty of cold water for 8 hours, or overnight. Drain the lentils, place in a saucepan, cover with fresh water and cook for 15–20 minutes, or until soft.

Heat the oil in a large frying pan over medium heat. Add the onion, celery, ginger, garlic, chilli, coriander, cumin and garam masala. Fry, stirring now and then, for about 3 minutes, until golden brown.

Stir in the remaining ingredients, along with the drained cooked or tinned lentils. Simmer over low heat, stirring regularly, until the tomatoes and cobbler's pegs are soft, and the lentils are heated through. Add some water if the curry is a little thick.

Serve with your favourite accompaniments.

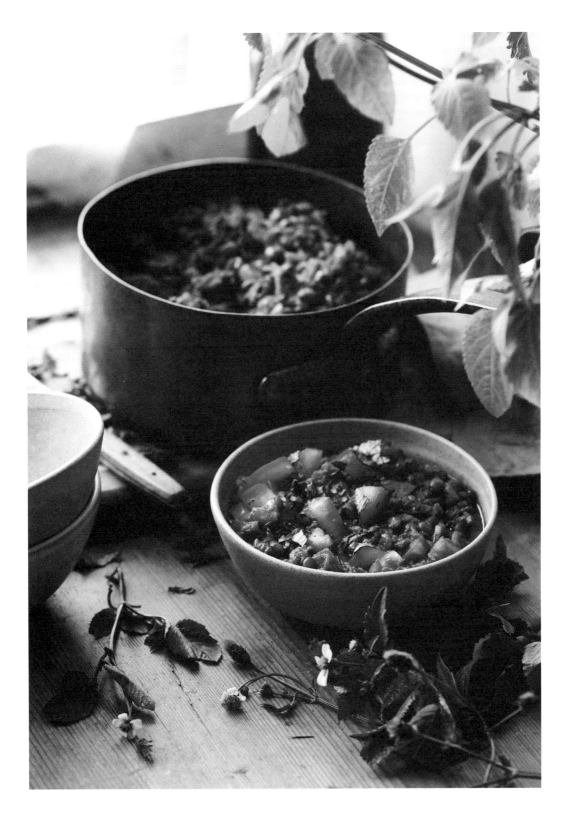

Wild greens powder

6 CUPS FRESH HERBS MAKES ABOUT 2 CUPS POWDER

15 MINUTES + 1–2 DAYS DRYING

3–6 handfuls of as many different wild plants as you can find — for example cobbler's pegs, nettle, nasturtium, purslane, nodding top, plantain, oxalis, chickweed, amaranth leaves, blackberry nightshade leaves, fat hen, cleavers, wild garlic, dandelion and bush basil/tulsi

1 tablespoon dried seaweed (see note)

Making this is like creating your own vitamin and mineral supplement and greens powder, all in one. For people who prefer to avoid synthetic supplements, this is an all-natural alternative, bursting with protein, fibre, vitamins and minerals. I like the main ingredient to be cobbler's pegs (farmer's friends), because of their protein content.

Adding seaweed boosts the mineral content and adds trace minerals that are often lacking in our food and soils. (Use seaweed with caution if you have an overactive thyroid, however.)

After a few weeks on this blend, you will often notice improvements in energy, mental clarity and stamina, and more stable blood sugar and hormonal regulation.

Dry the wild greens in a dehydrator. If you don't have a dehydrator, the best way I have found to dry herbs quickly is to leave them in the car for a day in a cardboard box, or on the dashboard — unless it's a rainy day, then they are probably better inside. You might want to turn them over during the day and make sure they're not burning. Alternatively, the herbs can be dried in the oven on the lowest setting with the door ajar for 3–4 hours, until crumbly.

When dry and crisp, discard the stalks and blitz or grind the leaves using a food processor, blender, coffee grinder or a mortar and pestle. (It can be good to put the greens in a food processor first, then a coffee grinder, to get them ground to a fine powder.)

Transfer to a sterilised glass jar (see page 23). Seal with the lid, then label the jar with the ingredients and date made.

Store in a dark cupboard or the freezer.

HOW TO USE WILD GREENS POWDER

Add 1–2 tablespoons to smoothies, water or milk of your choice as a protein powder, and enjoy once daily.

Note

If I'm using bought seaweed (rather than foraged), I like to use dulse or kombu. Nori isn't ideal because it isn't as rich in minerals as other seaweeds. Kelp is very strongly flavoured, so only add 1 teaspoon. If you have an overactive thyroid, use seaweed with caution.

Cobbler's pegs anti-inflammatory juice

SERVES 1; MAKES 1 CUP
15 MINUTES

3 handfuls of fresh cobbler's pegs leaves and stems

2 apples

½ cup (80 g) fresh diced pineapple

1 mint sprig

½ cup (125 ml) water (or a few ice cubes)

This delicious, refreshing juice is incredibly cooling and soothing when there is heat, pain and inflammation anywhere in the body. It also regulates blood sugar, curbs sugar cravings and helps support a healthy metabolism, particularly for those with metabolic syndrome, diabetes and obesity.

Pass all the ingredients through a juicer and drink straight away.

If you don't have a juicer, whiz them in a blender and drink the juice like a smoothie, or strain it through muslin (cheesecloth) if you prefer just the juice.

HOW TO USE COBBLER'S PEGS ANTIBACTERIAL SKIN JUICE

Fresh cobbler's pegs juice can also be used topically on the skin for bacterial or fungal skin infections or minor wounds. I've had great results with this for staph and other bacterial skin infections. Simply juice about 3 cups of coarsely chopped fresh cobbler's pegs leaves and stems. Apply the juice directly to the skin, or soak a gauze bandage in the juice, apply it to the skin and wrap with a crepe bandage. Change the dressing at least once daily or twice a day for wounds that have pus or weeping. I also recommend drinking ¼ cup (60 ml) of the juice. (You can also pour the fresh juice into ice cube trays and freeze for up to 3 months, and defrost as needed.)

Cobbler's pegs gel

MAKES ¼ CUP (60 ML)
10 MINUTES

2 teaspoons cobbler's pegs juice

¼ cup (60 ml) laponite gel (or aloe vera gel)

6 drops of citricidal (citrus seed extract)

As well as the antibacterial skin juice above, you can make a nice antibiotic gel to use on the skin for treating a minor skin infection or minor wound. This gel is cool and soothing and lasts longer than using the juice on its own. It can be stored in the fridge and used daily until the skin infection has cleared.

Mix all the ingredients into a nice green gel and store in a sterilised glass jar (see page 23) in the fridge. It will last for 3–5 days if made using aloe vera gel, and up to 3 months if made with laponite gel.

HOW TO USE THE GEL

Use directly on the skin 2–3 times a day for acne, minor skin infections and wounds. Aways wash your hands with soap before and after treating the wound, to prevent the spread of infection.

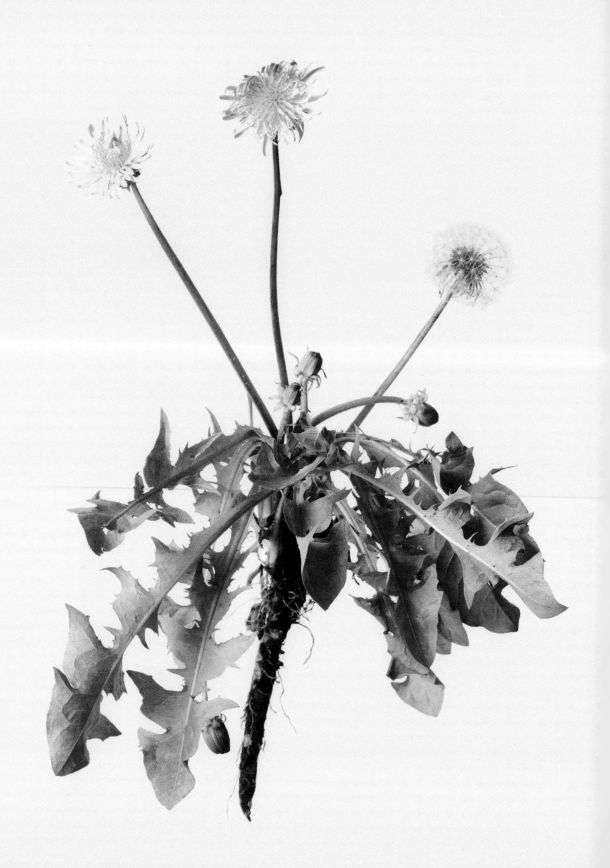

Dandelion

COMMON NAMES:

dandelion, pissenlit ('piss the bed' in French), clock flower

SPECIES:

Taraxacum officinale

GENUS:

Taraxacum

FAMILY:

Asteraceae

DISTRIBUTION:

Native to Europe and Asia. Naturalised throughout North and South America, Southern Africa, New Zealand, Australia and India.

PLANT SPIRIT QUALITIES:

Dandelion helps detoxify both your body and your life, to clear away obstacles and let go of that which no longer serves you. When you feel weakened or need extra energy for a big life change, it can strengthen the will and life force, bringing you the clarity and focus to eliminate jobs, houses or relationships you have outgrown, and to achieve large or small goals.
Key words — purpose, goals, life calling, decision-making.

How to identify it

- Dandelion has a basal rosette with serrated, deeply lobed leaves that generally point back towards the centre of the rosette.
- It produces bright yellow flowers on a leafless stalk, which are open in the daytime and closed at night.
- It has a straight hollow stem that is 1–10 cm (½–4 inches) high, with no branching or leaves.
- There is only one flower per stem.
- Stems and leaves have a white, milky latex sap.
- A rosette may produce several flowering stems at a time.
- The flower heads are 2–5 cm (¾–2 inches) in diameter and consist entirely of ray florets.
- Dandelion has a distinctive globe-shaped puffball seed head.
- The puffball is made up of many single-seeded fruits called achenes. Each achene is attached to a pappus of fine hairs.

How to harvest

Leaves
Leaves are best harvested in early spring when they are fresh and tender. Cut with scissors from the base, leaving the top leaves to keep growing so you can keep harvesting.

Flowers
Flowers appear in late spring to early summer and can be collected by cutting off the stalks. Flower stalks can be harvested and plunged into iced water for 5 minutes to use as drinking straws (see page 160).

Roots
Roots are best harvested in early spring before flowering, as this is when they will have the highest concentration of medicinal constituents. Dandelions have a long tap root that requires you to dig deeply in a circular motion around the plant to try to extract as much of the root as possible. Be sure to replace the earth you have disrupted, and make sure there are enough plants left to go to seed to maintain the dandelion population in that area. Leave the best and strongest plant for good genetic reproduction.

To use the root, remove the leaves, and spindly hairy bits. The leaves can be used in a salad, and hairy bits in a glycetract. Wash the thick part of the root with a scrubbing brush or metal scourer. Clean off any black stained bits with a paring knife. Cut the root into small pieces 1–2 cm (¾–½ inch) thick. If you have lots (more than 1 cup), you can chop them using a food processor; small amounts will just spin around the edges and not chop. Place in a dehydrator to dry, or on a baking tray in the oven at the lowest heat, or put in a cardboard box or over a drying rack in the sun.

Nutrients

Potassium, readily available magnesium, niacin, calcium, phosphorus, iron, sulphur, zinc, vitamins B1, B2, B6, B12, C, E, D and beta-carotene.

Culinary use

Young dandelion leaves are great in salads, juices, green smoothies and sandwiches. Older leaves can be used in soups and as a pot vegetable. The dried, ground-up root is used as a coffee substitute.

Folk medicine

Traditionally, dandelion has been used to treat disorders of the liver, kidneys and gallbladder. The root has traditionally been associated with effects relating to the liver, whereas the leaf has more of an affinity for the kidneys.

Dandelion breaks down fat by stimulating the flow of bile. This makes it beneficial for poor appetite, weak digestion, insulin disregulation and abdominal pain. It has been used to prevent gallstones, assist the liver with detoxification, and support kidney function as it has diuretic properties.

Due to its high calcium and magnesium content, it can also help maintain bone health.

Herbalist Juliette de Baïracli Levy recommends it for strengthening the enamel of the teeth, and also for diabetes and obesity.

It is also an excellent source of potassium, and is often used as a potassium-sparing diuretic.

Dandelion is regularly used in the treatment of skin disorders associated with sluggish liver and bowel conditions, and is a great herb for cleansing and detoxification. It is mildly laxative.

The latex is used on warts.

Research

Clinical trials have confirmed dandelion's use in the following areas: antioxidant,[1] diuretic,[2] improved liver detoxification and protection,[3] anti-inflammatory,[4] anti-diabetic[5] and metabolic syndrome.[6]

How to use it as a medicine

It can be used as an infusion (leaf), decoction (root), tincture (both root and leaf) or powder.

CAUTIONS + CONTRAINDICATIONS
Caution if allergic to the Asteraceae family. May cause excess acid in the stomach. Do not use if there are obstructions in the bile ducts or intestinal tract, or during acute gallbladder inflammation.

Dandelion can also be used in:

- Wild wilted greens
- Wild greens powder
- Dandelion glycetract
- Dandelion tea

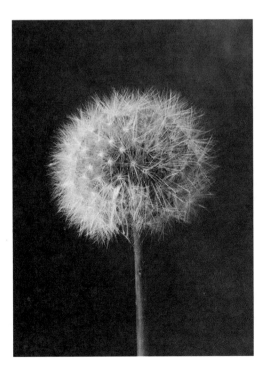

Bitter salad

SERVES 4
15 MINUTES

GF

I can wax lyrical for days about the benefits of bitters. They switch on the digestive system, causing the secretion of multiple digestive enzymes, saliva and bile, which enable your food to be fully broken down and properly digested — increasing the absorption of nutrients and decreasing the likelihood of bloating, gas and nausea after eating.

Bitters promote a healthy gut microbiome, supporting the growth of good gut bacteria, and leading to more effective elimination and detoxification via the bowels and liver. They also help regulate blood sugar and metabolism, and increase the feeling of fullness after eating, making it easier not to overeat.

Interestingly, bitters also have a mild antidepressant effect through their action on the gut–brain axis — a feedback loop whereby the health of the gut and our mental state impact each other.

They are also antioxidants, helping to prevent inflammation and reduce the risk of chronic diseases.

Most cultures understand the importance of bitter foods at the start of a meal, with bitter foods and drinks being staple fare in cuisines around the world.

This salad can be eaten regularly to maintain overall health and vitality. One handful of this salad at the start of a meal will be enough to get your digestion switched on and ready to roll. Chew slowly and thoroughly for maximum benefit.

1 handful of dandelion leaves

1 handful of chicory leaves

1 handful of endive

5 dandelion or chicory flowers, to garnish

1 handful of radicchio leaves

LEMON DRESSING

¼ cup (60 ml) lemon juice

2 tablespoons olive oil

1 garlic clove, crushed (optional)

Remove any stalky stems from the greens. Wash and thoroughly dry all the leaves, then roughly chop and place in a salad bowl.

In a small jug or bowl, whisk the dressing ingredients together. Season with salt and pepper to taste.

Just before serving, toss the dressing through the salad. Pull the petals off the dandelion flowers, sprinkle them over the salad and enjoy straight away.

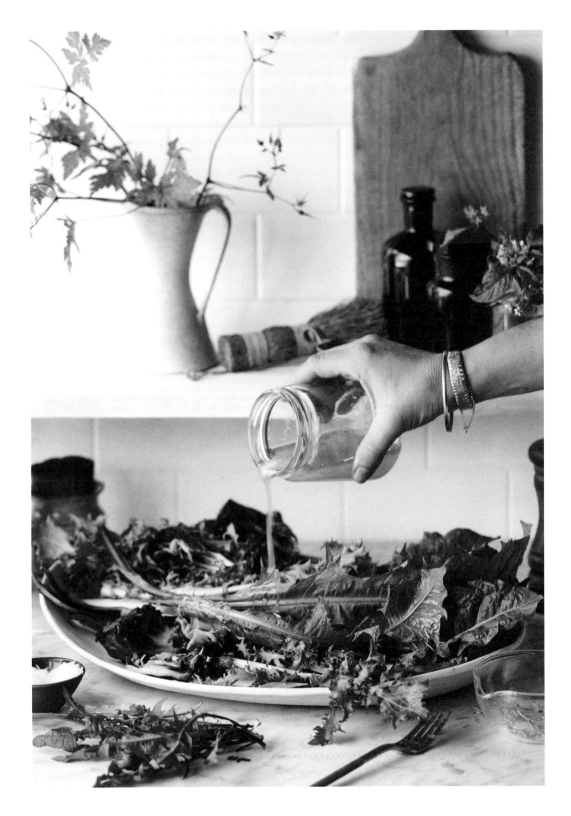

Deep-fried dandelion flowers

SERVES 2
25 MINUTES

GF

I have seen quite a few variations of this recipe — from Asian-style tempura versions to Appalachian ones deep-fried in butter. I have opted for a gluten-free Indian chickpea batter, made using no eggs, fried tempura style.

Dandelion flowers are nice and open in the day, but they close at night — so if you collect them during the day, make sure to cook them before nightfall so they don't close up on you. Make the dipping sauce first, so you can eat the flowers fresh and hot from the pan. If you don't want to make the dipping sauce, just use your favourite mayo or aioli.

You might think deep-fried dandelion flowers would be bitter and flowery, but they are a surprisingly delicious, soft and tender vegetable.

You can also use cat's ear flowers in this recipe — they are also delicious deep-fried.

1 cup (250 ml) ice-cold water

1 teaspoon salt

1 handful of large, open dandelion flowers

100 g (3½ oz) chickpea flour (besan)

1 teaspoon onion salt

1 teaspoon dried Italian herbs

1 cup (250 ml) sparkling mineral water

¼ cup (60 ml) rice bran oil, for frying

DANDELION DIPPING SAUCE

2 tablespoons tahini

2 tablespoons lemon juice

2 tablespoons maple syrup

1 small handful of dandelion leaves, coarsely chopped

2 tablespoons water

1 teaspoon capers or chopped preserved lemon rind

Put all the dipping sauce ingredients in a blender and whiz for 2 minutes, or until smooth. (Alternatively, put them in a jug and use a stick blender.) Season to taste and set aside.

Pour the icy water into a bowl and add the salt, stirring to dissolve. Plunge the dandelion flowers into water and let them soak for 10 minutes.

Sift the chickpea flour into a bowl. Mix in the onion salt and herbs, then gently stir in the mineral water to form a batter. (You want to keep as many bubbles as you can.)

Drain the flowers and pat dry with a tea towel.

Heat the rice bran oil in a cast-iron frying pan over medium heat.

Working in batches, dip the flowers into the batter, then place immediately in the hot oil; you can probably fry 5–10 flowers at a time. Cook for 3–5 minutes, turning every couple of minutes until golden brown.

Briefly drain on a plate lined with paper towel to absorb any excess oil.

Serve hot and crispy, with the dandelion dipping sauce.

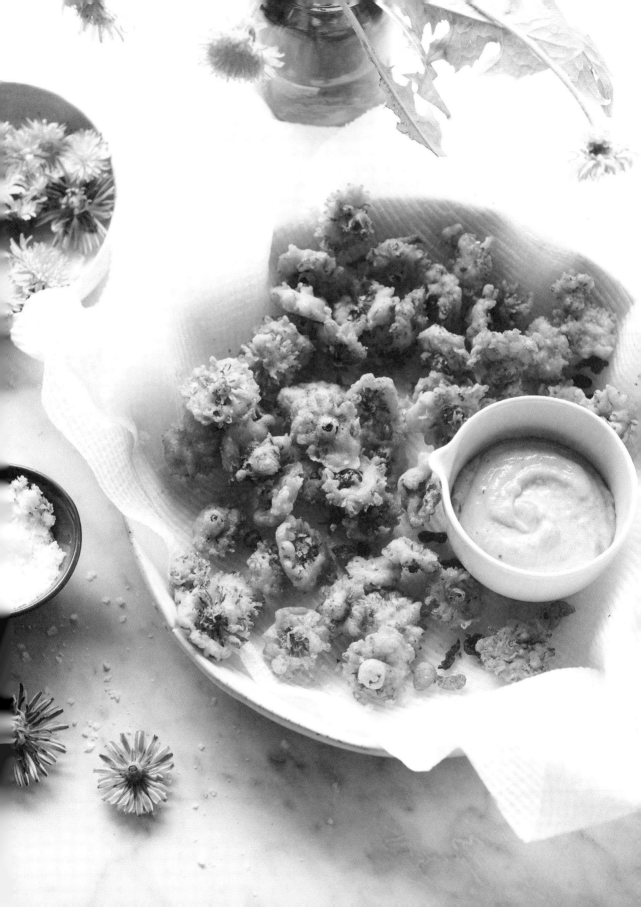

Dandelion root coffee

Dandelion roots are rich in minerals and have a detoxifying effect on the liver. They are also a good source of fibre and prebiotics, and make a delicious coffee-like beverage — without the caffeine. You can use either fresh or dried roots here.

SERVES 1; MAKES 1 CUP

15–30 MINUTES ROASTING + 5 MINUTES

GF

1 tablespoon roasted dandelion roots or powder (see note)

milk of your choice (optional)

sweetener of choice (optional)

If using roasted roots, place them in a saucepan with 1 cup (250 ml) water. Bring to the boil, then simmer for 5 minutes and strain into your cup.

If using powdered root, place it in a plunger or teapot, pour in 1 cup (250 ml) boiling water and let it sit for 3–5 minutes, depending on how strong you like it. Strain into your cup.

Enjoy your coffee either black, or with milk and/or sweetener.

Note

To roast dandelion roots, leave dried ones whole, and cut fresh roots into 1–2 cm (½–¾ inch) pieces. Spread on a baking tray and roast dried roots in a preheated 200°C (400°F) oven for 10–15 minutes, and fresh ones for 20–30 minutes. Check them every 5 minutes or so, to get the right roast — you want them to be dry and brown but not burned.

Steep the roasted chunks as directed above, or grind them into a powder using a coffee grinder. For a richer roast, you can roast the ground roots for another 5 minutes at 180°C (350°F).

Any excess roasted roots will keep in an airtight container in a dark cupboard for up to 12 months.

Dandelion straws

Dandelion straws are such a fun thing for outdoor parties, picnics or celebrations. Use the hollow stems once they have finished flowering and gone to seed.

If the puff balls are attached, you can blow these off and end enjoy counting the time (one puff for each hour).

When you are done, cut off the flower heads and place the stems in iced water for a minute or two. They are then ready to use in your favourite drink.

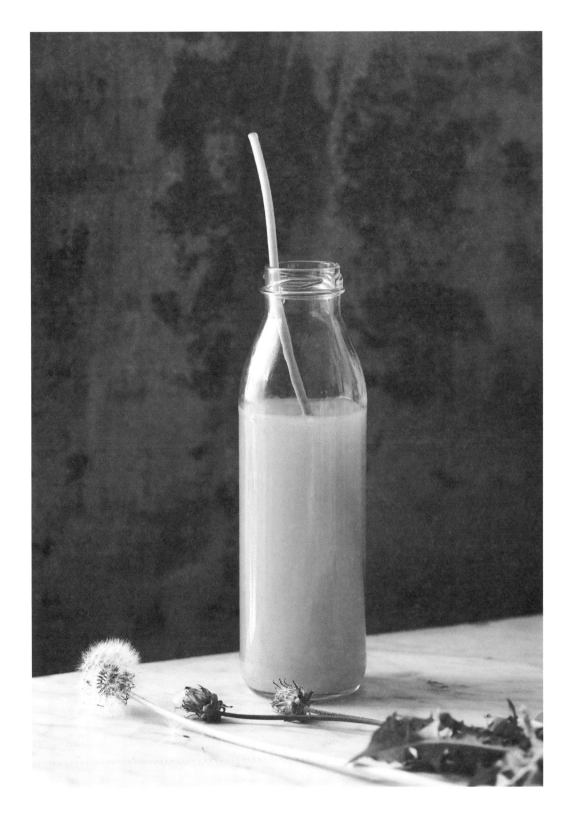

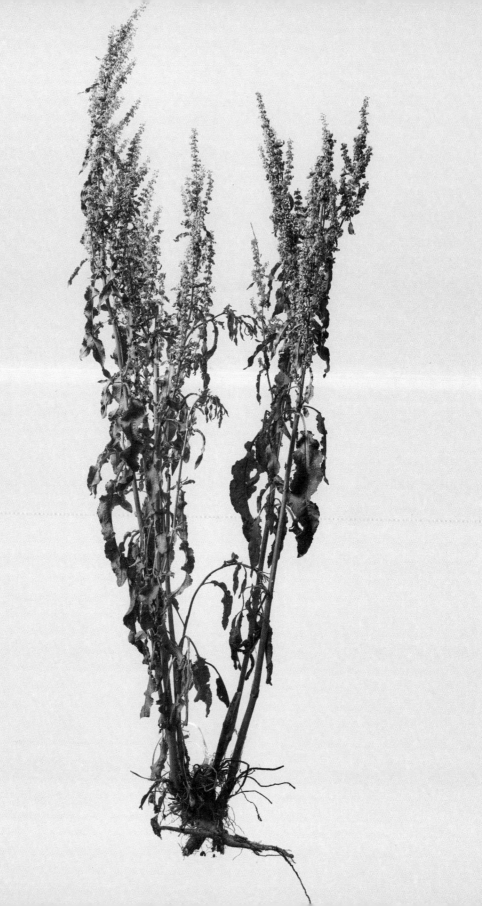

Dock

COMMON NAMES:

dock, yellow dock, curly dock, swamp dock

SPECIES:

Rumex crispus (dock, yellow dock, curly dock)

Rumex brownii (swamp dock)

GENUS:

Rumex

FAMILY:

Polygonaceae

DISTRIBUTION:

Native to Europe and Asia. Naturalised throughout the rest of the world.

PLANT SPIRIT QUALITIES:

Arcane knowledge must be made practical before it is valuable. Dock helps you to receive information from intuitive, divine or esoteric sources, then anchors that information in a deep inner knowing and practical wisdom. The plant reaches high into the air with its seed head, and deep into the earth with its long tap root, bringing the wisdom of heaven and earth together so that it can be embodied and used in everyday life. **Key words — deep knowledge, understanding, wisdom.**

How to identify it

Yellow dock (*Rumex crispus*)

- It has smooth, lance-shaped leaves shooting off from a large basal rosette, with distinctive waved or curled edges and sheathed bases.
- The plant produces an inflorescence (flower stalk) that grows to about 1 metre (3 feet) high.
- On the stalk, flowers and seeds are produced in clusters on branched stems, with the largest cluster being found at the apex.
- It has numerous greenish flowers on a tall panicle.
- The seeds are brown, and are encased in a paper-like sheath in the calyx of the flower that produced them.
- The root structure is a large, yellow, forking taproot.

Swamp dock (*Rumex brownii*)

- Also grows in a basal rosette.
- The leaves are long and oblong, and less curly on the margins than yellow dock.
- Long stalks can also have leaves growing off them.
- It has numerous flowering stalks, with seed heads that are more sparse and less dense than yellow dock.
- Fruits have hooked teeth that are dispersed by adhesion.
- The taproot is thinner and more branching than yellow dock, and is yellow inside.

How to harvest

Leaves

Dock leaves grow in early spring through summer, and die back in winter. The leaves are best harvested in spring when they are sour but not so bitter. Raw dock leaves are very stimulating to the digestion — eating more than 3 small leaves or 1–2 big leaves can make you vomit due to the high oxalate content, so only consume a small amount.

Cut leaves from the base of the plant so you can continue to harvest. Cooking the leaves neutralises the oxalates and makes them safe to eat without nausea or vomiting.

Seeds

Dock flowers in summer, and produces large seed heads from mid-summer through to late autumn. These seeds can be collected by cutting the seed stalks at the base and putting them upside down in a paper bag to dry. Once they are dried, you can run your hand along the stalk removing the seeds from the stalks.

It is very difficult to remove the seeds from the husks, so I generally use them with the husks still on (this just adds extra fibre.)

Roots

Roots are best harvested in spring before flowering, as this is when they have the highest concentration of medicinal constituents. Dock has a long yellow tap root, which can be hard to dig out. You will need a sharp shovel to dig all around the base, then try to get under it as much as possible, digging deep to get the root. You will probably need to excavate the root with your hands to remove the dirt.

Wash the root, then peel off any dark brown or black bits of skin using a sharp knife. Once you have a clean yellow root, you can chop it into 1–2 cm (½–¾ inch) pieces and dry them in a dehydrator or on a drying rack.

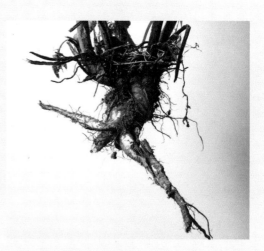

Nutrients

Vitamin A, beta-carotene, vitamin C, calcium, iron, zinc, manganese and selenium.

Culinary use

Dock leaves are tart and delicious when young and healthy, and lovely in salads and eaten as a raw green vegetable. When raw, only eat one or two leaves, as dock can cause vomiting due to the high oxalate content.

When older and rather bitter, the leaves can be cooked in soups and used like spinach or silverbeet. The cooking neutralises the oxalates, making it safer to eat.

Folk medicine

Yellow dock has a long history of use around the world. The main medicinal action comes from the root. In the digestive system, dock root has a laxative effect caused by its ability to increase the muscular contractions (known as peristalsis) that move food and faeces through the digestive tract. This makes it ideal for treating constipation.

It also tones and strengthens the bowel, and can be used for diarrhoea, colitis and Crohn's disease. It does this by stimulating the flow of bile from the liver and gallbladder. This makes it helpful for many disorders where digestion is weak or sluggish. It can be used for indigestion, constipation, liver stagnation and jaundice.

Because it helps improve elimination and detoxification via the bowel and liver, it takes the burden off the skin, which is forced to pick up the slack as an organ of elimination when the digestive system is not functioning effectively. As a result, it is often used to treat eczema, psoriasis and acne.

Swamp dock (*Rumex brownii*)

There is very little written about this species, but I have used the root as a laxative in the same manner as yellow dock, and found the leaves to be a digestive stimulant in small doses (1–2 leaves), and emetic (causing vomiting) when more than a couple of leaves are consumed.

Research

Clinical trials on yellow dock, *Rumex crispus*, have confirmed its use in the following areas: antimalarial,[1] antimicrobial,[2] antidiabetic,[3] antioxidant,[4] anti-inflammatory[5] and wound healing.[6]

How to use it as a medicine

It is used as a decoction, a tincture or a powder.

CAUTIONS + CONTRAINDICATIONS

Due to its laxative effect, dock should not be used for prolonged periods. It may cause spasmodic gripping pain in the abdomen, and too much eaten raw can make you vomit (cooking will neutralise the oxalates). Avoid if there is obstruction or inflammation in the gastrointestinal tract. Avoid in pregnancy.

Dock can also be used in:

- Dock root tea
- Dock root glycetract
- Wild grain bread

Dock & cannellini bean soup

SERVES 4–6
40 MINUTES

GF

When cooked, dock has a slippery — dare I say, slimy — texture. That doesn't sound appetising, but it is actually quite delicious. This soup is highly nutritious as dock is rich in the minerals calcium, iron, zinc, manganese and selenium. It is also rich in inflammation-reducing antioxidants. The cannellini beans add fibre and protein, rounding out a meal that makes a great menu staple. Simple to make for a hearty midweek meal, this tasty soup only gets better the next day.

2 tablespoons olive oil

1 brown onion, finely chopped

3 garlic cloves, finely chopped

1 teaspoon dried Italian herbs

2 celery stalks, finely chopped

¼ small white cabbage, shredded

2 small zucchini (courgettes), finely chopped

8 cups (2 litres) vegetable stock

1 tablespoon tamari or soy sauce

400 g (14 oz) tin of chopped tomatoes, or a 500 g (1 lb 2 oz) bottle of your favourite pasta sauce

400 g (14 oz) tin of cannellini beans, rinsed and drained

2 handfuls of fresh dock leaves, finely chopped

Heat the oil in a large heavy-based saucepan over medium–high heat. Add the onion, garlic and dried herbs and cook, stirring, for 2 minutes, or until the onion is translucent.

Add the celery, cabbage and zucchini, stirring for 5 minutes to lightly cook the vegetables.

Pour in the stock and bring to the boil.

Add the tamari and chopped tomatoes. Turn the heat down to a simmer and add the cannellini beans. Continue to cook over medium–low heat for 20 minutes.

Stir in the dock and continue cooking for 10 minutes.

Season with salt and pepper to taste, then serve.

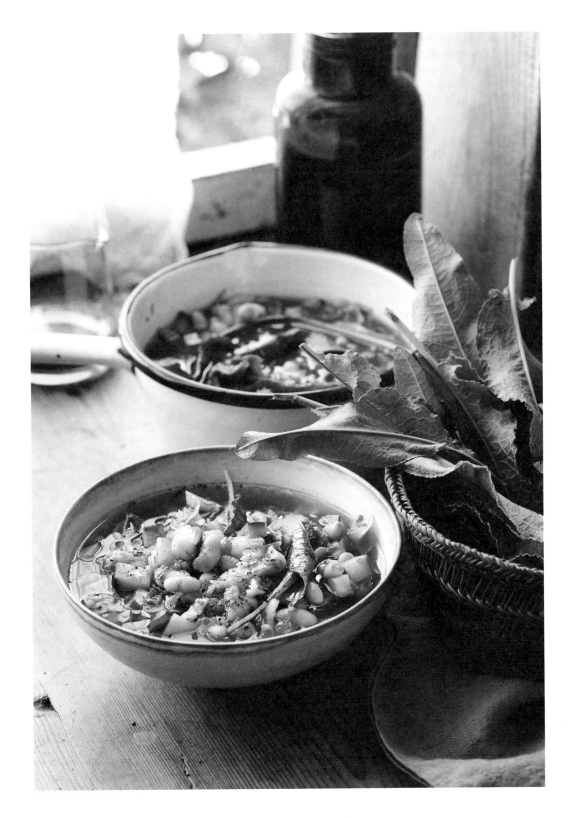

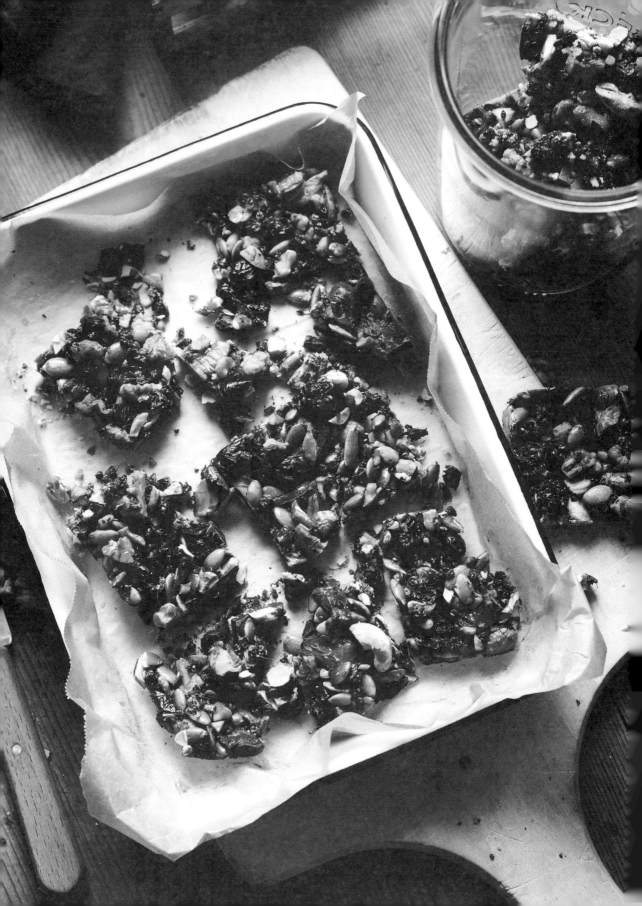

Dock scroggin fruit & nut bars

**MAKES 12 SMALL BARS
1 HOUR**

GF

¼ cup (40 g) almonds or walnuts

¼ cup (40 g) cashews

¼ cup (35 g) chopped dark chocolate (or cacao nibs)

¼ cup (8 g) dried dock seeds

¼ cup (40 g) dried pepitas (pumpkin seeds) and/or sunflower seeds

¼ cup (40 g) dried cranberries

¼ cup (60 ml) maple syrup

I know 'dock scroggin' sounds like the name of a nutty professor in a novel, but it's actually a high-protein trail mix that will help to stabilise your blood sugar and keep your energy levels up throughout a busy or physically demanding day, whether you're hiking, bushwalking or running about town.

You can easily vary this recipe to suit your taste, budget and what's available. The basic gist is a blend of nuts, seeds and dried fruits, coated in maple syrup and baked in the oven. If the maple syrup is too much sugar for your body, just leave it out, mix the ingredients together loosely in a jar or small container and eat it like a trail mix.

Preheat the oven to 150°C (300°F) and line a baking tray with baking paper.

Coarsely chop the nuts and chocolate. Toss in a bowl with all the other ingredients and mix to combine, coating everything in the maple syrup.

Spread the mixture over the baking tray, in an even layer about 1 cm (½ inch) thick.

Bake for 30 minutes, then remove from the oven. Leave on the tray to cool for another 30 minutes before touching it.

Once completely cooled, it should be solid. You can now cut it with a sharp knife into 12 equal portions. It will crumble at the edges, but you should have nice clean squares in the middle.

The scroggin will keep in an airtight container in the pantry for up to 2 weeks.

Dock seed banana bread

MAKES 1 MINI LOAF
45 MINUTES

This recipe uses dock seed flour mixed with spelt, which is rich in protein and minerals, giving you a banana bread that will keep you feeling full and happy and your blood sugar much more stable for longer than one made with only grain-based flour. It's surprisingly light for a seed cake (although admittedly denser than a grain-flour cake). It's really good with cultured vegan butter, or on its own with a cup of tea. Perfect in lunch boxes, it makes a great mid-morning or afternoon snack.

1 cup (25 g) dock seeds

1½ cups (210 g) plain (all-purpose) spelt flour

1 teaspoon ground cinnamon

¼ teaspoon grated nutmeg

½ teaspoon ground ginger

½ cup (85 g) rapadura or coconut sugar

2 teaspoons baking powder

½ teaspoon bicarbonate of soda (baking soda)

a pinch of salt

3 ripe bananas (plus extra banana slices to decorate if desired)

¼ cup (60 ml) rice bran oil

¼ cup (60 ml) water

½ cup (45 g) sultanas (optional)

¼ cup (30 g) roughly chopped walnuts (optional)

Preheat the oven to 160°C (315°F). Grease a small loaf (bar) tin, about 1 litre capacity, measuring about 18–19 cm (7–7½ inches) long, 10 cm (4 inches) wide and 7.5 cm (3 inches) deep. Line the tin with baking paper.

Grind the dock seeds into a flour using a coffee grinder, then tip into a bowl. (You'll need ⅓ cup dock seed flour.) Add the spelt flour, spices, sugar, baking powder, bicarbonate of soda and salt. Mix to combine.

Mash the bananas in another bowl, then pour in the rice bran oil and water and mix to form an oily paste. Gently fold the mixture through the dried ingredients in a figure-eight movement.

If using sultanas and/or walnuts, gently stir them through the batter.

Spoon the batter into the loaf tin, and decorate the top with banana slices if desired. Bake for 40–45 minutes, checking regularly during the last 10 minutes. Test with a skewer to make sure the loaf is cooked in the middle; the skewer should come out clean.

Turn the loaf out onto a wire rack to cool.

Serve with your favourite butter, or enjoy plain with a cup tea.

The loaf will keep in an airtight container in the pantry for 5 days.

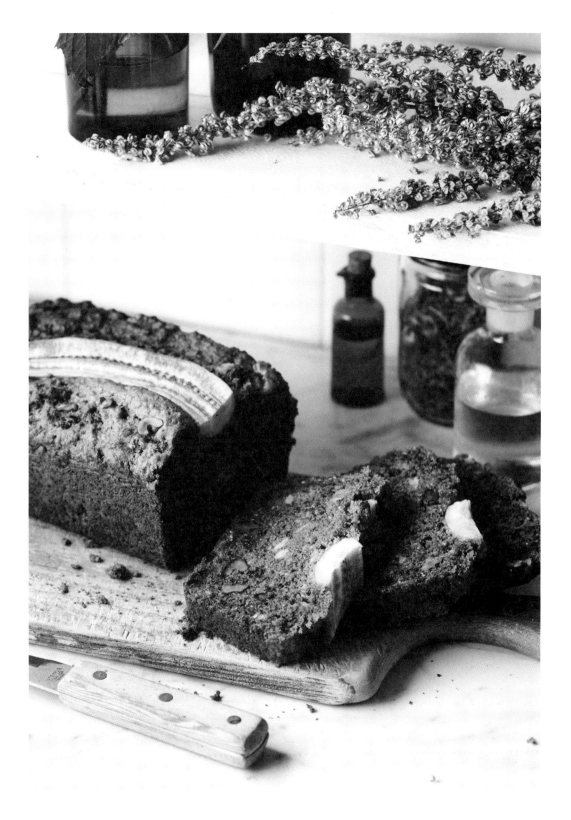

Wild seed crackers

MAKES 24 SQUARE CRACKERS

40 MINUTES

GF

4 tablespoons dock flour (from 1 cup/25 g seeds)

4 tablespoons amaranth flour (from 4 tablespoons amaranth seeds; you'll have a bit of extra flour)

4 tablespoons pepita (pumpkin seed) flour (from 2 tablespoons pepitas)

1 tablespoon chia flour (from 2 teaspoons chia seeds)

½ teaspoon salt

1 teaspoon baking powder

1 teaspoon olive oil

1 teaspoon fat hen seeds

1 teaspoon plantain seeds

These rustic seed crackers are made with seeds instead of grains. They are packed with protein and minerals and have a stabilising effect on blood sugar and metabolism. They are also loaded with fibre and are good for regular bowel movements. They are light and easy to take hiking, biking or camping or on any outdoor adventure, and are also perfect for keeping by your desk at work for a mid-morning or afternoon snack. You can add any topping or eat them on their own.

If you don't have plantain or fat hen seeds, you can use sesame, hemp or chia seeds instead.

The seeds can be collected and stored throughout the year in glass jars as you find them. (This may mean being a patient forager!) Be sure to label them with the name of the seeds and date collected, and also where they were collected from. They should last around 12 months in a dark cupboard.

When grinding the seeds into flour, start with the quantities given below, then measure again after grinding to get the right amount of flour. The ratios will vary depending on your grinder. Some seeds such as amaranth and pepitas (pumpkin seeds) expand, whereas dock, which has quite a lot of husk, shrinks.

The dock, fat hen and plantain seeds give these crackers a rustic, earthy flavour that make it easy to imagine eating something similar hundreds or even thousands of years ago. They taste like 'original' food. If there is such a thing, these must come pretty close.

Preheat the oven to 180°C (350°F).

Sift the seed flours, salt and baking powder into a large bowl. Rub the oil in with your fingers until the mixture is soft and crumbly.

Add ⅓ cup (80 ml) water and mix into a dough that holds together when pressed.

Roll or press the dough into an oiled baking tray, measuring about 22 x 32 cm (8½ x 13 inches). To stop the dough bubbling during baking, use a fork to push air holes along the whole length of the dough, in several rows.

Sprinkle the fat hen and plantain seeds over the top, pressing them in gently so they stick to the dough. Cut into squares using a sharp knife.

Bake for 20 minutes, then remove from the oven and leave to cool on the tray, then a wire rack. The crackers will become harder as they cool.

Eat on their own, or with your favourite toppings. The crackers will keep in an airtight container in the pantry for 2–3 weeks.

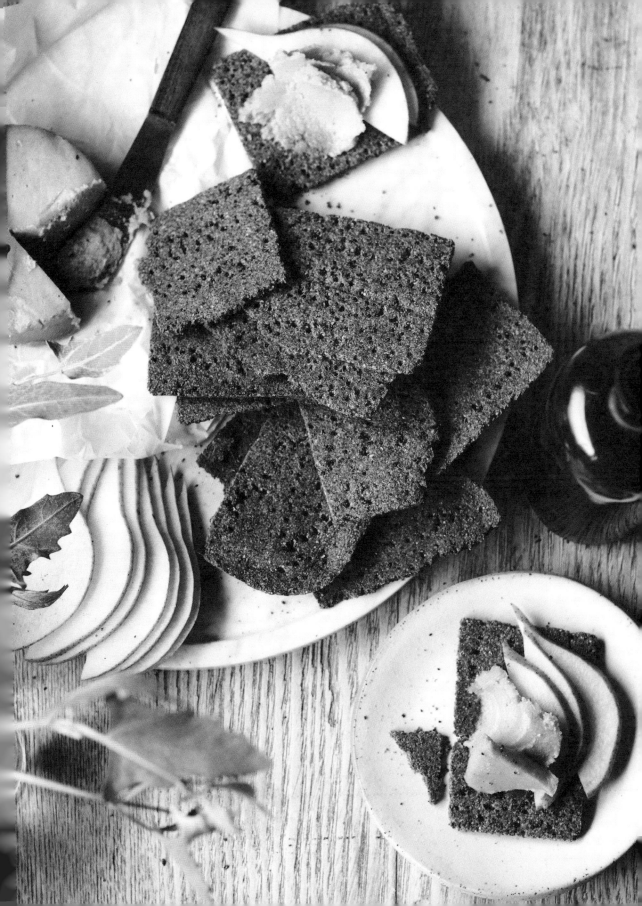

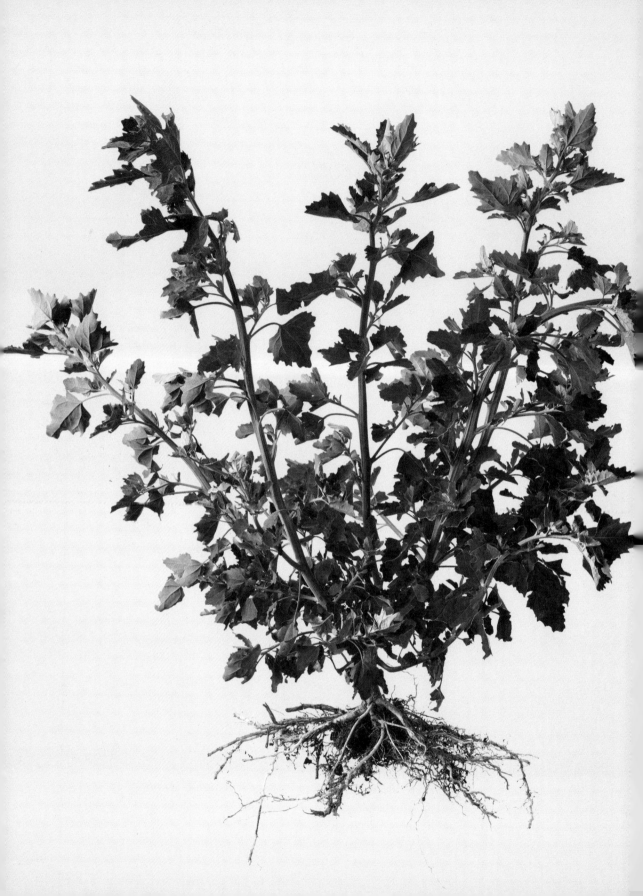

Fat hen

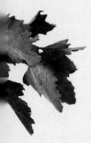

COMMON NAMES:

fat hen, pigweed

SPECIES:

Chenopodium album

GENUS:

Chenopodium

FAMILY:

Amaranthaceae

DISTRIBUTION:

Native to Europe. Naturalised in Africa, Asia, the Americas, Australia and New Zealand.

PLANT SPIRIT QUALITIES:

Fat hen helps you feel nourished and supported, especially when there have been repeated rejections and disappointments in life. It gives you the strength and moral support to keep going when it seems all the odds are against you. It helps actors, musicians, writers or athletes persist with their work.
Key words — nourished, supported.

How to identify it

- The most distinctive feature of fat hen is the irregular leaf shape. The lower leaves are diamond shaped (rhombic) to ovate, with irregular margins.
- The leaves are 3–5 cm (1½–2 inches) long, but can be up to 10 cm (4 inches). The upper ones are oval or lance-shaped, and can look quite different from the lower ones.
- The leaf surface has a powdery coating that is more noticeable on the lower leaves, which look whitish, greyish or bluish-green.
- The stems are angular, branched, erect and grow 1.5–2.5 metres (5–8 feet) high. They are brownish-yellow with parallel reddish or green stripes.
- The flower heads are in panicles (dense clusters of tiny flowers with many branches), the larger ones being leafy but not obscuring the flowers.
- Flowers are whitish-grey or green, clustered, bisexual or female, with five parts fused in the lower half and five stamens.
- The seeds are tiny, black, smooth and 1–1.5 mm in diameter.
- Fat hen has an extensive fibrous root system.

How to harvest

Leaves

Fat hen leaves grow in early spring through summer, and die back in winter. Cut leaves from the base of the plant so you can continue to harvest.

Seeds

Fat hen flowers in summer, and produces large seed heads from mid-summer through to late autumn. The seeds can be collected by cutting the seed stalks at the base and putting the seed heads upside down in a paper bag to dry. Once dried, you can run your hand along the stalk removing the seeds from the stalks.

Husks can be removed by rubbing them through your hands, then gently blowing away the husks.

Nutrients

High in nutrients. A good source of protein, fibre, calcium, magnesium, potassium, vitamin C, vitamin A and trace elements.

Culinary use

Fat hen is commonly eaten around the world. The young shoots are used as a vegetable in many dishes, or dried for later use. In Europe, the seeds have been ground into flour for breads, cakes, gruel or porridge; it is also used this way in the Americas and the Himalayas. In India, they call fat hen *bathua* and make a raita yoghurt sauce from it. Fat hen can also be used to make a fermented alcoholic drink.

It is also a common livestock feed.

Folk medicine

Chenopodium album has anti-inflammatory, analgesic, gastroprotective, liver protective, antioxidant, antimicrobial, antiparasitic and insecticidal effects. It has been used in Ayurvedic medicine for disorders of the liver or spleen. The Zulus used it externally as a powder for rashes and irritation. The leaf juice is used for burns. The seeds are used to improve appetite, get rid of roundworms, hookworms and parasites, and as a laxative, aphrodisiac and a tonic. The whole plant has also been used for stomach pain, eye and throat problems and diseases of the blood.

A decoction of aerial parts mixed with alcohol is rubbed on the body part affected by arthritis and rheumatism.

Research

Clinical trials have confirmed its use in the following areas: antioxidant,[1] antimicrobial,[2] antibacterial,[3] antiviral,[4] anti-parasitic and insecticidal,[5] useful for muscle pain,[6] protective against liver damage,[7] male fertility (intravaginal spermicidal effect in women),[8] itching and pain management.[9]

How to use it as a medicine

It is used internally as a food or infusion, and externally as a powder or a poultice of seeds or leaves.

CAUTIONS + CONTRAINDICATIONS

Avoid if pregnant or trying to get pregnant (has anti-fertility effects). Contains oxalates that can build up if consumption is prolonged; cooking minimises this risk. May cause asthma and rashes in sensitive individuals.

Fat hen can also be used in:

- Wild weed pesto
- Wild wilted greens
- Wild greens powder
- Wild grain bread

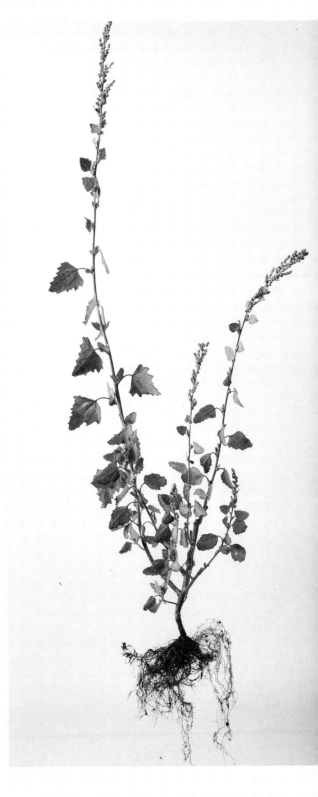

Fat hen & cashew cheese tart

SERVES 8
1 HOUR

GF

A commonly foraged vegetable throughout the world, fat hen is a good source of protein, fibre, calcium, magnesium, potassium, vitamin C, vitamin A and trace elements, making this vegan tart — which uses both the seeds and leaves of the plant — highly nutritious. It is a lovely light lunch or dinner option, and smaller individual tarts are great in lunchboxes or to take on picnics. Add any savoury toppings you fancy. Some options are suggested below, but feel free to choose your own.

1 large handful of fresh fat hen leaves

DOUGH

¼ cup (20 g) fat hen seeds

1 cup (100 g) almond meal

2 tablespoons coconut oil

1 tablespoon psyllium husk

1 tablespoon water

CASHEW CHEESE

2 cups (310 g) raw cashews, soaked in cold water for 30 minutes

1 garlic clove, crushed

1 tablespoon nutritional yeast

1 tablespoon apple cider vinegar

½ teaspoon salt

½ teaspoon black pepper

POSSIBLE TOPPINGS

fresh fat hen leaves (blanched)

roasted zucchini (courgette)

roasted capsicum (pepper)

sautéed mushrooms

sliced tomato

pitted olives

capers

vegan feta

fresh herbs

Preheat the oven to 160°C (315°F).

Blanch the fat hen leaves by placing them in a heatproof bowl and pouring boiling water over them, then straining them immediately, pressing the water out of them. Set aside.

Place all the dough ingredients in a food processor and blend until they form a dough that pulls away from the sides. (You can also mix them together by hand if you don't have a food processor.) The dough should stick together.

Press the dough into a loose-based flan (tart tin), or a shallow tray lined with baking paper.

Blind-bake the dough for 15 minutes, then remove from the oven and leave to cool.

Turn the oven up to 180°C (350°F).

Using a food processor, blend all the cashew cheese ingredients to a paste, adding a tablespoon of water if the mixture is too dry. Pour or spoon the cashew cheese over the cooled tart base.

Arrange the blanched fat hen leaves over the tart, then add your choice of toppings.

Bake for a further 20 minutes, until the crust is golden.

Remove from the oven and leave to cool in the tin for 30 minutes, before cutting into eight slices for serving.

The tart will keep in an airtight container in the fridge for 3–5 days.

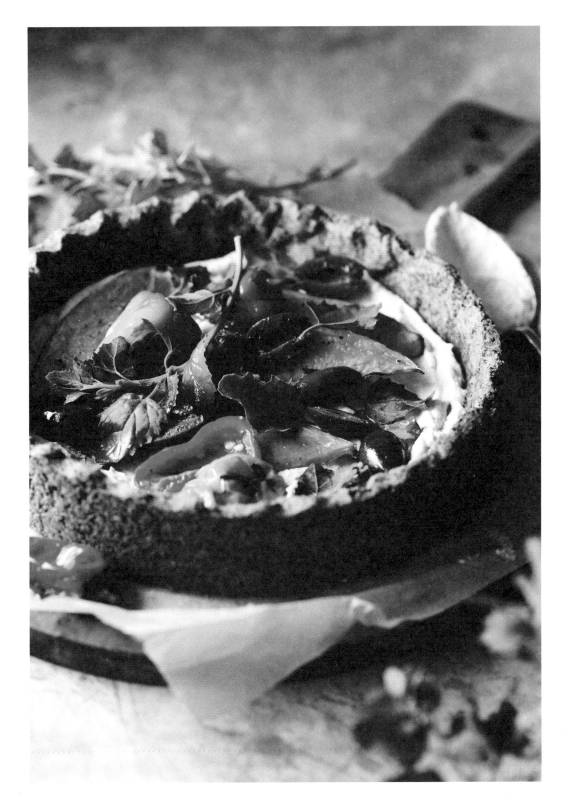

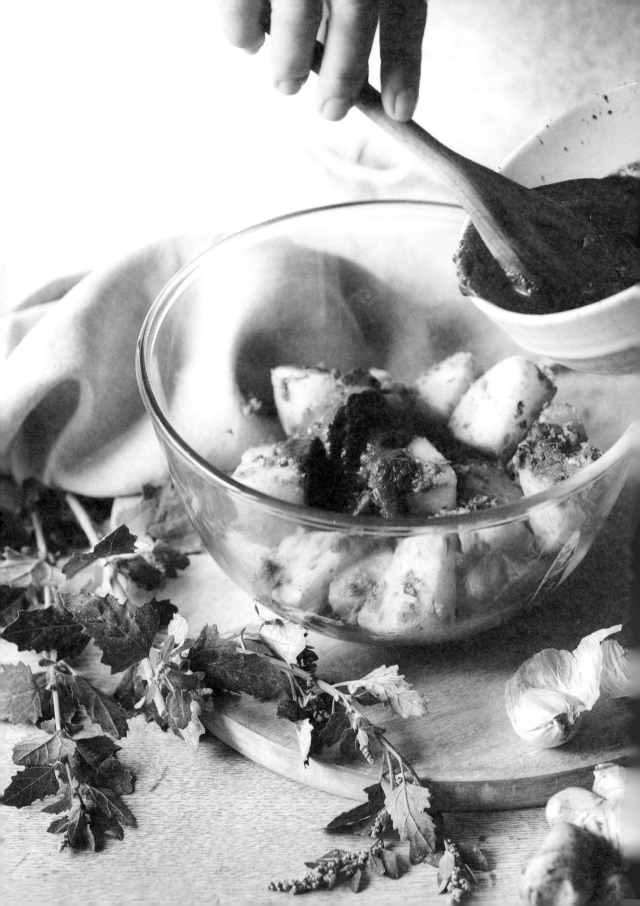

Bathua saag aloo

SERVES 4
50 MINUTES

GF

2 large waxy potatoes

6 handfuls of fresh fat hen leaves (if you can't forage the whole amount, replace the shortfall with spinach)

1 tablespoon olive oil

1 onion, chopped or sliced

1 teaspoon fresh ginger, finely chopped or grated

3 garlic cloves, crushed

2 teaspoons ground coriander

1 teaspoon garam masala

1 teaspoon ground cumin

½ teaspoon cumin seeds

½ teaspoon chilli powder or sweet or hot paprika (or ¼ teaspoon chilli powder if you prefer less spice)

½ teaspoon ground turmeric

½ teaspoon salt

Bathua ('fat hen') *saag* ('dark leafy greens') *aloo* ('potato') is a traditional Indian dish usually made with spinach. Simple but flavourful, it is easily made into a wild, foraged meal by substituting fat hen leaves for the spinach — either completely, or even half and half, depending on how much fat hen you can harvest.

By adding some fat hen, you end up with a higher nutritional profile than from just spinach alone. This is the power of adding wild edibles to everyday meals.

Any leftovers will keep for lunch the next day, or can be frozen for later. For a lower-carb, higher-protein variation, you can replace the potatoes with tofu or paneer.

Peel the potatoes and dice into 2 cm (¾ inch) cubes. Place in a saucepan with 2 cups (500 ml) water and bring to the boil. Reduce the heat and simmer for 15–20 minutes, until soft but not mushy.

Meanwhile, bring another saucepan of water to the boil. Add the fat hen and blanch for 1 minute, then strain through a colander in the sink.

Purée the fat hen, either back in the pan using a stick blender, or using a jug blender (in which case you may need to add a tiny bit of water). Set aside.

Heat the oil in a heavy-based saucepan over medium–high heat. Add the onion, ginger, garlic, all the spices and the salt. Fry for 1–2 minutes, stirring often. Add the potatoes and puréed fat hen and cook for another 5 minutes, stirring in ¼–½ cup (60–125 ml) water if the mixture is too dry.

Taste and add more salt or chilli if needed.

Serve with your favourite accompaniments — rice, naan bread, salad and a dollop of coconut cream or yoghurt.

Fat hen vegan brownies

MAKES 16
1 HOUR

3 tablespoons activated fat hen seeds (see note)

3 tablespoons flaxseeds

1¾ cups (250 g) plain (all-purpose) spelt flour (or gluten-free flour)

1½ cups (160 g) unsweetened cocoa powder, plus extra for dusting

3 teaspoons baking powder

½ teaspoon salt

185 g (6½ oz) vegan butter (the hard, cultured type, not margarine)

2 cups (300 g) coconut sugar

1½ tablespoons pure vanilla extract

1½ cups (240 g) vegan choc chips or broken chocolate bits

These brownies are chewy, fudgy, rich and chocolatey — everything you want a brownie to be. You can't taste the seeds, but they're full of protein, fibre, calcium, magnesium and omega-3 fatty acids. Sure, some of that goodness is negated by the coconut sugar and flour, but really, these are so good I'm taking the win and running with it!

You can harvest fat hen seeds yourself (see page 176) or buy them online (look for 'bathua' or 'Chenopodium seeds'). You'll need to activate them first (see note), which may seem like a lot of mucking around, but it makes the seeds more digestible and palatable, giving you yummier brownies.

Grind the fat hen and flaxseeds using a coffee grinder. Tip into a bowl, add ¾ cup (185 ml) water and leave to thicken for 10 minutes.

Preheat the oven to 180°C (350°F). Grease a shallow 24 cm (9½ inch) square baking dish or tin and line with baking paper.

Sift the flour, cocoa powder, baking powder and salt into a mixing bowl. Set aside.

Gently melt the butter in a saucepan. Add the soaked seeds, coconut sugar and vanilla and stir over low heat until you have a thick, gooey mixture.

Tip the mixture over the dry ingredients and mix until combined into a thick batter. Mix the choc chips through, then pour the batter into the baking dish.

Bake for 25–30 minutes, or until a skewer poked in the centre of the loaf comes out clean.

Remove from the oven and leave to cool, before removing from the dish. Turn out onto a board and cut into squares using a sharp knife. Dust with cocoa powder if desired.

The brownies will keep in an airtight container in the pantry for 3–4 days, in the fridge for 1 week, or freezer for up to 3 months.

Note

To activate fat hen seeds, wash them, place in a bowl with 2 cups (500 ml) fresh water and leave overnight. Next day, drain and rinse your seeds. Place in a saucepan with 2 cups (500 ml) water and bring to the boil, then reduce the heat and simmer for 20 minutes. If the water is very brown and dirty, rinse the seeds, add fresh water and bring to the boil again. (With fresh, hand-picked seeds, you may not need to do this.) When cooked, the seeds will still be quite gritty, but softer and easier to eat. Spread the seeds on a baking tray and bake in a preheated 140°C (275°F) oven for 20–30 minutes, until dry. Your seeds are now ready to grind and use.

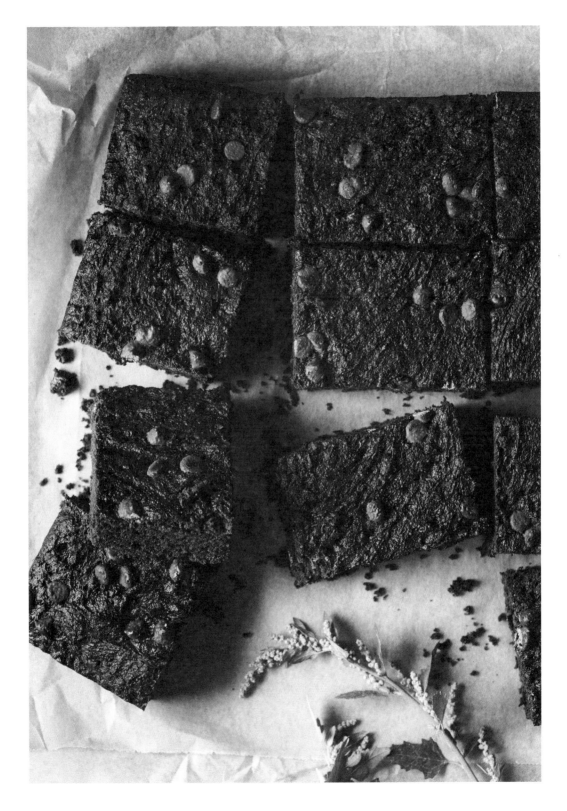

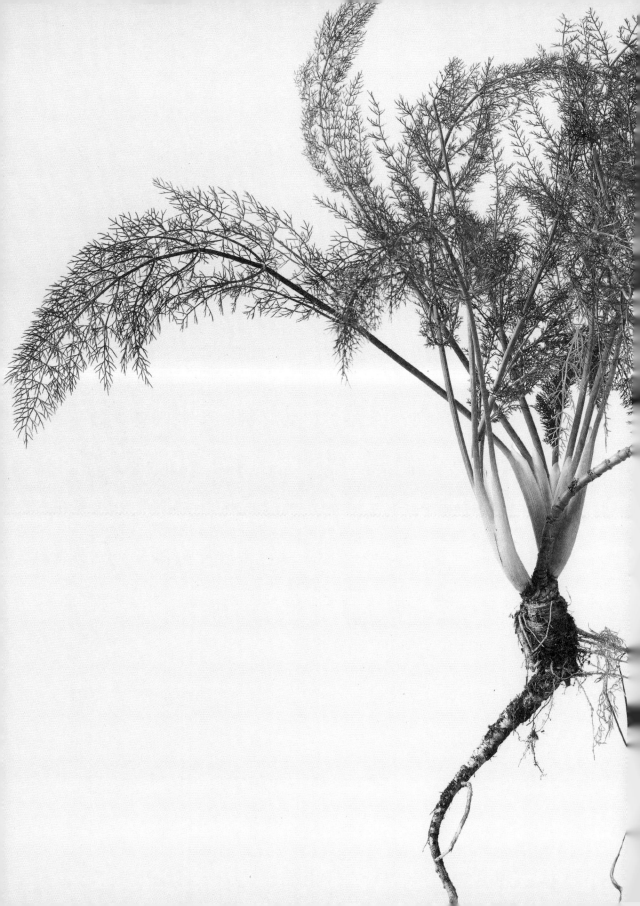

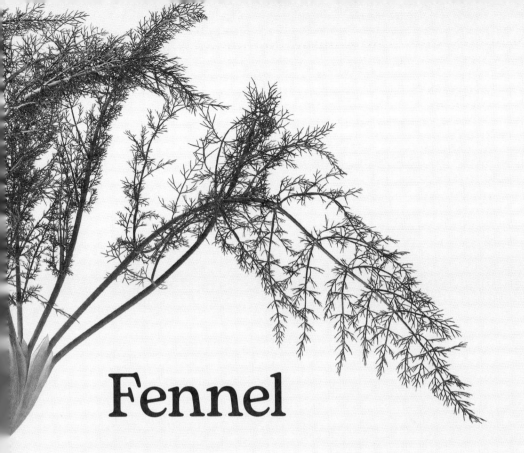

Fennel

COMMON NAMES:

Fennel

SPECIES:

Foeniculum vulgare

GENUS:

Foeniculum

FAMILY:

Apiaceae

DISTRIBUTION:

Native to the Mediterranean, but has become widely naturalised in many parts of the world.

PLANT SPIRIT QUALITIES:

You can use fennel to overcome shock, trauma or fear after injury, nightmares, fights or stress. It helps calm the nervous system and restore a feeling of safety. It can be good for insomnia, calming the mind and helping to go to sleep or relax.

Key words — soothing and calming.

How to identify it

- The leaves of fennel comprise thin filiform (thread-like) segments about 0.5 mm thick, which give a distinctive feathery appearance.
- The flowers are on terminal umbels (flower clusters in which stalks of nearly equal length come from a common centre and form a flat or curved surface).
- The flowers are yellow, with each umbel having 20–50 tiny yellow flowers on short pedicels (stems that attach to a single flower).
- The stems are upright and hollow, and can reach heights of up to 2.5 metres (8 feet).
- The fruit is a dry, green to brown seed, 4–10 mm ($\frac{3}{16}$–$\frac{1}{2}$ inch) long, with grooves along it. It has a characteristic liquorice-like taste.
- Fennel roots are fibrous, white and spindly.
- Fennel bulbs are cultivated from the swollen stem; they are not found like that in the wild.

How to harvest

Leaves
Wild fennel grows in spring and summer and is often very abundant. Using scissors, the feather-soft leaves can be cut from the stalk below the branching leaves.

Flowers
The bright yellow flowers appear mid-summer. They can be cut below the cluster and added to salads.

Seeds
Seed clusters turn brown in late summer to autumn, and can be collected by cutting below the clusters and leaving them in a paper bag to dry out. Once dried, give them a good massage into the paper bag to get the seeds off the stalks.

Nutrients

Rich source of beta-carotene, vitamin C, and B vitamins. A good source of fibre, potassium, calcium, magnesium, iron and trace elements.

Culinary use

Around the world, fennel is a culinary staple. The bulb, foliage and seeds are all used in a variety of dishes. The small flowers of wild fennel (known as fennel pollen) are the most potent and expensive form of fennel. The cultivated bulb is a crisp vegetable that is used in sautés, stews, salads or with grilled fish. Young tender leaves are used for garnishes and in salads, puddings, sauces and soups.

Fennel is used in Indian, Afghani, Iranian, Middle Eastern, Kashmiri, Pandit and Gujarati cooking. It is an essential ingredient of the Assamese/Bengali/Oriya spice mixture *panch phoron*, and in Chinese five-spice powders. In India, sugar-coated fennel seeds, called *mukhwas*, are used as an after-dinner digestive and breath freshener.

In Syria and Lebanon, the young leaves are used to make a special kind of egg omelette (along with onions and flour), called *ijjeh*. Florence fennel is used in Italian and German salads, with chicory and avocado, or braised and served as a warm side dish. The Italians also blanch or marinate it, or cook it in risotto or sausages. In Spain, the stems are used with pickled eggplants, in a dish called *berenjenas de Almagro*. In Israel, fennel salad is made of chopped fennel bulbs and parsley, flavoured with salt, black pepper, lemon juice, olive oil and sometimes sumac.

Fennel is a popular ingredient of herbal teas or tisanes for its flavour and digestive properties.

Folk medicine

Herbalists around the world use fennel for its carminative (gas-reducing) properties to relieve bloating, flatulence and indigestion, as well as to promote appetite in those who have no desire to eat. It was a popular remedy of the 12th century German mystic nun Hildegard of Bingen, whose medical treatments have survived to the present day. Fennel is often used with laxatives to reduce the gripping pains that laxatives can cause.

It is also one of the ingredients of the well-known compound, liquorice powder.

Fennel water has properties similar to anise and dill water, which is often mixed with sodium bicarbonate and syrup to make 'gripe water' for babies' flatulence or colic.

It is also commonly used to promote the flow of breast milk, along with fenugreek seeds.

In India, it has been said anecdotally to improve eyesight.

Research

Clinical trials have confirmed its use in the following areas: antibacterial,[1] antifungal,[2] antioxidant,[3] reduces blood clotting,[4] allergies and inflammation,[5] oestrogenic,[6] period pain,[7] menopause,[8] protective against liver damage[9] and antidiabetic.[10]

How to use it as a medicine

Used as an infusion or decoction, a powder or a tincture.

CAUTIONS + CONTRAINDICATIONS

The essential oil should not be used during pregnancy or lactation, but the tea is considered safe under supervision. The essential oil should not be given to young children and infants, but teas are considered safe.

The fruit and the essential oil can cause irritation in the digestive tract. People with allergies to anethole or plants in the Apiacaeae family should avoid using fennel.

Fennel can also be used in:

- Fennel glycetract
- Fennel tea
- Fennel and pear salad (see chickweed)

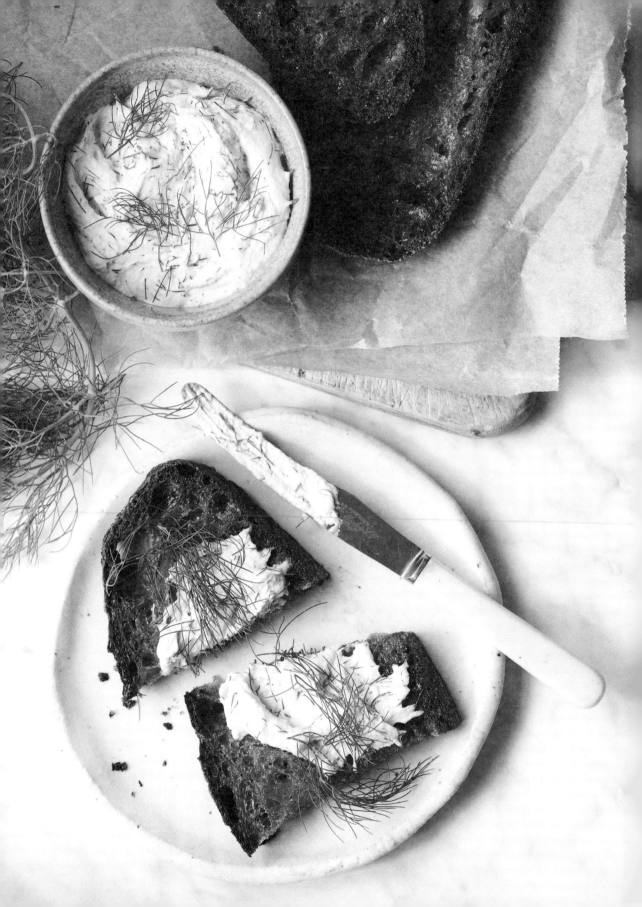

Sweet fennel cream cheese

Here's a delicious way to use your wild fennel leaves. This sweet fennel cream cheese is great on crackers, toast or cheese platters. It's a good base layer for building lots of wild greens on (like the Chickweed, Cashew and Caper Toasts on page 116), as the sweetness of the fennel balances the pepperiness of hotter plants, such as nasturtiums. Experiment by adding other wild plants from your garden to make a wild weed cheese with fennel as the star.

MAKES 250 G (9 OZ)

3–12 HOURS SOAKING + 20 MINUTES

GF

1 cup (155 g) raw cashews

1 tablespoon nutritional yeast

2 tablespoons sauerkraut brine or apple cider vinegar

1 tablespoon lemon juice

½ teaspoon salt

2 tablespoons chopped fresh fennel leaves

Soak the cashews in 2 cups (500 ml) cold water for 3–12 hours.

Strain and rinse the cashews, then place in a blender with the nutritional yeast, sauerkraut brine, lemon juice, salt and ¼ cup (60 ml) water.

Blend on high speed for 4–5 minutes, stopping every minute to scrape down the sides and remove the mixture from under the blades to get it super smooth.

Scrape the mixture into a bowl and mix the fennel leaves through.

The cheese will keep in a sterilised glass jar (see page 23) in the fridge for up to 1 week.

Ayurvedic CCF tea blend

MAKES 18 SERVES
5 MINUTES

GF

CCF tea is classical Ayurvedic tea that combines equal parts cumin, coriander and fennel seeds. Rich in minerals including iron, as well as medicinal compounds and antioxidants, it is traditionally used to stimulate digestion; reduce gas, bloating and indigestion; soothe the lining of the digestive tract; and improve elimination of waste through the digestive and lymphatic systems. It is also used to help clear sinuses and relax bronchial spasms, which may reduce symptoms of asthma, bronchitis and congestion. This tea can be drunk regularly to help support overall digestion and wellbeing.

With this amount of seeds in your tea storage jar, you should be able to make 18 cups of tea.

2 tablespoons fennel seeds
2 tablespoons cumin seeds
2 tablespoons coriander seeds

Place all the seeds in a storage jar or tin, mixing or shaking to distribute them evenly.

Label with the ingredients used and the date made.

This tea will last in a dark, cool cupboard for 12 months.

To use, add 1 teaspoon of the CCF blend per 1 cup (250 ml) boiling water and let it steep for 5 minutes.

Gripe water

MAKES 2 CUPS (500 ML)
40 MINUTES

GF

Gripe water is a traditional syrup used for gas, bloating and indigestion. It may help soothe the smooth muscle of the digestive tract, and promote the movement of gases and waste through the digestive tract so they can be eliminated. It may also reduce the number of gas-forming bacteria, which can also ease pain. It has a calming effect on the nervous system.

2 tablespoons crushed fennel seeds
2 tablespoons chamomile tea (or 2 chamomile tea bags)
½ teaspoon ground cinnamon
3 cloves
2 teaspoons maple syrup or coconut sugar (optional)

Add the fennel seeds, chamomile, cinnamon and cloves to 2 cups (500 ml) hot boiled water. Cover and let it steep for 30 minutes.

Strain through a fine sieve or muslin (cheesecloth), into an airtight container. Stir in the maple syrup or coconut sugar, if using, until dissolved.

The gripe water will keep in the fridge for up to 4 days, and can also be frozen in ice cube trays to be used as needed.

Can be taken 3–4 times daily, or as needed; in some cases only 1–2 doses are required.

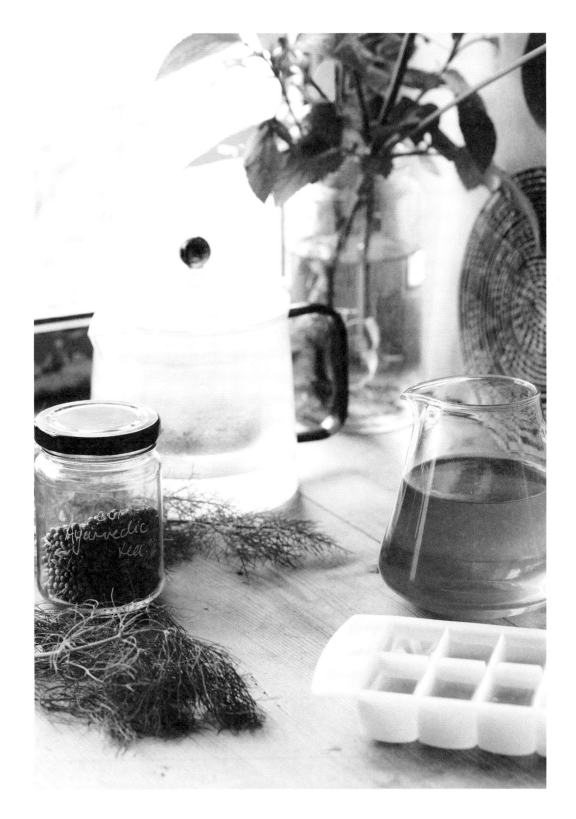

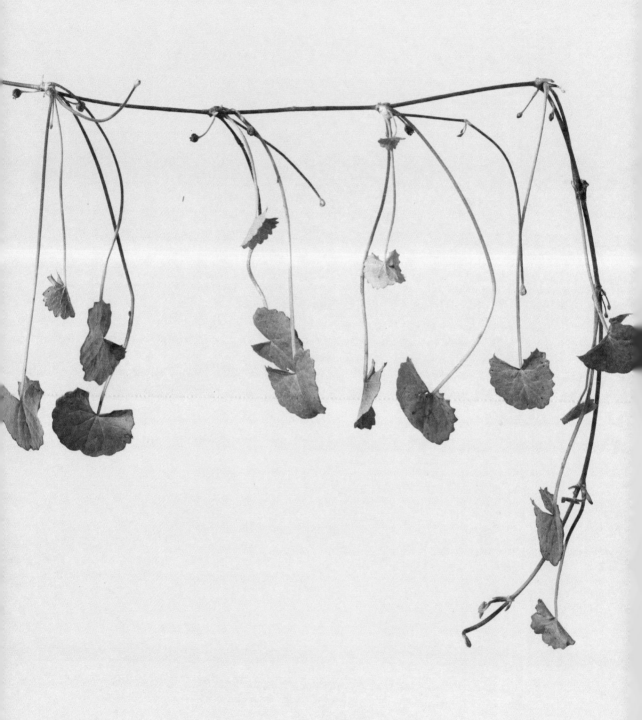

Gotu kola

COMMON NAMES:

gotu kola

SPECIES:

Centella asiatica (syn. *Hydrocotyle asiatica*)

GENUS:

Centella

FAMILY:

Apiaceae

DISTRIBUTION:

Originated in Asia, India and south-east US, but is now pantropical. Naturalised in tropical Africa, Asia, Australia, South America and some Pacific islands.

PLANT SPIRIT QUALITIES:

Instead of working with an individual person or issue related to this lifetime, gotu kola works with the soul, and can help us to see and heal deep karmic patterns that span many lifetimes. In Hindu philosophy, we are born again in order to resolve or perfect these karmic imprints until we reach a state of enlightenment and are free from the cycle of births and deaths. Gotu kola helps with this process. **Key words — order, karma, relationships.**

How to identify it

- Gotu kola is a perennial, creeping groundcover.
- The leaves are 2–4 cm (¾–1¼ inches) wide and kidney-shaped, with a V-shaped slot where the leaf joins the stem.
- The leaves have serrated margins; the edges look as if they have been cut with pinking shears. They also have distinct palmate veins (branching out from a single point).
- The leaves are borne on petioles or stems, about 2–4 cm (¾–1¼ inches) long.
- The stems are slender stolons (creeping horizontal plant stems or runners that take root at points along its length to form new plants).
- Stems are green to pink in colour, connecting plants to each other.
- The root is a cream-coloured rhizome, covered with root hairs that grow vertically down.
- The flowers are white or pinkish to red, and found in small, rounded bunches (umbels) near the soil surface. They are almost invisible, being less than 3 mm (⅛ inch) in size. Unless you look carefully, they are easy to miss.
- Each flower bears five stamens and two styles.
- The fruit are densely reticulate (form a cluster), distinguishing it from species of *Centella* that have smooth, ribbed or warty fruit.

There are many plants that look similar, such as swamp pennywort (*Centella cordifolia*), kidney weed (*Dichondra repens*), native violet (*Viola hederacea*), coast pennywort (*Hydrocotyle bonariensis*), alehoof (*Glechoma hederacea*), several ranunculus species and other *Centella* species. Before using gotu kola, it is important to make sure you have the correct plant.

How to harvest

Leaves

Gotu kola can grow year round in temperate climates, but will die off in winter in cold regions. It is a very delicate plant with fine, hair-like roots, so harvest leaves gently with a pair of scissors, cutting the leaves near the base of the stem to avoid damaging roots. Leaves can be used fresh, or dried for future use.

Nutrients

Vitamins A, B, C and D, and the minerals calcium, chromium, cobalt, magnesium, manganese, phosphorus, sodium, potassium, selenium, silica and zinc.

Culinary use

Gotu kola is used as a leafy green in Sri Lankan cuisine. It is most often prepared as *malluma*, a traditional accompaniment to rice and curries. In addition to finely chopped gotu kola, *malluma* almost always contains grated coconut, and may also contain finely chopped green chillies, chilli powder, ground turmeric and lime (or lemon) juice.

A nutritious porridge known as *kola kenda* is made with gotu kola by the Sinhalese people of Sri Lanka. *Kola kenda* is made with very well boiled red rice (with extra liquid), coconut milk and puréed gotu kola. The porridge is accompanied with palm sugar (jaggery) for sweetness.

Gotu kola leaves are also used in sweet 'pennywort' drinks, popular in Asia. In Indonesia, the leaves are used for *sambaioipeuga-ga*, a type of salad, and are also made into a pickle in Bogor. In Vietnam and Thailand, it is made into a drink, or eaten raw in salads or cold rolls. In Bangkok, vendors in the famous Chatuchak Weekend Market sell it as a health drink. In Malay cuisine, the leaves of this plant are used for *ulam*, a type of salad. It is one of the constituents of the Indian summer drink *thandaayyee*. In Bangladeshi cuisine, mashed gotu kola is eaten with rice.

Folk medicine

Centella asiatica has a centuries-long history of use in Ayurvedic and Chinese traditional medicines. Monographs of *C. asiatica*, describing its wound healing and memory enhancement effects, are found in the European Pharmacopoeia, Commission E of the German Ministry of Health, and the World Health Organization (WHO).

A wide range of actions have traditionally been attributed to gotu kola, including wound healing, anti-inflammatory, antipsoriatic, anti-ulcer, liver protective, anticonvulsant, sedative, immunostimulant, cardioprotective, antidiabetic, cytotoxic and anti-tumour, antiviral, antibacterial, insecticidal, antifungal and antioxidant.

Gotu kola has been used medicinally for a multitude of complaints. Today it is mainly used to treat skin conditions and to speed the healing time of wounds, burns and bruises.

The 19th century Indian pharmacopoeia recommends it for skin conditions such as leprosy, lupus, varicose ulcers, eczema and psoriasis, as well as diarrhoea, fever, amenorrhoea and diseases of the female urogenital tract.

It is also used as a tonic for longevity, to strengthen digestion and increase overall metabolism. It has a particular effect on brain function, revitalising nerve and brain cells, promoting calmness and clarity, helping poor memory and lack of concentration, increasing meditation ability, and balancing the left and right hemispheres of the brain. It is used to improve intelligence and reflexes, renewing mental alertness, clarity and energy levels. It is also used for rheumatism and arthritis.

Gotu kola is one plant to which the longevity of the t'ai chi ch'uan master Li Ching-Yuen has been attributed. Depending on which account you read, he was said to have lived to be either 197 or 256, due in part to his usage of traditional Chinese herbs, including gotu kola.

Research

Clinical trials have confirmed gotu kola's use in the following areas: anti-inflammatory,[1] wound healing,[2] atopic dermatitis,[3] stretch marks in pregnancy,[4] scar reduction,[5] cognitive function,[6] mood enhancing,[7] reducing the effects of ageing,[8] reducing anxiety[9] and cardiovascular benefits.[10]

How to use it as a medicine

Internally it can be used as an infusion, a juice, a powder or a tincture; externally as a cream, ointment or poultice.

CAUTIONS + CONTRAINDICATIONS
Centella asiatica has no known toxicity in recommended doses. Avoid 2 weeks before surgery.

Gotu kola can also be used in:

- Gotu kola glycetract
- Gotu kola tea

Gotu kola iced tea

MAKES 1 CUP (250 ML)
15 MINUTES

GF

1 handful of fresh gotu kola leaves, or 2 tablespoons dried leaves

2 tablespoons maple syrup

juice of ½ lemon

1 mint sprig

ice cubes, to serve

Throughout Asia, gotu kola drinks are popular due to their refreshing taste and many healing benefits. Gotu kola adds zest to your brain — perfect for getting though work deadlines or study when it's hot and you need to keep concentrating.

You can scale up the recipe to make a 1 litre (4 cup) batch and store it in the fridge so it's nice and cool. It will last 3–5 days in the fridge.

Add the gotu kola leaves to 1 cup (250 ml) hot boiled water and leave to infuse until cool.

Stir in the maple syrup and lemon juice until dissolved. Add the mint and a few ice cubes and serve.

Gotu kola sambal

MAKES 3 CUPS
20 MINUTES

GF

3 handfuls of fresh gotu kola leaves

1 small fresh chilli

3 shallots or spring onions (scallions)

1 tomato

¼ cup (25 g) desiccated coconut

2 teaspoons coconut sugar

2 teaspoons tamari or vegan fish sauce

juice of 2 limes

½ teaspoon salt

This flavoursome sambal is a clever way to get all those health benefits of gotu kola in one delicious little side dish. It's spicy, tart and tangy, and you can almost feel yourself getting healthier and smarter as you eat it.

Wash and dry the gotu kola leaves, then finely chop, along with the chilli, shallots and tomato. Place in a bowl.

Add the remaining ingredients and mix together. Taste to see if you need to adjust any of the flavours.

The sambal is ready to use straight away, but will keep for 1 week in an airtight container in the fridge to enjoy with a variety of dishes. It is especially good with vegetable curries.

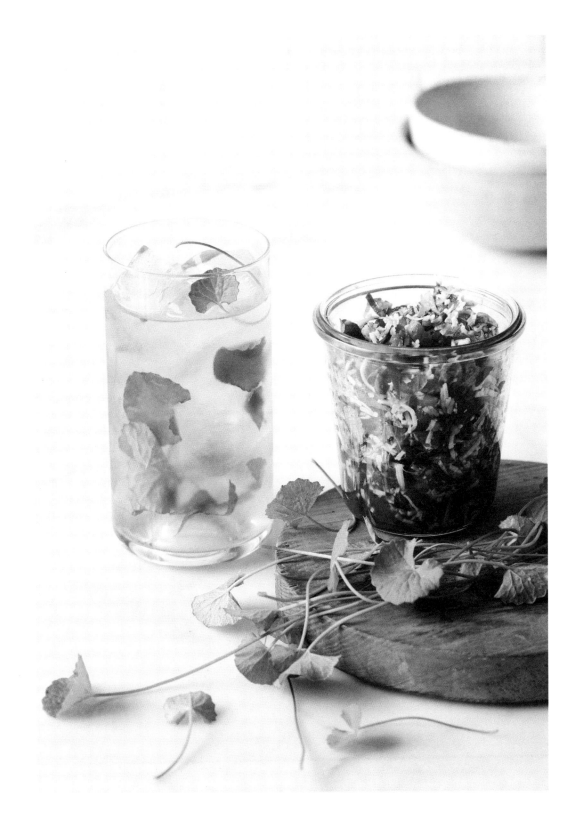

Gotu kola capsules

MAKES 100 CAPSULES
20–30 MINUTES

Taking a medicinal compound in capsule form is ideal for healing wounds when you can't use a topical application because a dressing covers the wound. Capsules can also be used in conjunction with topical applications for a stronger healing action.

These capsules are ideal for burns, wounds and surgical incisions. Gotu kola works best in the first 24–48 hours after an injury or surgery, so the sooner you can get onto it the better. Do not use it before surgery, however, as it may increase bleeding.

I always have a jar of gotu kola capsules in the cupboard in case of injury so they can be taken straight away.

See the section on powders and capsules on page 21 in the Herbal Medicine-making Fundamentals chapter.

1 cup (20 g) coarsely chopped dried gotu kola leaves and stems

100 x 000 size vegetable capsules

Grind the dried herbs using a coffee grinder or mortar and pestle.

Pull the capsules apart, scoop the powder into one half of the capsule, then put the other half back on.

If you plan to make lots, you might want to invest in a capsule maker, which can be bought cheaply online.

You can take 2 capsules, 3 times per day. Store in a sealed airtight container or glass jar with a screw-top lid. They will last for up to 12 months in a cool, dark cupboard.

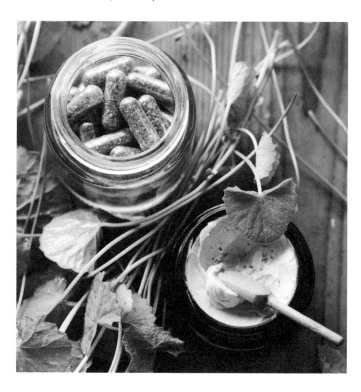

Gotu kola healing cream

This cream may help speed the healing time of burns, wounds, bruises and surgical incisions. It can also be used as a face cream to deal with fine lines and wrinkles.

Before starting this recipe, read the section on making creams on page 34. This recipe uses two saucepans — one for your water infusion, and the other for your waxes and oils.

MAKES ½ CUP (125 ML)

40 MINUTES + 30 MINUTES INFUSING

2 tablespoons dried gotu kola, or 1 handful of fresh gotu kola leaves

1½ tablespoons olivem 1000

1 teaspoon vegetable glycerine

3 tablespoons gotu kola infused oil (see note)

12 drops of citricidal (citrus seed extract)

Note

Make your gotu kola infused oil either by slow method (2 weeks) on page 30, or the fast method (1–2 days) on page 31.

Soak the dried or fresh gotu kola in ½ cup (125 ml) water overnight, or for a minimum of 30 minutes. (A longer soaking creates a stronger herbal infusion.)

Pop some ice cubes in a large bowl half filled with water, to have an ice bath ready for when you are mixing your cream. (You can leave the ice bath in the fridge or freezer until needed.)

Strain and compost the gotu kola, then pour the rich green infusion into a small saucepan, but leave it off the heat.

In a Pyrex or other heatproof glass jug, combine the olivem 1000, glycerine and gotu kola oil. Place the jug in another saucepan, then pour about 5 cm (2 inches) water into the pan to make a water bath. Bring the water to the boil, then reduce the heat to a slow boil. Stir the mixture in the jug until the wax has melted, about 8–10 minutes.

Add the citricidal to the jug.

Heat the green gotu kola infusion in the other pan until close to boiling point — but take it off the heat as soon as bubbles start to form. This is important because the oil and water component of the cream need to be at the same temperature to incorporate smoothly.

Pour the oil mixture into your green gotu kola infusion and, while pouring, mix with a fork or whisk until incorporated. Place the saucepan in the ice bath (this will help the mixture thicken much more quickly) and continue mixing with a fork or whisk. (If making a large batch, a stick blender will be much faster.)

Stop mixing when the mixture forms nice stiff peaks like whipped cream.

Spoon into sterilised amber glass jars (see page 23). Seal with the lid, then label with the ingredients, date made, and an expiry date of 3 months.

Best stored in the fridge.

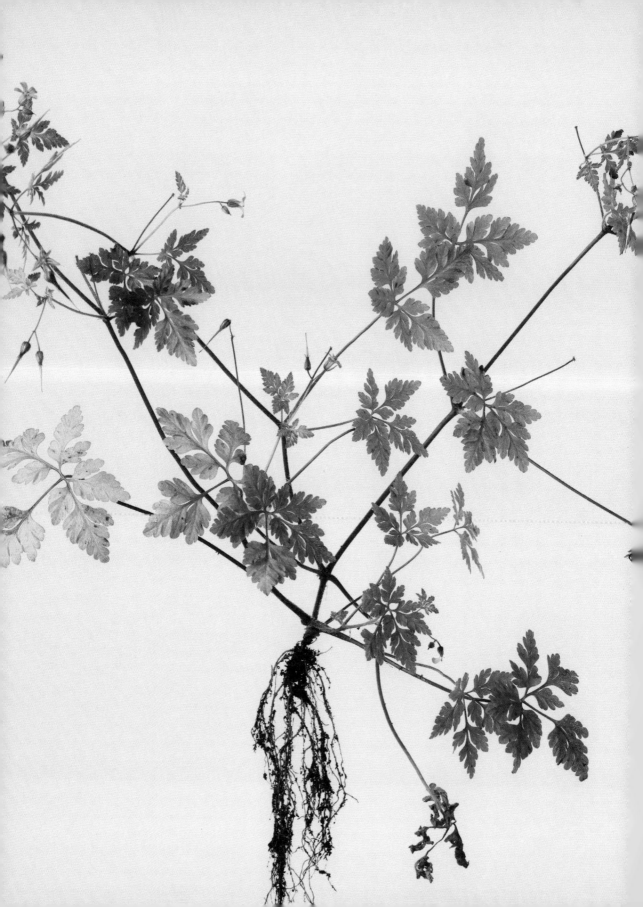

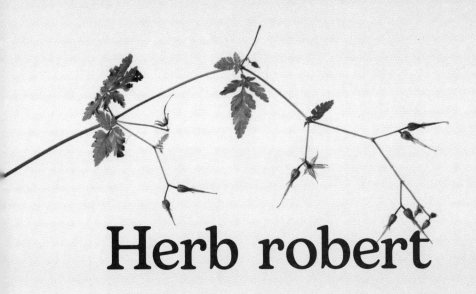

Herb robert

COMMON NAMES:

herb robert, cranesbill, storksbill

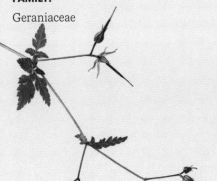

SPECIES:

Geranium robertianum

GENUS:

Geranium

FAMILY:

Geraniaceae

DISTRIBUTION:

Native to Europe and parts of Asia, North America and North Africa, and now found in temperate regions around the world.

PLANT SPIRIT QUALITIES:

Throughout history there have been people who have been able to forgive unspeakable acts of cruelty through the power of unconditional love. No matter what has happened to us in the past, herb robert helps us release anger, resentment, pain and guilt, to make room for miracles and healing to occur in our bodies and transform our lives. **Key words — unconditional love, forgiveness.**

How to identify it

- The leaves are dark green, palmately divided and about 6 cm (2½ inches) long, with light green, purple-edged leaflets with irregular borders. The leaves can turn red after flowering. Some people think the crushed leaves smell like burning tyres.
- The stems and leaves are covered with very fine hairs.
- It is a groundcover, and only grows to an average height of 30–40 cm (12–16 inches).
- Herb robert flowers are star-shaped, measuring 1.5–2 cm (⅝–¾ inch) across. They have five petals, usually dark rose-red or pale pink, with paler veins and round tips.
- The flower has 10 stamens and five sepals, and the pistil has five carpels.
- Flowers usually grow on the stem, from axillary nodes in pairs, or on terminating stems.
- Herb robert flowers in spring into early autumn, depending on location.
- The stems are green or red.
- The plant has weak, shallow roots.

How to harvest

In temperate areas, herb robert grows from late spring through summer, into early autumn. In subtropical areas it can grow year round, depending on location.

It is very easy to harvest as it pulls out with little effort. In order to not pull up the roots accidentally, you may want to harvest with scissors, or else gently pull up sections only, leaving enough for the patch to regenerate. The whole plant — but mainly the leaves, stems and flowers — can all be eaten and used medicinally.

Nutrients

Calcium, potassium, magnesium, iron, phosphorus, germanium, vitamins A, B and C, protein, carbohydrate, fatty acids, tocopherols.

Culinary use

Fresh leaves can be eaten in soups or salads. The are furry and bitter, so small amounts are recommended if eating it fresh. The flowers, leaves and roots can be dried and stored to be used as a tea.

Folk medicine

Herb robert, or St Robert's herb, was named after a French monk, Saint Robert of Molesme, who was born around 1027 AD. He healed people suffering from a variety of conditions using this plant. Native Americans used this plant both internally for many conditions, and externally for healing wounds, herpes and skin eruptions. It was often used for pain or bleeding. Rubbing fresh leaves on the skin is said to repel mosquitoes.

Traditionally, it was thought to bring good luck and enhance fertility.

In traditional herbalism, herb robert was used for the treatment of wounds, ulcers, diarrhoea, toothache and nosebleeds.

This herb always makes me think of the Australian herbalist Isabell Shipard, who was so passionate about it and used it extensively in her work. She recommends it to enhance the immune system, and attributes its effectiveness to the fact that it is a good source of germanium. She used it as a wound healer, antibiotic, antiviral and antioxidant, and also recommended it for chronic fatigue and other chronic inflammatory diseases.

Research

Clinical trials have confirmed its use in the following areas: antimicrobial,[1] antioxidant,[2] anti-inflammatory,[3] anti-ulcer,[4] ear aches,[5] diabetes,[6] cold sores,[7] anxiety[8] and gastric ulcers.[9]

How to use it as a medicine

Herb robert can be used as a tincture, an infusion, a powder or a poultice.

Herb robert can also be used in:

- Herb robert tea
- Herb robert glycetract
- Wild weed pesto
- Wild wilted greens
- Wild greens powder

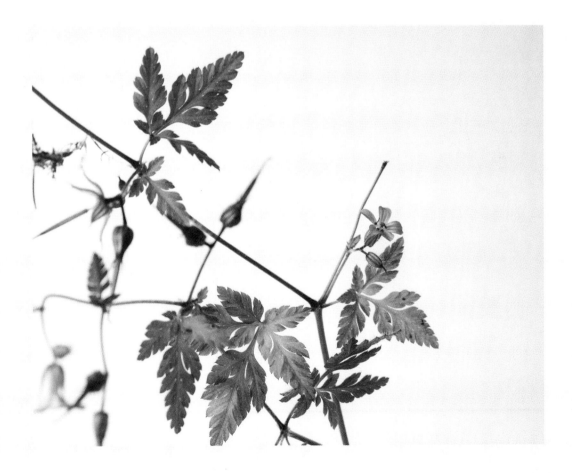

Herb robert & radish salad

Eating herb robert regularly is a lovely way to use your food as medicine for overall health. It is so delicate and so healing it deserves a beautiful salad like this. Herb robert is a little bit furry, but used in small amounts is still pleasant. It has a very mild flavour that combines wonderfully with the tart, sweet, peppery and light flavours of cranberries, apple, radish and cucumber.

SERVES 2 AS A SIDE SALAD
15 MINUTES

GF

2 radishes

juice of 1 lemon

1 handful of salad greens

¼ cucumber, very thinly sliced

¼ green apple, very thinly sliced

¼ cup (40 g) dried cranberries

1 small handful of fresh herb robert leaves

1 teaspoon olive oil

Very thinly slice the radishes using a mandoline or sharp knife. Place in a bowl with the lemon juice, six of the cranberries and a pinch of salt. Mix gently and leave to sit for 10–15 minutes.

Arrange the salad greens on a plate and top with the cucumber and apple slices.

Reserving the pink lemon juice for the dressing, arrange the radish slices over the salad, then the herb robert. Sprinkle the salad with the remaining dried cranberries.

Add the olive oil to the pink lemon juice and adjust the flavour as needed with more salt, lemon juice or oil.

If the sweetness of the cranberries has not infused the dressing, you can gently warm it to release the sweetness. Let it cool before using.

Pour the dressing over the salad just before serving.

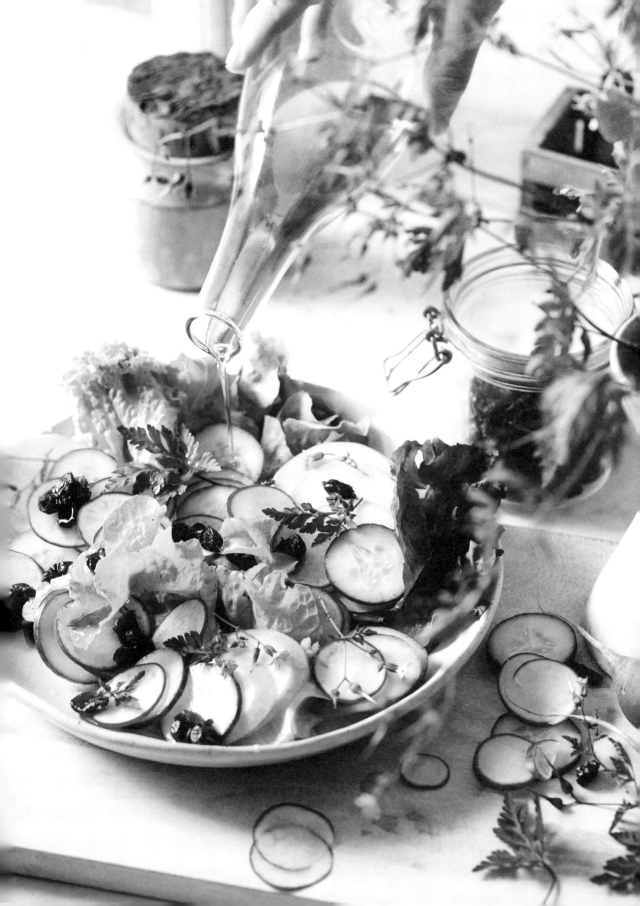

Herb robert capsules

MAKES 100 CAPSULES
20 MINUTES

1 cup (25 g) dried herb robert leaves and stems

100 x 000 size vegetable capsules

Herb robert has traditionally been used for chronic fatigue, fibromyalgia and other long-term debilitating illnesses characterised by pain and fatigue.

See the section on powders and capsules on page 21 in the Herbal Medicine-making Fundamentals chapter.

Grind the dried herbs using a coffee grinder or mortar and pestle.

Pull the capsules apart, scoop the powder into one half of the capsule, then put the other half back on.

If you plan to make lots, you might want to invest in a capsule maker that can be bought cheaply online.

Take 1–2 capsules daily. Store the capsules in an airtight container in a cool dark cupboard. They will last for up to 12 months.

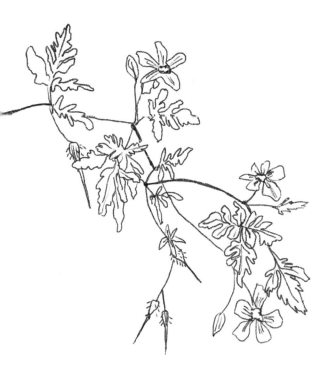

Herb robert healing balm

Herb robert has anti-inflammatory, antibacterial, antiviral and wound-healing properties. This salve has traditionally been used for wounds, cold sores, genital herpes, ulcers and skin eruptions such as acne and boils. Always consult a doctor with any concerns.

MAKES 30 ML (1 FL OZ)
20 MINUTES

20 ml (¾ fl oz) herb robert infused oil (see note)

5 ml (⅛ fl oz) castor oil

5 g (⅛ oz) sunflower wax

5 drops of tea tree essential oil

In a Pyrex or other heatproof glass jug, combine the herb infused oil, castor oil and sunflower wax. Place the jug in a saucepan, then pour about 5 cm (2 inches) water into the pan to make a water bath.

Bring the water to a slow boil, then reduce the heat to a simmer. Stir the mixture in the jug until the wax has melted, about 8–10 minutes.

Take off the heat and add the tea tree essential oil.

Pour into a sterilised amber glass jar (see page 23), or recycled lip balm pot, and allow to set.

Seal with the lid, then label with the ingredients, date made, and an expiry date of 12 months. If making multiple batches, add a batch number.

I generally put a 12-month expiry date on balms to be conservative, but they will often last much longer than this, especially if they contain essential oils.

HOW TO USE THE BALM

Apply directly to wounds, herpes, ulcers and skin eruptions such as acne and boils. To avoid creating or spreading infection, use a fresh cotton bud for each application. Be very careful with hygiene and wash your hands thoroughly before and after application.

Apply 2–3 times a day.

Note
Make your herb robert infused oil, either by the slow method (2 weeks) on page 30, or the fast method (1–2 days) on page 31.

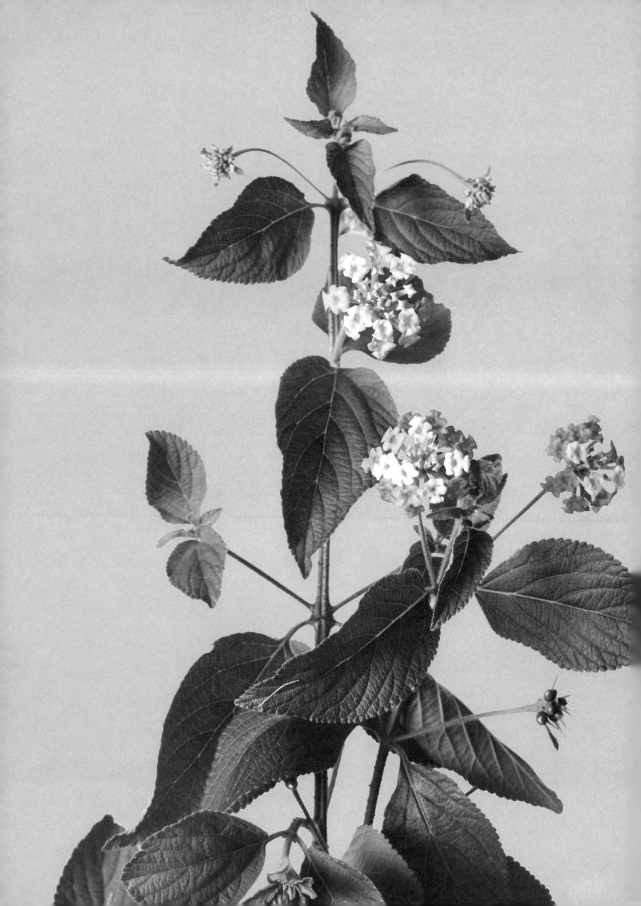

Lantana

COMMON NAMES:

lantana

SPECIES:

Lantana spp. There are over 150 *Lantana* species. Most research focuses on *Lantana camara*.

GENUS:

Lantana

FAMILY:

Verbenaceae

DISTRIBUTION:

Originated in Central and South America, but has now spread to over 50 countries around the world.

PLANT SPIRIT QUALITIES:

Lantana protects you from any kind of negative influence, whenever you are in a difficult environment, in crowds, or with people who have a very dark, heavy or unpleasant energy. It can protect you from overwhelm and intentional or unintentional psychic attacks from others. If you have had a traumatic experience, lantana can soften the physical, psychological and energetic effects of the incident. Lantana helps you maintain your light, and keep your energy field strong. **Key word — protection.**

How to identify it

- Lantana is a small tree or shrub.
- The leaves are simple, opposite or whorled, with toothed margins. They are usually quite rough on top, with soft, hairy undersides.
- The leaves are fragrant when crushed.
- It has spiny, square stems.
- It flowers in flat-topped clusters on a long stalk. Each flower is small and tubular, with four sections.
- The flowers are white, pink or yellow, or change to orange or red.
- A sweet nectar can be tasted in the bottom of the flowers, making them attractive to birds and butterflies.
- The fruit is fleshy and green, becoming bluish-black.

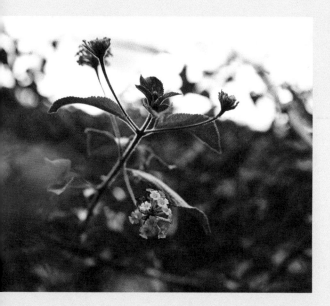

How to harvest

Lantana can be harvested all year round. The leaves, stems and flowers can all be used. It is prickly, so you might want to use gloves. I recommend cutting with a sharp pair of secateurs. Collect outer branches that have plenty of leaves and flowers and are not too woody.

Nutrients

Seeds
Protein, fatty acids (oleic acid), potassium, phosphorus, sodium, zinc, iron and copper.

Leaf
Protein, potassium, phosphorus, calcium, manganese, sulphur, iron, magnesium and copper.

Toxicity
There is much controversy around the toxicity of lantana to animals and humans. This may arise from the variations in toxicity associated with different species. Red-flowering species are often considered to be more toxic. There have been many reports of fatal toxicity to cattle, sheep, buffalo and guinea pigs.

Lantana camara is generally safe in humans, despite often being regarded as toxic, particularly to children. This seems to be based on a 1964 report on 17 children that suggested it could be harmful. Other articles mention cases of fatal poisoning in children; however, strong documentation for this is hard to find. The most compelling research on lantana's safety in kids comes from an article in the US journal *Pediatrics*, which reviewed 641 patients aged 1–16 years. The article stated:

> Ingestion of *L. camara* (including unripe berries) was not associated with significant toxicity; patients who ingested unripe berries did not exhibit more frequent or more severe symptoms than did patients who ingested ripe berries or other plant parts. Most patients displayed no or minimal symptoms. Children with asymptomatic ingestions and those with mild symptoms can be treated at home.[1]

To err on the side of caution, do not eat green berries, and no more than a small handful of black ones. Cooking further reduces the toxicity that is due to the presence of volatile oils, tannins and oxalates, making an infusion a safer option. If in doubt, consult your medical practitioner.

Culinary use

Lantana is not a common food source.

Folk medicine

Lantana spp. have traditionally been used in Africa as a mosquito repellent.

In traditional medicine, lantana has been used as a treatment for asthma, ulcers and tumours. It has been used in folk medicine as a carminative, antispasmodic and antiemetic, and to treat respiratory infections, rheumatism, wounds, asthma, biliary fever, bronchitis, tumours, ulcers, high blood pressure and epilepsy.

Healers in Asia and South America have used *Lantana* spp. for skin conditions, gastrointestinal diseases, malaria and tumours. Parts of *L. camara* are traditionally used for itches, cuts, ulcers, swellings, fever from jaundice, catarrh, eczema, tumours and rheumatism.

Research

Clinical trials have confirmed its use in the following areas: antibacterial,[2] gastroenteritis,[3] pest and tick control,[4] antioxidant[5] and antiepileptic.[6]

How to use it as a medicine

Lantana is used as a powder, an infusion, or externally as a poultice.

CAUTIONS + CONTRAINDICATIONS

L. camara has been associated with poisoning in cattle, sheep, buffalo and guinea pigs, with photosensitivity and liver and kidney damage being the most common symptoms. Poisoning is dose dependent and occurs with high or prolonged consumption.

There is mention of cases of fatal poisoning of children; however, these seem to be rare and poorly documented.

Lantana is generally safe in humans. However, side effects have been reported and include vomiting, abdominal pain, agitation, diarrhoea, throat and mouth irritation, tachycardia, drowsiness, nausea, dilated pupils and skin irritation. Mild side effects are safely treated at home. Serious side effects are rare but warrant medical attention.

Due to the presence of volatile oils, lantana should be avoided during pregnancy.

Caution is advised in liver and kidney disease.

Lantana can also be used in:
- Insect repellent
- Lantana gastro tea

Lantana itch balm

Clinical studies have confirmed lantana can help with pest and tick control. This balm can be used as an insect repellent and for itches, insect bites and tick bites. It's a great balm to take bushwalking and apply to exposed areas of skin (avoiding the face and eyes).

MAKES 30 ML (1 FL OZ)
20 MINUTES

20 ml (¾ fl oz) infused lantana oil (see note)

5 ml (⅛ fl oz) castor oil

5 g (⅛ oz) sunflower wax

5 drops of lantana essential oil (available online)

In a Pyrex or other heatproof glass jug, combine the infused oil, castor oil and sunflower wax. Place the jug in a saucepan, then pour about 5 cm (2 inches) water into the pan to make a water bath.

Bring the water to a slow boil, then reduce the heat to a simmer. Stir the mixture in the jug until the wax has melted, about 8–10 minutes.

Take off the heat and add the essential oil. Pour into a sterilised amber glass jar (see page 23) or recycled lip balm pot, and allow to set.

Seal with the lid, then label with the ingredients, date made, and an expiry date of 12 months. If making multiple batches, add a batch number. I generally put a 12-month expiry date on balms, but they often last much longer, especially if they contain essential oils.

Note

Make your infused lantana oil by the slow method (2 weeks) on page 30, or fast method (1–2 days) on page 31.

HOW TO USE THE ITCH BALM

Apply directly to itchy skin as often as needed. Apply a small amount to arms, legs and feet to keep mosquitoes away. **Do not use on the face or eyes.**

Room & travel spray

Any time you feel you need protection from the world around you, use this spray and feel lantana's love embrace you like a mother's hug. This oil is used for energetic and psychic protection from strong, unpleasant or overwhelming energies. It is ideal for travel, especially on airplanes, or even a busy day at a shopping centre.

MAKES 1 CUP (250 ML)

OVERNIGHT INFUSING
+ 10 MINUTES

1 handful of lantana leaves, stems and flowers

10 drops of lantana essential oil (available online)

Infuse the lantana in 1 cup (250 ml) hot boiled water overnight.

Strain the herbs and add the essential oil. Pour into a spritzer bottle. Pop the lid on, then label with the ingredients, date made, and an expiry of 12 months. The spritzer bottle can live in your handbag or on your desk for whenever you need it.

Any leftovers will keep in a sterilised glass jar (see page 23) in a dark cupboard for 12 months or more.

HOW TO USE THE SPRAY

Shake the bottle well before spraying. If a room needs a change in energy, spray around it. Hold it at arm's length and spray around the body. **Do not spray near the eyes and mouth.**

Natural insect repellent & itch spray

This insect repellent works really well and not only keeps insects and mosquitoes away, but also takes away the itch if you've already been bitten — a repellent and itch treatment all in one.

MAKES 2 CUPS (500 ML)

OVERNIGHT INFUSING + 10 MINUTES

1 cup (20 g) fresh lantana leaves, or ½ cup (5 g) coarsely chopped dried leaves (see notes)

1 cup (20 g) fresh blue top leaves, or ½ cup (3 g) coarsely chopped dried leaves (see notes)

1 cup (20 g) fresh fleabane leaves, or ½ cup (3 g) coarsely chopped dried leaves (see notes)

30 ml (1 fl oz) lemon eucalyptus essential oil (see notes)

Make a strong infusion of the herbs by steeping them in 2 cups (500 ml) water for 6–8 hours.

Strain the herbs and add the lemon eucalyptus essential oil.

Pour into a glass bottle with a spray top and seal with the lid. Label the bottle with the ingredients and date made and store safely in a dark, cool cupboard or drawer. It will keep for 1–2 years.

HOW TO USE THE REPELLENT

Shake the bottle before use. Spray onto bare skin to prevent new bites, and to soothe itching from old bites. **Avoid the eyes and close your mouth to avoid inhaling the mist.**

Notes

Lantana (*Lantana camara*) species have traditionally been used in Africa as a mosquito repellent. Extracts from the leaves of *L. camara* were tested and found to possess antimicrobial, fungicidal, insecticidal and nematicidal activity. A South African study found a 40% concentration of *L. camara* to have a 57% efficacy rate against cattle ticks.

Blue top (*Ageratum conyzoides*) is used for fevers, and tick and insect bites. Crushing the leaves and rubbing on the bite rapidly reduces pain and swelling.

Fleabane (*Conyza canadensis*) has demonstrated insecticidal activity against fleas, flies, mosquitoes and agricultural pests.

Lemon eucalyptus (*Corymbia citriodora*; also known as *Eucalyptus citriodora*) is the only essential oil that has consistently passed scientific tests for its ability to ward off mosquitoes. Protection at 30% is said to last up to 7 hours, whereas citronella only showed 30 minutes protection.

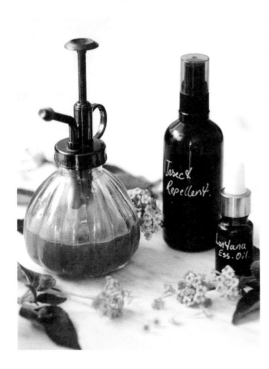

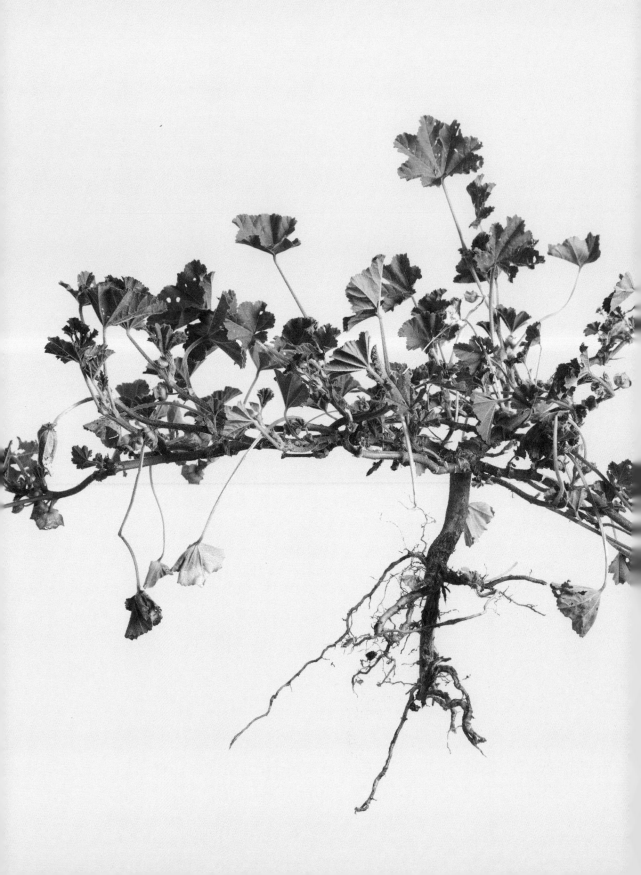

Mallow

COMMON NAMES:

common mallow, cheeseweed, wild mallow

SPECIES:

Malva sylvestris

OTHER SPECIES:

Malva parviflora (small-flowered mallow),
Malva neglecta (dwarf mallow). There
are about 25–30 species of mallow. The
most well known is *Althaea officinalis*
(marshmallow), which is more common
in Europe.

GENUS:

Malva

FAMILY:

Malvaceae

DISTRIBUTION:

Native to Europe and the Mediterranean.
Now also found in Asia, America, Canada,
Mexico, Africa, Siberia and Australia.

PLANT SPIRIT QUALITIES:

Mallow helps to soothe anger and
irritation, so you can be calmer and kinder
to yourself, and to others. It also helps
soften and loosen emotions that are trapped
in the body, helping you to cry or express
your pain through sound or movement,
releasing it from your body and energy
field. It is useful in dealing with emotions
around traumatic experiences, as well
as guilt or shame — helping you make
amends as part of your recovery process.
**Key words — emotional soothing,
expression.**

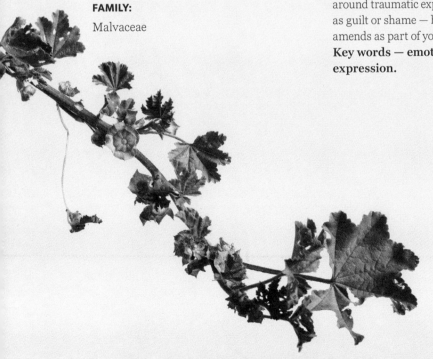

How to identify it

- The leaves are rounded, palmate and compound, with irregular toothed margins, characteristic soft hairs, and prominent veins on the underside.

- *Malva sylvestris* grows 1–1.5 metres (3–5 feet) high. The flowers are reddish-purple to bright pinkish-purple with dark stripes. Two to four flowers arise at the junction of the stem and form irregularly along the main stem, with the flowers at the base opening first.

- *M. parviflora* grows to about 50 cm (20 inches). The flowers are pink, white or occasionally pale purple. I have seen mostly white ones. The tiny flowers are only 5–6 mm (¼ inch) in diameter, and not much bigger than the green calyx.

- *M. neglecta* grows to about 50 cm (20 inches). The flowers are white to light pink to light purple, with five petals. The petals are notched at the tip, so the flowers may appear to have 10 petals.

- The fruits are also called 'cheeses' or 'peas', as they are shaped like a cheese wheel or a little green segmented pea. They are brown to brownish-green when ripe, about 2.5 mm (¹⁄₁₆ inch) long and 5–7 mm (¼ inch) in diameter.

- Wild mallow has a central tap root, with fibrous secondary roots – unlike marshmallow (*Althaea officinalis*) there is more musilage in the fruit (peas) than the root.

How to harvest

Leaves

Mallow leaves can be harvested during spring and summer, and are highest in nutrients and medicinal compounds before flowering and fruiting. You can cut the leaves with scissors, or pluck them off with your hands. Unlike the famous 'marshmallow' (*Althaea officinalis*) that is traditionally used to make marshmallows, wild mallow is mainly used for its leaves and fruit, as the root tends to be very small and fibrous and has very little mucilage.

Fruit (peas)

Wild mallow fruits from summer to autumn. The little pea-shaped fruits can be prised off by gently pulling your hand up the stem, or by plucking them off with your fingers. The fruit contains the most mucilage and is the best part for using in food and medicine. Use them at any stage while they are green. Once they turn brown, they are no good to use anymore.

Nutrients

Fibre, protein, sugars, fatty acids, niacin, folic acid, vitamin A, vitamin C and vitamin E.

Culinary use

The use of *M. sylvestris* is thought to have originated around 3000 BC in Syria, where archaeological studies have found the seeds in human teeth. Another reference to its use in antiquity comes from the Roman lyric poet Horace (c. 65–8 BC), who said of his diet: *Me pascunt olivae, me cichorea levesque malvae*, meaning, 'As for me, olives, endives and mallows provide sustenance.'

The leaves of all common mallow species are used to thicken soups. They can be used like okra, and can also be eaten raw in salads.

The mucilage from the fruits can be used to make marshmallow and other desserts.

Folk medicine

The use of *M. sylvestris* and other mallows in folk medicine is extensive around the world. It is helpful for the entire digestive tract, from the mouth to the anus, for any kind of irritation or inflammation. It is also used for irritation and inflammation in the respiratory tract, urinary tract and reproductive organs, and any 'itis' anywhere in the body, such as gingivitis, tonsillitis and cystitis.

Externally, it is used on the skin for any kind of wound, bite, burn or rash.

It is usually combined with other antimicrobial herbs in cases of infection.

It is also used in both constipation and diarrhoea.

Research

Clinical trials have confirmed the use of *M. sylvestris* in the following areas: antioxidant,[1] anti-inflammatory,[2] antibacterial,[3] wound healing and chronic skin conditions,[4] ulcerative colitis,[5] liver and kidney protection[6] and cardiovascular protection.[7]

How to use it as a medicine

The mucilage from mallow is extracted better in water than alcohol, so it is often used as a decoction (root and fruits).

Externally, the leaves make an excellent poultice and can be used in creams and ointments.

CAUTIONS + CONTRAINDICATIONS
Use with caution during pregnancy; otherwise generally very safe.

Wild mallow can also be used in:
- Mallow tea
- Mallow glycetract

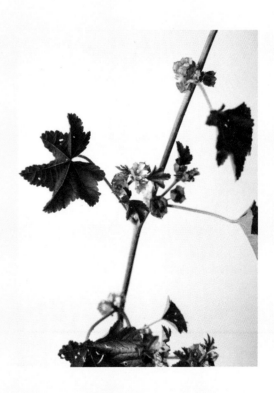

Mallow salad

SERVES 2
30 MINUTES

GF

4 handfuls of fresh mallow leaves and stems

2 tablespoons olive oil

2 garlic cloves

1–2 tablespoons chopped parsley and/or coriander (cilantro)

¼ teaspoon sweet paprika

¼ teaspoon ground cumin

2 teaspoons chopped preserved lemon rind, plus extra to garnish

a splash of lemon juice

5 olives, pitted and cut in half

Common mallow grows wild in Morocco, where it is known as *khoubiza or bakoula*, and is commonly gathered as a vegetable. It is also sold in large bunches in the *souks* (food markets). This dish is often eaten as a dip served with bread, inspired me to cultivate wild mallow plants in my garden because it is so delicious, and feels so soothing to my gut and digestion. Wild mallow leaves are helpful for the entire digestive tract and for easing any kind of irritation or inflammation throughout the body.

Set a steamer basket or pan over a saucepan of boiling water. Wash the mallow, then chop the leaves and stems and steam them for 20 minutes, or until soft. Carefully tip the mallow into a sieve in the sink. When cool enough to handle, squeeze out any excess water.

Heat the olive oil in a frying pan. Fry the garlic, herbs and spices over medium heat for 1 minute, or until the garlic has softened and browned. Add the mallow and preserved lemon and cook for another 5 minutes, stirring gently.

Remove from the heat and taste, adding as much or as little lemon juice and salt as you prefer.

Place in a dish and garnish with the olives, cut side facing down, and some more preserved lemon rind. It's nice with an extra drizzle of olive oil and an extra pinch of paprika.

Mallow lung tea

MAKES 1 CUP (250 ML)
25 MINUTES

GF

2 tablespoons chopped fresh mallow leaves

2 tablespoons fresh mallow peas

1 teaspoon dried thyme leaves

1 teaspoon fennel seeds

½ teaspoon dried liquorice root (optional)

1–2 teaspoons honey or maple syrup (optional)

Use this tea for a rattling cough with lots of mucus. Mallow soothes irritation, liquorice helps bring up mucus, and fennel helps to clear sinuses and relax bronchial spasms. It's traditionally used to reduce symptoms of asthma, bronchitis and congestion. Thyme's antibacterial effects may help fight infection. Enjoy this tea hot or cold. You can scale up the recipe to make a 750 ml–1 litre (3–4 cup) batch and leave it in the fridge.

Pour 2 cups (500 ml) water into a saucepan. Add the mallow leaves, mallow peas, thyme and fennel seeds, and dried liquorice if using. Bring to the boil, then keep boiling for 15–20 minutes, or until the water has reduced to 1 cup (250 ml) and has thickened with the marshmallow.

Strain out the herbs and stir in the honey or maple syrup, if using, until dissolved. Pour into a sterilised glass bottle or jar (see page 23). Seal with the lid, then label with the ingredients and date made.

Store in the fridge, where it will keep for up to 3 days.

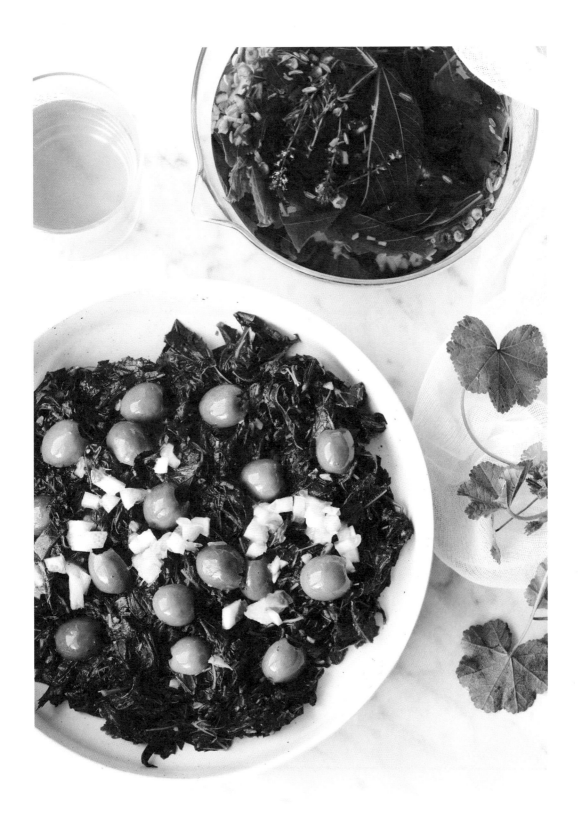

Wild vegan marsh-mallows

MAKES 12–15
1½ HOURS

½ cup (60 g) cornflour (cornstarch), plus extra for dusting

½ cup (125 ml) aquafaba

¼ teaspoon cream of tartar

⅓ cup (80 ml) pure vanilla extract

½ cup (30 g) fresh wild mallow peas

1½ cups (375 ml) water

1 tablespoon agar agar powder

1 cup (185 g) caster (superfine) sugar (see note)

Note
Use white caster sugar rather than golden or raw caster sugar if you want white (rather than slightly off white) marshmallows.

I tried a few times to make marshmallows from the roots of wild mallow, thinking it would be the same as the classic marshmallow plant (*Althaea officinalis*). It was John Kallas' book *Edible Wild Plants* that solved the mystery by explaining that it's actually the wild mallow peas (or fruits) that provide the mucilage in the wild mallow plant. Here I use mallow peas and a recipe inspired by Monica Davis, from her blog 'The Hidden Veggies', to make these beautiful vegan wild marshmallows.

Line a shallow baking dish with baking paper and dust it with one-third of the cornflour.

Using a stand mixer or an electric hand mixer, whip the aquafaba and cream of tartar in a bowl for about 6 minutes, until stiff peaks form. (I have tried using a hand whisk, stick blender and a normal blender, and the results are not as good.)

Add the vanilla and mix for another 3 minutes to incorporate. (Depending on the power of your mixer, you might need to mix for a good 10 minutes in total.)

It's ready when the aquafaba forms stiff peaks and doesn't fall out when you turn the bowl upside down. Set aside.

Place the mallow peas in a saucepan with 1½ cups (375 ml) water. Bring to the boil, then allow to boil rapidly for 5 minutes. The water should thicken as the mucilage comes out of the peas, and be reduced by about half.

Scoop the peas out and pour the water into a measuring jug. Pour ⅔ cup (170 ml) of the water back into the saucepan, stir in the agar agar and boil for another 3 minutes.

Add the sugar and boil for another 3 minutes, until the sugar has dissolved. Remove from the heat.

While mixing at low speed, slowly and carefully pour the mixture into the whipped aquafaba. As soon as it is incorporated, quickly pour it into your baking dish. It will start to set quickly, and if you mix it for too long you will have hard lumps!

Dust the top of the marshmallow with more cornflour, then place in the fridge for 30–60 minutes to fully set.

Once cooled, cut into squares. If it's a bit wet, you can dry it with a paper towel before cutting. Dust the marshmallows with more cornflour to coat them.

Store in an airtight container, but not too tightly packed, or they will stick together. They will keep in the pantry or fridge in an airtight container for 7 days. If they get sticky, simply pat dry with paper towel and recoat with cornflour.

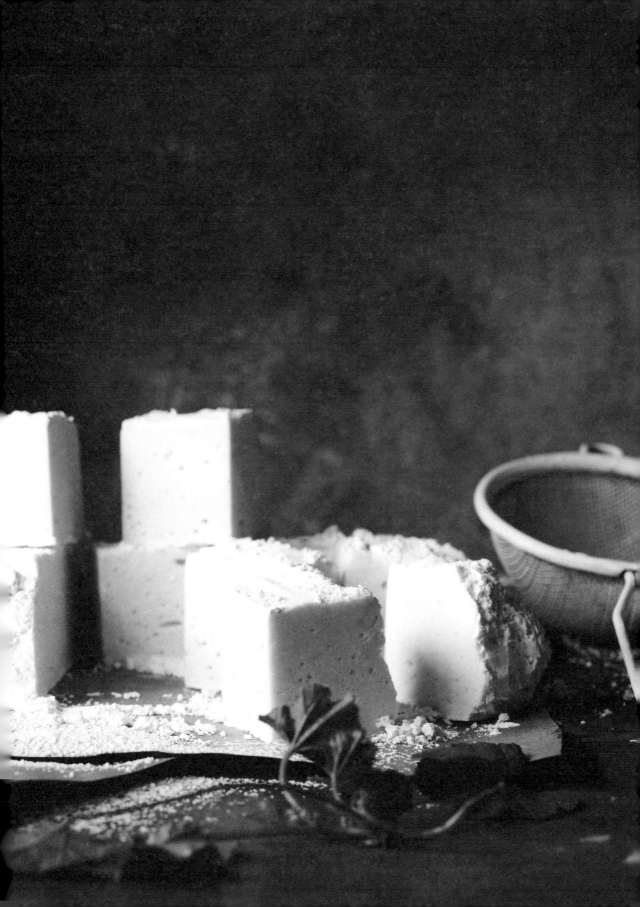

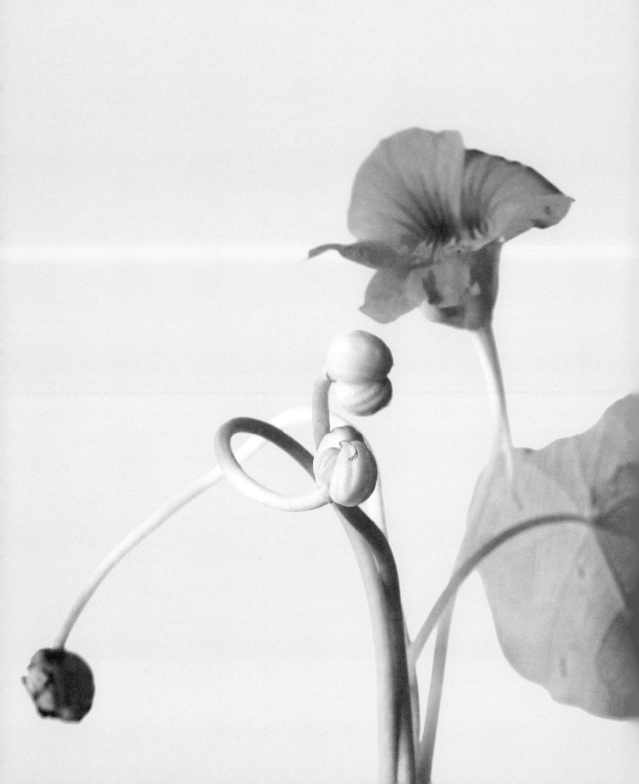

Nasturtium

COMMON NAMES:

nasturtium

SPECIES:

Tropaeolum majus

GENUS:

Tropaeolum

FAMILY:

Tropaeolaceae

DISTRIBUTION:

Native to South America. Naturalised in North America, Europe, Africa, Australia and New Zealand.

PLANT SPIRIT QUALITIES:

Energetically, nasturtium has a fiery quality that will burn up any dross or stagnant energy in your body and life — giving you the 'fire in the belly' to get things done when you're feeling exhausted, uninspired, creatively or emotionally stuck, indecisive, lacking in energy or motivation, or when your 'fight' or creative fire has died. It can help if your work has become overly analytical and intellectual, and the passion or joy has gone out of it, or when you have a lot of mental chatter but your body feels exhausted. It can also reignite your passion for a spiritual practice or exercise regime. **Key words — action, decision-making, creative spark.**

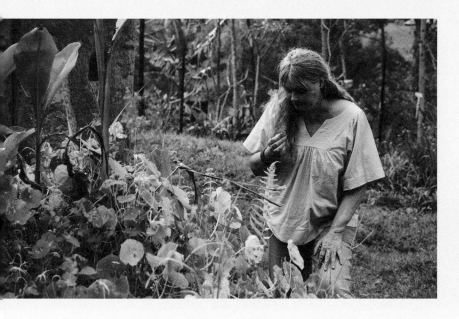

How to identify it

- Nasturtium is recognised by its bright yellow, orange and red flowers.
- The flowers have five petals and a funnel-shaped nectar spur at the back, formed by modification of one of the five sepals.
- It flowers in spring and summer.
- Another key feature is its spirally arranged, round, umbrella-like (peltate) leaves with radiating veins.
- The young leaves have a peppery, watercress flavour, and drops of water bead on the surface like mercury.
- The top of the leaf is hairless, but the under-surface is rough, with small warts, and can be bluish.
- The smooth stems branch from the base and are circular, weak, soft and fleshy.
- Nasturtiums scramble or climb to usually about 1 metre (3 feet) long, and occasionally up to 10 metres (32 feet) long, and have a watery sap.
- The seeds are green and succulent, until they drop and turn light brown.
- The plant has a taproot.

How to harvest

Leaves
Nasturtiums grow from spring through summer and into late autumn. In warmer climates, they can sometimes grow year round. Leaves can be harvested throughout the growing season. Use scissors to cut the leaves at the stems so the plant can keep growing.

Seeds
Pick the seeds while they are still green and succulent. The seeds can be hard to see, so you need to gently move the leaves aside to look for them growing on the stalks. Harvest gently with scissors, or by pinching them off with your fingers.

Flowers
Flowers can be harvested throughout the growing season by gently picking them off with your fingers.

Nutrients

Protein, vitamin C, beta-carotene, quercetin, lutein, potassium, phosphorus, calcium, magnesium, zinc, copper, iron, sulphur and iodine — with 100 g (3½ oz) of fresh nasturtium flowers providing 73–100% of the adult recommended dietary allowance of zinc. Nasturtium flowers contain up to 45 mg of lutein per 100 g — the highest amount found in any edible plant.

Culinary use

The flowers and leaves have a strong peppery taste and are used most commonly in salads or stir-fries. The unripe seed pods can be harvested and dropped into spiced vinegar to produce a condiment and garnish that can be used in place of capers.

Folk medicine

Nasturtium was first introduced to Europe from Peru in the 1600s. The Peruvian Indians used the natural antibiotic qualities of nasturtium leaves to treat coughs.

Traditionally, it has been used as an antibiotic to treat various infections, particularly those of the lungs and the urinary tract, but also upper respiratory tract infections, sinusitis and rhinitis.

It was used as a remedy against scurvy, due to its high vitamin C content. In folk medicine it has a history of use in the common cold and influenza.

It has traditionally also been used externally for muscular pain, bacterial infections and minor scrapes and wounds.

Research

Clinical trials have confirmed nasturtium's use in the following areas: diuretic,[1] urinary tract infections,[2] circulation,[3] blood pressure lowering,[4] respiratory infections,[5] antibiotic[6] and antioxidant.[7]

How to use it as a medicine

Nasturtium can be used as a powder, a vinegar, as a syrup, macerate, infusion or tincture. Fresh flowers and immature green seeds can be eaten raw or pickled.

CAUTIONS + CONTRAINDICATIONS

The volatile mustard oil in nasturtium causes skin irritation and should not be used during pregnancy or breastfeeding. It should be avoided by people with kidney diseases, or ulceration of the stomach or intestinal tract.

Nasturtium can also be used in:

* Chickweed, cashew and caper toasts

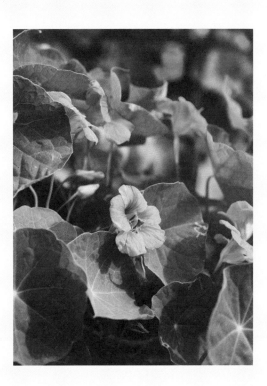

Nasturtium salad

SERVES 4
25 MINUTES

GF

This is a beautiful, colourful salad for parties and special events, or you can make a simple one to accompany any meal. The nasturtium flowers are really high in lutein, which is good for your eyes. Feel free to vary the ingredients based on your preferences and seasonal availability, so you can make a simple salad to accompany any meal.

1 small carrot

1 small zucchini (courgette)

1 red capsicum (pepper)

1 avocado

3–6 large fresh nasturtium leaves, plus a handful of smaller leaves to garnish

2 handfuls of salad greens

6 or more nasturtium flowers

6 or more viola flowers (or any other edible flowers)

1 tablespoon nasturtium capers (page 229), or regular capers

GOLDEN SALAD DRESSING

2 tablespoons lemon juice

1 tablespoon maple syrup

1 teaspoon olive oil

1 teaspoon creamy dijon mustard

¼ teaspoon salt

In a small bowl or jug, combine the dressing ingredients and set aside.

Peel the carrot, then shave the carrot and zucchini with a vegetable peeler. Finely slice the capsicum and avocado.

On a large tray or board, spread out the nasturtium leaves. Cover them with the salad greens.

Roll up the slices of carrot and zucchini and arrange them over the salad leaves, along with the capsicum and avocado.

Top with all the flowers and the nasturtium capers.

Serve the dressing on the side, so people can add it to their own plate as they help themselves to the salad.

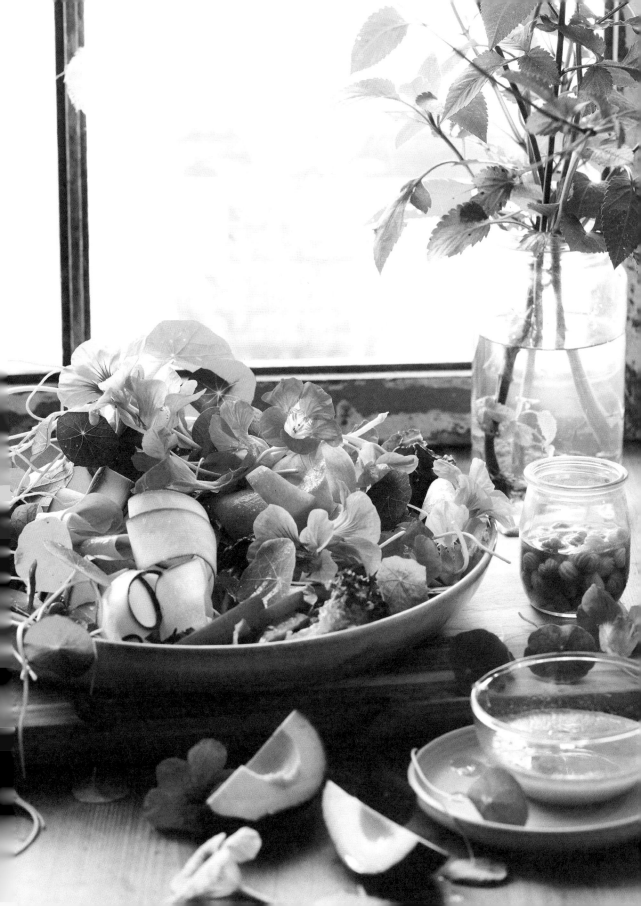

Nasturtium cold & flu tonic

MAKES 2 CUPS (500 ML)

20 MINUTES + 2 WEEKS INFUSING

1 handful of fresh nasturtium leaves and flowers

1 cup (250 ml) apple cider vinegar

3 garlic cloves, peeled

1 thumb-sized piece of fresh ginger

1 thumb-sized piece of fresh turmeric

1 lemon

This is one of the best winter tonics I know of. It's an all-round immune booster to help fight off winter viruses and bacteria. You can take it throughout cold and flu season as a preventative, or at the first sign of a cold or sore throat.

Roughly chop the nasturtium leaves and flowers and place in a sterilised glass jar (see page 23). Pour in the vinegar.

Coarsely chop the garlic, ginger and turmeric and add to the jar.

Leaving the skin on, slice the lemon into rounds and add the slices to the jar as well.

If your jar has a metal lid, place baking paper between the jar and the lid to stop it rusting.

Cap tightly, label with the ingredients and date made, and leave in a cool, dark place for at least 2 weeks. It will then keep in the fridge for up to 6 months.

HOW TO USE THE TONIC

Take 1 tablespoon in ¼ cup (60 ml) warm water. If desired, you can sweeten the tonic with a teaspoon of honey or maple syrup. Take daily for prevention, or up to 3 times a day at the first sign of infection.

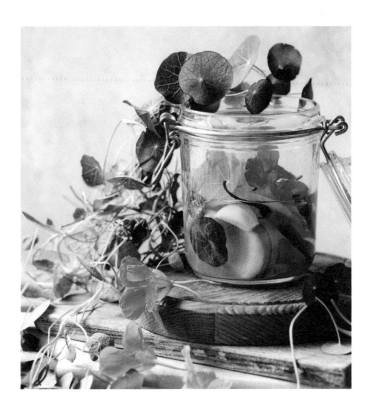

Nasturtium capers

These delicious little flavour bombs taste much like normal capers, but have a bit more crunch and pepperiness, and come with all the antibiotic benefits of nasturtium leaves, plus some good probiotics. The hard part can be gathering enough of them, so just keep adding them to a jar as you find more seeds in your nasturtium patch.

I've given two versions below. One simply pickles the seeds in apple cider vinegar, while the lacto-fermented method uses a brine and is the traditional and probiotic way to ferment vegetables.

15 MINUTES + 2½ WEEKS FERMENTING

MAKES 1 CUP CAPERS

GF

VINEGAR CAPERS

1 cup (160 g) green nasturtium seeds

1 cup (250 ml) apple cider vinegar

1 teaspoon salt

Place the nasturtium seeds in a sterilised glass jar (see page 23). Fill with the apple cider vinegar and add the salt.

If your jar has a metal lid, place baking paper between the lid and the jar to stop it rusting.

Cap tightly and leave on the bench or in a cupboard for at least 2 weeks. The nasturtium capers will then last 3 months in the fridge.

LACTO-FERMENTED CAPERS

1 teaspoon salt

1 cup (250 ml) water

1 cup (160 g) green nasturtium seeds

Combine the salt and water in a sterilised glass jar (see page 23). Add the nasturtium seeds and put a lid on lightly, so air can escape.

Leave on the bench or in a cupboard for 3–5 days, until bubbles appear.

Once bubbles appear, leave the jar in the fridge for 2 weeks before eating the capers.

If bubbles appear after only a day or two on the bench, keep taste testing until the capers are nice and sour, then store them in the fridge, where they will keep for 3 months.

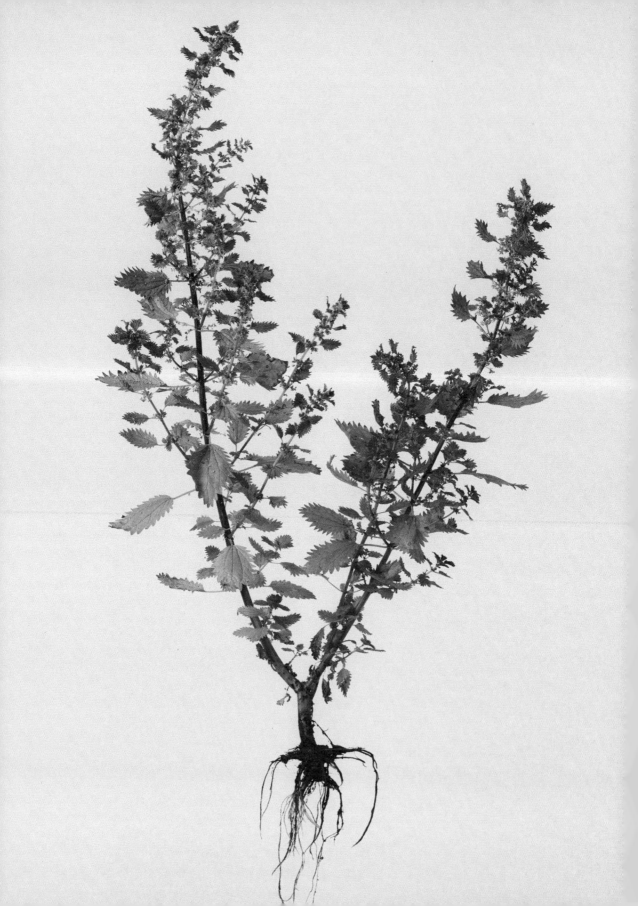

Nettle

COMMON NAMES:

tall nettle, common nettle, large-leaf stinging nettle, English nettle, dwarf nettle, native nettle, small-leaf stinging nettle, scrub nettle

SPECIES:

Of the 30–45 *Urtica* species, the literature and research focus on *Urtica dioica* (tall, common, large-leaf) and *Urtica urens* (English, dwarf, native, small-leaf). South-eastern Australia and New Zealand have *Urtica incisa* (scrub nettle) as well as *Urtica dioica* and *Urtica urens*.

GENUS:

Urtica

FAMILY:

Urticaceae

DISTRIBUTION:

Native to Europe, Asia, northern Africa and western North America, and introduced throughout the world.

PLANT SPIRIT QUALITIES:

Nettle helps to bring back joie de vivre. Its sting shocks us out of self-doubt, self-loathing and complacency, and helps us smile and laugh again. It strengthens our life force when we are stuck, and helps us feel there is light at the end of the tunnel and that life is worth living. It can be used for depression and hopelessness, or during a 'dark night of the soul', or to give the strength and insight to break free of toxic situations that no longer serve us. Nettle is a bright light in the darkness, like a firework exploding in the night sky, bringing joy to everyone who sees it.
Key words — joy, creative spark.

How to identify it

- Nettles are erect, upright plants, most easily identified by the small stinging hairs of silica that cover the leaves and stems.

- Tall nettle (*Urtica dioica*) is perennial and can grow to 1 metre (3 feet) or more. It is tall in the summer and dies off in winter, except in Queensland, where it can grow throughout winter.

- Nettle has opposite ovate leaves, with strongly serrated margins, a heart- shaped base, and a tip that tapers to a point. The tip is longer than the serrations on the sides of the leaves.

- It has numerous green to brown flowers in dense axillary inflorescences, with male and female flowers found on separate plants.

- It has widely spreading yellow rhizomes, stolons and roots.

- English or dwarf nettle (*Urtica urens*) differs from *U. dioica* in the following ways:

  - it is an annual, rather than perennial

  - it is a smaller plant (10–50 cm/4–20 inches)

  - the stem is upright, with branches and four sides, and covered in stinging hairs

  - the leaves are 2–4 cm (¾–1¼ inches) long, but more deeply toothed

  - male and female flowers are found on the same plant

  - the flower spikes are short and stumpy

  - it has a milder sting.

- Scrub nettle (*U. incisa*) is similar to *U. dioica*, being both perennial and growing up to 1 metre (3 feet) or more. It can have large leaves up to 10 cm (4 inches) long and, like *U. dioica*, it has male and female flowers on separate plants.

How to harvest

Leaves

Make sure you wear gloves when harvesting nettles. If you don't have them handy, your best chance to not get stung is to put your fingers on the underside of the leaf (which doesn't have stinging hairs), fold it in on itself and pinch it off. If you are careful, it works. Generally, though, wear gloves and cut off the leaves using scissors or secateurs. Cutting the top 5–10 cm (2–4 inches) off the stems allows the lower stems to continue growing.

Seeds

Nettle flowers and goes to seed in the warmth of late spring and early summer. Shake the flower heads and see if the seeds fall into your hand; if they do, they're ready to harvest. Cut the flower heads and gently shake and massage them over a large bowl. There are often little insects in the flower heads — be careful not to harm them, so they can return to their work in the garden, as butterflies breed on nettles. You can also hang the seed heads upside down with a bag wrapped around them for a few days.

Roots

If you have a large enough population of nettles (ensuring there are enough to regrow), you can dig up the whole plant to obtain the roots. A small gardening trowel is generally enough to dig them out. Roots are best harvested either before or after flowering, when there is more energy, nutrition and phytochemicals in them.

Nutrients

High in protein, chlorophyll, beta-carotene, vitamins B1, B2, B9, C, E and K, as well as silica, phosphorus, potassium, calcium, magnesium and sulphur.

Culinary use

There are many recipes for nettle. The leaves and stems can be used in place of spinach, and as a cooked green in a large variety of dishes, including soups, stews, pastas and pesto. It is commonly drunk as a tea, and is used in tonic preparations with other nutritive herbs and foods. It should not be eaten raw due to the stinging hairs, but can be juiced.

The seeds can be eaten on their own or with other seeds in culinary seed mixes.

Folk medicine

Nettle has a long history of use around the world as a food, a medicine and a fibre for textiles. It is traditionally picked in early spring, and used as a steamed vegetable tonic to help rejuvenate the body after winter. The renowned yogi, Milarepa, is said to have turned green after eating nothing but nettles during his long periods of meditation.

It has also been used for a variety of lung complaints, including asthma, cough and bronchitis. On the hair it is a scalp tonic, said to cure everything from dandruff to baldness, and to speed hair growth.

Many cases have been reported of arthritic pain being removed by applying the stinging hairs of nettle directly to the affected areas.

It is also said to affect the kidneys and act as a diuretic, helping reduce oedema and promote uric acid excretion, making it beneficial in gout and arthritis.

Nettle (apart from the roots) is also used for anaemia and to stimulate milk flow, so is often recommended for pregnant and breastfeeding mothers.

The juice of the nettle is said to act as an antidote to the plant's own sting, providing instant relief. The juice of dock, which is often found growing near nettle, is also an effective remedy for nettle stings — hence the old rhyme, 'Nettle in, dock out. Dock rub nettle out!'

Research

There is a considerable amount of research on *Urtica dioica* and *U. urens*, but a very limited amount on *U. incisa*. I have simply highlighted major areas of research relating to *U. dioica*, although compounds and levels of constituents may vary.

Clinical trials have been done on *U. dioica* in the following areas: diabetes, metabolic syndrome and cardiovascular benefits,[1] benign prostatic hyperplasia[2] and allergic rhinitis and arthritis.[3]

How to use it as a medicine

Both the leaf and root can be used as a tincture, tea, tablet or powder.

CAUTIONS + CONTRAINDICATIONS

Apart from the obvious discomfort of being stung by nettles, which causes stinging pain, rash and itching, nettle leaf is considered safe during all stages of life. It is recommended that the root be used with caution medicinally during pregnancy, lactation and childhood, due to its effects on androgen and oestrogen metabolism. However, it is considered safe as a food.

Nettle can also be used in:

- Nettle tea
- Nettle glycetract
- Wild wilted greens
- Wild greens powder
- Wild weed pesto

Mushroom, thyme, garlic & nettle soup

SERVES 4–6
30 MINUTES

GF

6 handfuls of fresh nettle leaves, stems removed

1 tablespoon extra virgin olive oil

2 shallots, or 6 garlic cloves, chopped

1–2 celery stalks, chopped

3 potatoes, peeled and chopped

2–3 thyme sprigs, plus extra to garnish

2–3 bay leaves

4 cups (1 litre) vegetable stock

½ cup (20 g) dried medicinal and culinary mushrooms, soaked (reserving the soaking water), or 1 cup (125 g) fresh mushrooms (see note)

Nettles are rich in protein, vitamin K and minerals including iron, calcium, magnesium, potassium and zinc. You can use medicinal mushrooms such as reishi, shiitake or lion's mane, or flavourful ones such as porcini, Swiss brown, oyster or chanterelles — all of which have their own list of benefits for either the nervous system or immune system, or both. Thyme is used in traditional herbal medicine for all kinds of infections. You can be as light or as heavy handed with the garlic as you wish; for a medicinal soup for a cold or as an anti-inflammatory meal, use plenty. The potato can be replaced with sweet potato or omitted if you are sensitive to starch or Solanaceae vegetables, or prefer a lighter broth. Play with your own variations until you find your perfect potion!

Prepare a large bowl of iced water.

Bring a large saucepan of lightly salted water to the boil. Wearing protective gloves, drop the nettles into the boiling water and blanch for 2 minutes. Use tongs to lift the wilted nettles out of the pan and into the bowl of iced water to refresh them. Drain the nettles in a colander in the sink.

Cut away and discard any large stems from the nettles. (This should be easier now that they've lost their stingers due to the blanching.) You should have 3–4 cups of blanched tender nettles for this recipe. Any left-over blanched nettles can be frozen for future use.

In a large saucepan, heat the olive oil over medium heat. Add the shallot and celery and cook for about 5 minutes, until softened.

Add the potatoes, thyme, bay leaves and stock, along with the mushrooms (and soaking water, if using dried mushrooms). Season with salt and black pepper to taste. Bring to a simmer, then cook for 20 minutes, until the potatoes are tender. Remove the bay leaves and thyme sprigs and season to taste.

Purée the blanched nettles and divide among the soup bowls. Ladle the soup over the top, garnish with extra thyme and serve.

Note
If using dried mushrooms, soak them in 2 cups (500 ml) water and ½ teaspoon salt for at least 1 hour, or even overnight.

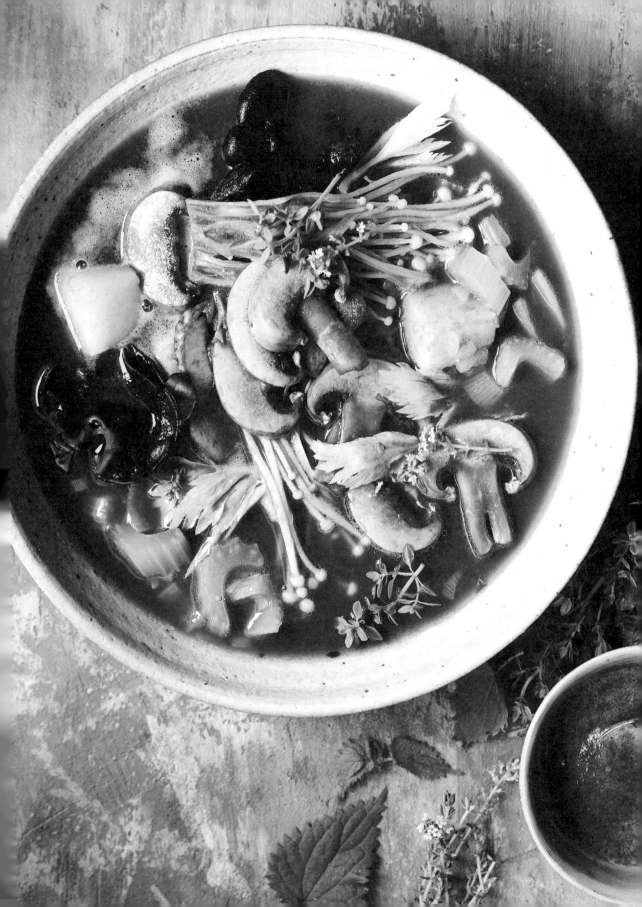

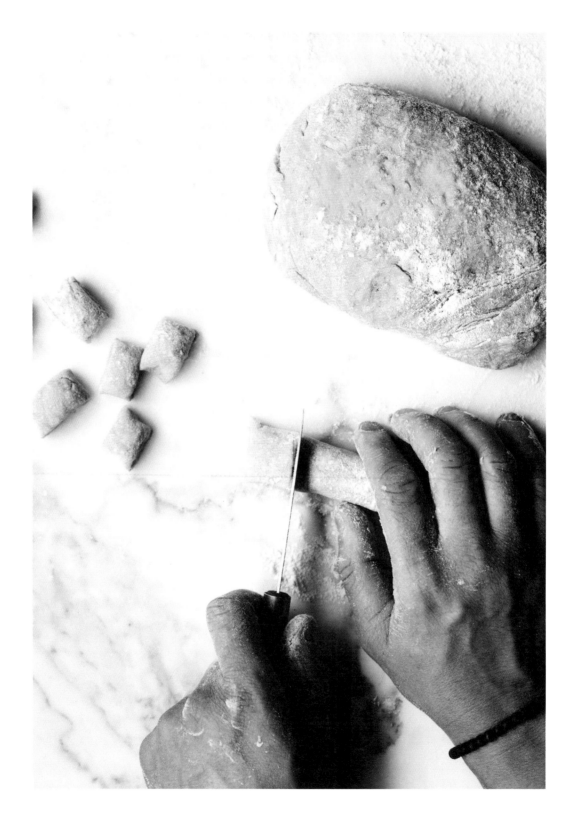

Nettle gnocchi verdi

SERVES 4
1 HOUR

---

450 g (1 lb) floury potatoes, peeled and cut into 4 cm (1½ inch) chunks

100 g (3½ oz) fresh nettle leaves and stems

275 g (9½ oz) plain (all-purpose) white spelt flour, plus extra for dusting

½ teaspoon fine sea salt

2 tablespoons olive oil, plus extra for tossing the gnocchi

2 garlic cloves, crushed

a pinch of ground black pepper

a pinch of flaky sea salt

chilli flakes, to taste

These little gnocchi are a labour of love. They can be fun to prepare for a special event if you can make them together with friends, music and a few nice drinks. They should not be attempted when you are stressed or tired or overwhelmed. If you're feeling any of those things, turn to page 60 and make the Wild Wilted Greens instead.

To make gnocchi, you need to get into the ZONE. You need to be peaceful and equanimous and Zen. Then you will find great joy and much reward in fiddling with small pieces of green dough. It's the nettles that add the beautiful green colour, as well as the health benefits of extra protein and minerals.

Bring 2 cups (500 ml) water to the boil in a saucepan. Add the potatoes and boil for 15 minutes, until just cooked. Using a slotted spoon, remove the potatoes to a bowl, reserving the cooking water. Let the potatoes steam for 10 minutes, then mash well and set aside.

Prepare a large bowl of iced water, and return the potato water to the boil. Add the nettles and blanch for 30 seconds, then use tongs to transfer the nettles to the bowl of iced water to refresh them.

Purée the nettles using a stick blender, or a blender jug. Set a sieve over the bowl of mashed potato and push the nettle purée through with the back of a spoon, until only the fibre remains in the sieve. (The fibre can go into a green smoothie, or the compost.)

Mix the puréed nettles through the mashed potato until well combined. Add the flour and salt, and mix well until you have a sticky ball of dough. Wrap the dough in plastic wrap and leave to rest in the fridge for 30 minutes.

Dust a wooden board or smooth surface with extra flour. Slice the dough into quarters. Working in batches, roll each portion out into a long snake, then slice into pieces about 2 cm (¾ inch) long. If you like, you can roll the pieces down the back of a fork to give them lovely ridges. Gently toss the gnocchi in flour.

Bring a saucepan of salted water to the boil. Add one-quarter of the gnocchi and cook for a few minutes, until they float to the top. Remove using a slotted spoon and toss in a little olive oil to stop them sticking together. Repeat with the remaining gnocchi.

Heat a large frying pan over medium heat and add the olive oil. Fry the garlic for 30 seconds, making sure it doesn't burn. Add the gnocchi to the pan and fry, tossing occasionally, for a few minutes, until the gnocchi are starting to brown. Add the pepper, sea salt and chilli flakes and stir to coat.

Serve straight away, with toppings such as sautéed mushrooms, or your favourite parmesan or pasta sauce.

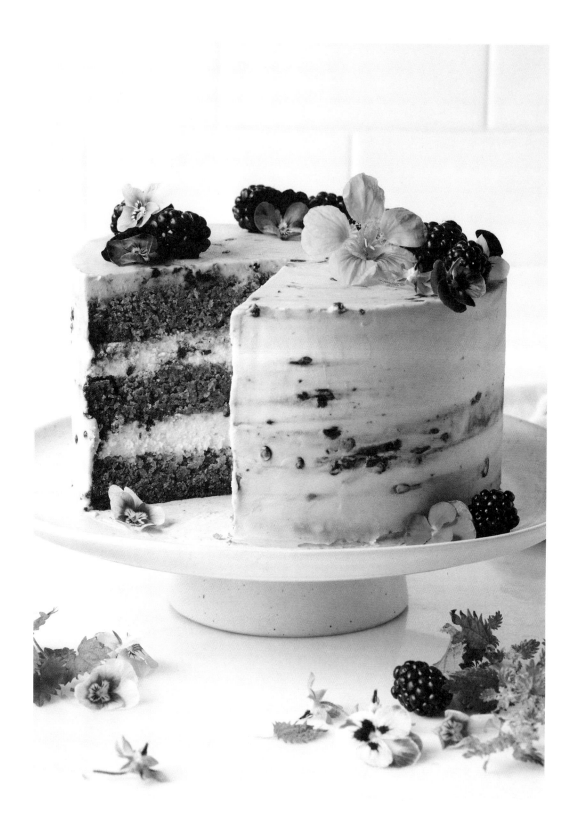

Nettle & blackberry forest cake

SERVES 8
2½ HOURS

'Must be the season of the witch' sang Donovan in 1966. This song comes to mind when creating this witchy, magical cake with nettles and blackberries from the heart of the forest. Light and fluffy, this vegan sponge is fun at any gathering and feels really nourishing, with the nettle in the batter adding extra protein, minerals and iron.

This recipe makes one cake with two layers. You can double all the ingredients to make a fancy four-layered cake, as we've done, except we've only shown three layers in the photo (and used the left-over cake for other goodies). You'll need to make the icing the day before.

LEMON & BLACKBERRY ICING

1 cup (155 g) raw cashews, soaked in cold water for 2 hours

½ cup (125 ml) maple syrup

½ cup (125 ml) lemon juice

1½ tablespoons lecithin

1 teaspoon pure vanilla extract

a pinch of salt

½ cup (80 g) coconut oil, melted

¼ cup (60 ml) blackberry juice or purée (made from squashed blackberries)

NETTLE CAKE

2 handfuls of fresh nettle leaves

1¼ cups (310 ml) rice bran oil

¾ cup (185 ml) orange juice

2 teaspoons pure vanilla extract

2 cups (300 g) plain (all-purpose) white spelt flour

1 cup (185 g) raw caster (superfine) sugar

2 teaspoons baking powder

1 teaspoon bicarbonate of soda (baking soda)

BLACKBERRY FILLING

2½ cups (325 g) fresh, fully ripe blackberries

½ cup (110 g) raw sugar

3 teaspoons lemon juice

TO GARNISH

fresh ripe blackberries

fresh edible leaves and flowers

To make the icing, put the cashews, maple syrup, lemon juice, lecithin, vanilla and salt in a blender and blend for 3 minutes. Add the melted coconut oil and blend for another 2 minutes. Tip into a shallow bowl, then cover and leave in the fridge overnight.

Preheat the oven to 180°C (350°F). Oil a 20 cm (8 inch) cake tin and line with baking paper. To make the cake, blanch the nettles in a pan of boiling water for 5 minutes, until soft and bright green. Drain and cool slightly, then purée using a stick blender, or in batches using a jug blender. Set a sieve over a bowl and push the purée through with the back of a spoon, to give you about ½ cup (125 ml) of nettle purée. Stir in the oil, orange juice and vanilla until combined.

Sift all the dry ingredients into a large bowl. Add the nettle purée. Using a figure-eight motion, fold gently to remove the lumps, but don't overmix; you want to keep in the air bubbles for a fluffy cake.

Pour the batter into your cake tin and bake for 40–45 minutes, until a skewer poked in the centre comes out clean. Remove from the oven and leave in the tin for 10 minutes, then turn out onto a wire rack to cool. Chill in the fridge for 30 minutes before icing and filling.

To make the filling, lightly mash the berries in a saucepan with a fork to release some juice. Add the sugar and lemon juice. Bring to the boil, then reduce the heat and simmer for 10–15 minutes (or a little longer if making a double batch), stirring so they don't stick. To check they're ready, dip a cold spoon into the mixture, wait a few seconds, then wipe your finger across the spoon. Your finger should leave a clean streak across the spoon. Cool completely before using.

To assemble the cake, mix the icing using an electric hand mixer or stand mixer. Add the blackberry juice, teaspoon by teaspoon, for a softer consistency and a lovely colour; you may not need it all. The icing should be spreadable, but still hold its shape in peaks and waves, and shouldn't fall out of the bowl when tipped upside down.

Using a long sharp knife, cut the cake in half horizontally. Spread a 1 cm (½ inch) thick icing layer over the bottom cake half, then the blackberry filling. Top with the other cake half, spread the remaining icing over the top and garnish as desired.

Nettle tea

MAKES 4 CUPS (1 LITRE)
10 MINUTES

GF

Nettle tea has a long history of use around the world — mainly for sinus problems and seasonal allergies, difficult urination, inflammation and joint pain associated with arthritis, muscle spasms and high blood sugar. It has high concentrations of protein, and minerals, including iron, calcium, magnesium, potassium and zinc, as well as vitamin K. It is beneficial for strengthening hair, skin and nails. The simplest way to use nettles is to make them into a tea.

a large handful of fresh nettle leaves, or 4 tablespoons (25 g) dried nettles

sweetener to taste (optional)

In a saucepan, bring 4 cups (1 litre) water to the boil, then turn the heat off.

Add the nettles and allow the tea to brew for 5–10 minutes before drinking.

If you like a sweet tea, stir in your favourite sweetener.

Nettle tea blends

AMOUNTS PER 4 CUPS
(1 LITRE) OF WATER

CAUTIONS + CONTRAINDICATIONS

Salix alba contains natural aspirin, so people with sensitivity to aspirin, bleeding disorders, surgery coming up in 2 weeks or less, and pregnant women are advised not to use this arthritis herb blend. Also not recommended for children.

FOR STRONGER HAIR, SKIN AND NAILS

Nettle leaf (*Urtica dioica*) – 4 tablespoons dried leaf
Horsetail leaf (*Equisetum arvense*) – 4 tablespoons dried leaf
Comfrey leaf (*Symphytum officinale*) – 2 tablespoons dried leaf

FOR ARTHRITIS

Nettle leaf (*U. dioica*) – 4 tablespoons dried leaf
White willow bark (*Salix alba*) – 4 teaspoons dried bark
Turmeric root (*Curcuma longa*) – 1 thumb-sized piece of freshly grated turmeric, or 4 teaspoons ground turmeric
Frankincense resin (*Boswellia carteri*) – 4 teaspoons

FOR ALLERGIES

Nettle leaf (*U. dioica*) – 4 tablespoons dried leaf
Elder flowers (*Sambucus nigra*) – 4 tablespoons dried
Blue top (*Ageratum conyzoides*) – 4 tablespoons dried

FOR ENLARGED PROSTATE

Nettle leaf (*U. dioica*) – 4 tablespoons dried leaf
Saw palmetto berries (*Serenoa repens*) – 2 tablespoons dried

FOR BLOOD SUGAR REGULATION

Nettle leaf (*U. dioica*) – 4 tablespoons dried leaf
Fenugreek (*Trigonella foenum-graecum*) – 2 tablespoons seeds

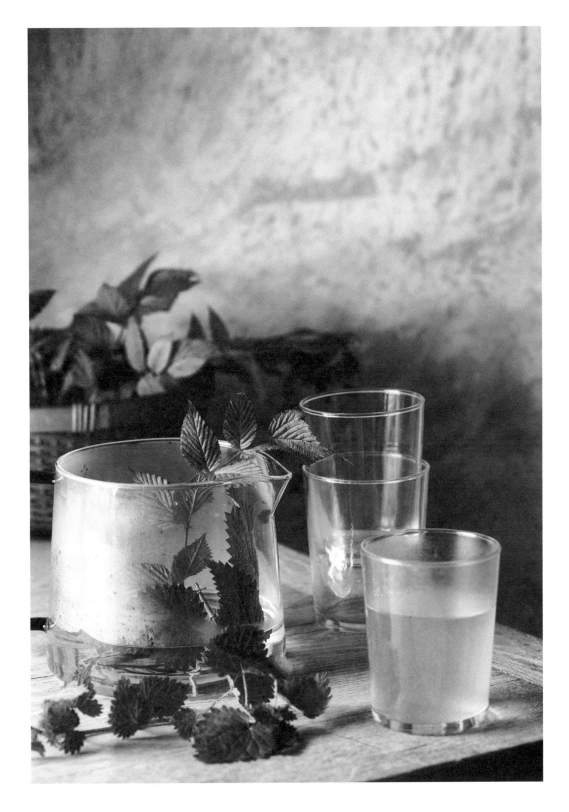

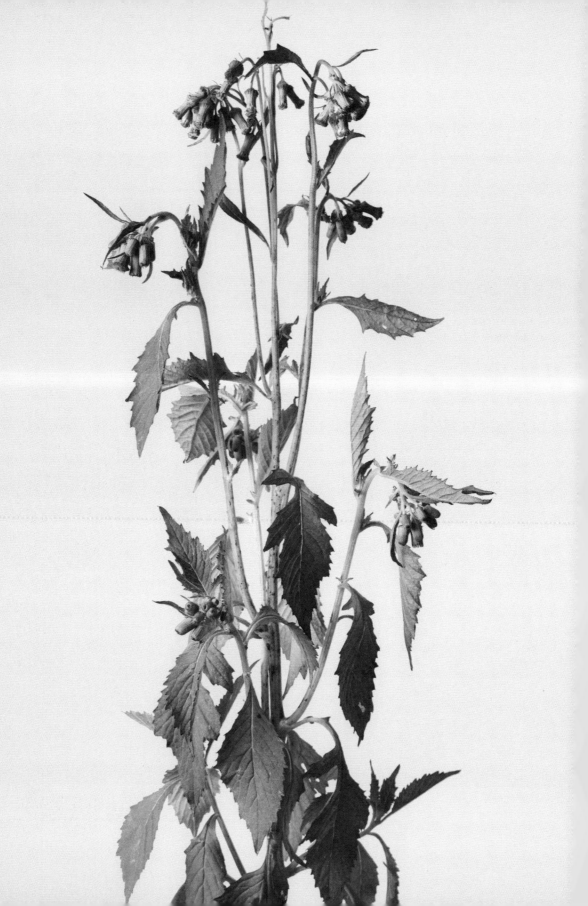

Nodding top

COMMON NAMES:

nodding top, thickhead

SPECIES:

Crassocephalum crepidioides

GENUS:

Crassocephalum

FAMILY:

Asteraceae

DISTRIBUTION:

Possibly originated in Africa. Naturalised throughout tropical and subtropical Asia, Australia, the Oceanic islands and the Americas.

PLANT SPIRIT QUALITIES:

Nodding top helps us to accept things as they are. In the body it is protective against toxins in the liver; in our lives it protects us from the toxic emotions of resistance, anger and frustration that cause us so much pain and suffering. When we surrender to what is and 'go with the flow', we can overcome obstacles and transform painful situations with ease and grace, rather than having to fight against them. **Key words — acceptance, surrender, going with the flow.**

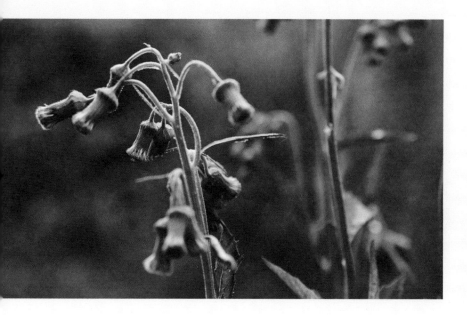

How to identify it

- Recognised by clusters of pinkish/orange flowers (cymes), which initially droop down in clusters of four or more before becoming erect.
- Seed heads (achenes) develop white, fluffy thistledown (pappus) that is tinged reddish or mauve.
- Leaves are elliptic to ovate in shape, with coarsely toothed margins.
- Upper leaves are smaller, not lobed, or with a lobe each side towards the base.
- Nodding top has the distinctive smell and taste of carrots.

How to harvest

Nodding top grows from spring through to autumn, and in some places all year. It prefers a warm tropical climate and does especially well during the wet season.

Leaves, stems and flowers can all be used as food and medicine.

Leaves
Harvest leaves near the bottom so that the plant can keep growing. You can gently pick them off with your fingers, or snip stems with leaves with a pair of scissors.

Flowers
Flowers can be harvested along with the leaves and stems by picking them off with your fingers or snipping with scissors.

Seeds
Seeds can be collected for regrowing by pulling the fluffy heads off the plants and putting them in a paper bag.

Nutrients

Amino acids (especially tyrosine), calcium, magnesium, potassium, iron and vitamin C.

Culinary use

The leaves have a carrot-like taste and are quite pleasant eaten raw in salads or lightly cooked. Young plants are a common food in Japan, especially in the Okinawa Islands, where the population is renowned for its health and longevity, and where it is known as 'Okinawan spinach'.

It is used as a vegetable in soups and stews, especially in West and Central Africa. In south-western Nigeria, the leaves are lightly blanched, then cooked with peppers, onions, tomatoes, melon and sometimes fish or meat, to make soups and stews. In Sierra Leone, the leaves are popular and are made into a sauce with groundnut paste.

In Australia, it is eaten as a salad green, either cooked or raw.

In Thailand, the roots are eaten with chilli sauce.

Folk medicine

In Africa, the leaf sap is given to soothe indigestion and an upset stomach, and a leaf infusion is used for headaches. The leaf sap is also combined with *Cymbopogon giganteus* and used orally and externally to treat epilepsy. Applied externally, the leaf sap is also used on fresh wounds. The dried leaf powder is applied as a snuff to stop nose bleeding, and smoked to treat sleeping sickness. Tannin found in the roots of the plant is used to treat swollen lips.

In China, decoctions of the whole plant are used internally for colds, fevers, dysentery, gastroenteritis and urinary tract infections. Externally it is used for mastitis.

Research

Clinical trials have confirmed its use in the following areas: antioxidant,[1] liver protective,[2] neuroprotective,[3] anticoagulant,[4] antidiabetic[5] and wound healing.[6]

How to use it as a medicine

Mainly it is eaten as a food, but medicinally it can be used as a maceration to extract the sap, as an infusion (leaves) or decoction (roots), as a tincture, or as a powder that is eaten, snuffed or smoked.

CAUTIONS + CONTRAINDICATIONS
Due to the presence of pyrrolizidine alkaloids, *Crassocephalum crepidioides* should not be used by those with liver disease or by pregnant women. Discontinue use 2 weeks before surgery due to anticoagulant effects.

Nodding top can also be used in:
- Wild weed pesto
- Wild wilted greens
- Wild greens powder

Nodding top chimichurri

MAKES ABOUT 2 CUPS (500 G)

20 MINUTES

GF

1 handful of fresh nodding top leaves
¼ cup coriander (cilantro)
¼ cup fresh oregano
1 small handful of flat-leaf parsley
1 shallot
1 fresh red chilli
3 garlic cloves, crushed
½ cup (125 ml) red wine vinegar or lemon juice
1 cup (250 ml) olive oil
1 teaspoon salt

This addictive chimichurri sauce is based on the Argentinian classic, but uses the delicious carroty taste of nodding tops, along with oregano, coriander and parsley. You can add it to just about anything. Use it on tacos, pizza, roast vegetables, sautéed mushrooms or fresh crusty bread ... or anything else your heart desires.

This is a great sauce for detoxification because the nodding top can be protective and healing for the liver, the coriander can help draw out heavy metals, the parsley may help improve detoxification via the kidneys, and the garlic and chilli can help kill off parasites and improve circulation.

Very finely chop all the herbs and put them in a bowl or jar.

Finely chop the shallot and chilli, removing the chilli seeds if you prefer a milder heat. (Remember to wash your hands after chopping chilli, so it doesn't end up in your eyes or on your face!)

Stir the shallot and chilli through the herbs with the remaining ingredients. Cover and leave to sit at room temperature for 30 minutes or more, to let the flavours infuse.

The chimichurri will keep for up to 2 weeks in an airtight container in the fridge.

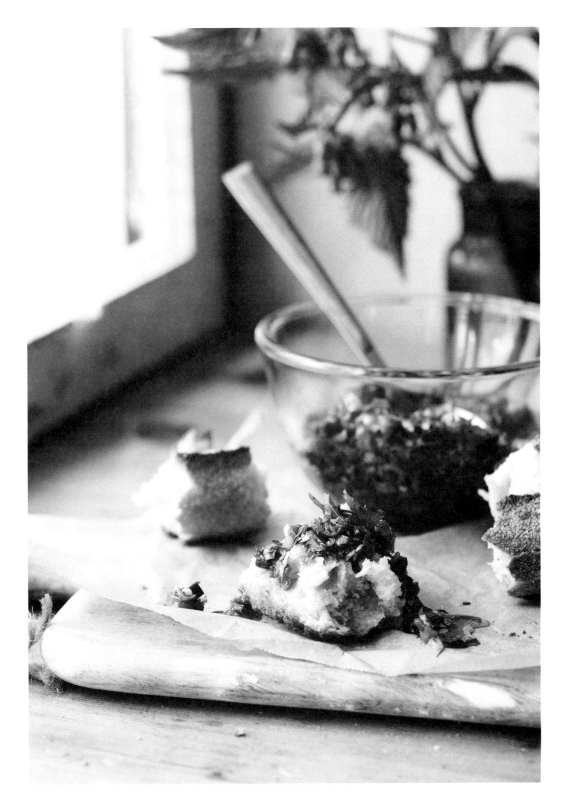

Maple roast carrots with nodding top sauce

Sweet carrots with a tangy nodding top sauce deliver a real carroty punch. It's a simple way to boost your use of wild greens and get all the liver protective benefits of the nodding tops, as well as the beta-carotene from the carrots, which is beneficial for the eyes, skin and immune system. But at the end of the day, health benefits aside, it's just plain yummy!

SERVES 2–4
40 MINUTES

10–15 baby carrots, green tops trimmed

2 tablespoons maple syrup

2 tablespoons olive oil

¼ teaspoon salt

NODDING TOP SAUCE

1 handful of fresh nodding top leaves and stems

juice of ½ lemon

2 tablespoons maple syrup

2 tablespoons hulled tahini

¼ teaspoon salt

¼ cup (60 ml) hot water

Preheat the oven to 200°C (400°F).

Spread the carrots on a baking tray. Drizzle the maple syrup and olive oil over the carrots and sprinkle with the salt.

Bake for 30–40 minutes, or until soft and tender, turning the carrots every 10–15 minutes so they brown evenly.

To make the sauce, wash the nodding tops and place in a blender. Add the other ingredients and blend for 2 minutes, stopping to scrape down the sides, until you have a nice smooth green sauce. (You might find it easier to put it all in a jug and blend with a stick blender.) Taste and adjust any flavours as needed.

Spoon the sauce over the maple carrots before serving, or serve on the side.

Liver tonic powder

Nodding top is a potent antioxidant. In conjunction with your medical practitioner's advice, this liver tonic blend may be helpful for anyone with liver conditions. As the liver also plays a role in weight loss, this tonic can be beneficial for people who are trying to lose weight. It can be added to juices or smoothies on a regular basis to help maintain liver health.

MAKES 25 SERVES;
ABOUT 40 G (1½ OZ)
10 MINUTES

10 g (¼ oz) dried nodding top leaves

15 g (½ oz) dried dandelion root

15 g (½ oz) St Mary's thistle seeds

Grind all the ingredients to a fine powder using a coffee grinder.

Transfer the powder to a glass jar and cap tightly. It will keep in a cool, dark cupboard for up to 12 months.

HOW TO USE THE POWDER

Add 1 teaspoon daily to juices and smoothies, or simply mix with ¼ cup (60 ml) water and drink on its own.

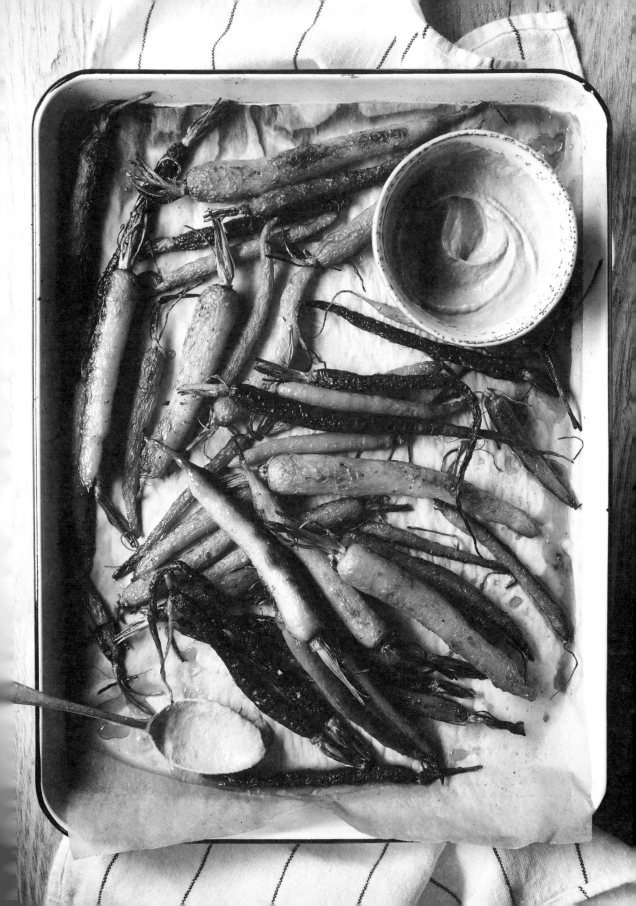

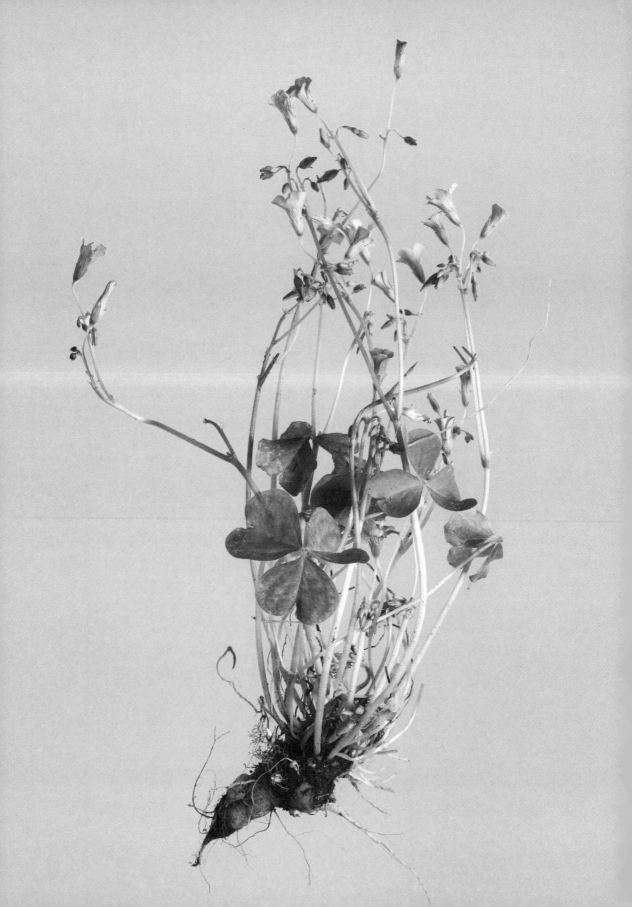

Oxalis

COMMON NAMES:

oxalis, wood sorrel

SPECIES:

There are about 570 *Oxalis* species. *Oxalis pes-caprae* and *Oxalis corniculata* (creeping wood sorrel) are common in Australia and have a yellow flower. The pink-flowering *Oxalis debilis* is also common.

GENUS:

Oxalis

FAMILY:

Oxalidaceae

DISTRIBUTION:

Originated in South Africa, South America and tropical America. The genus occurs throughout most of the world, except for the polar areas; species diversity is particularly rich in tropical Brazil, Mexico and South Africa.

PLANT SPIRIT QUALITIES:

Oxalis brings fun and joy. If you have become overly sour, stuffy or serious, oxalis will lift your spirits and help you let go and be silly, fun and playful. Children naturally love oxalis and will often find it in the garden and include it in their games and 'potions'. Oxalis helps you connect with your inner child. Use oxalis if you are healing your inner child from an unhappy childhood, or if you just need to feel more joy and fun in your life. It can also be used for children who have had too much screen time and have forgotten how to play.
Key words — fun, joy.

How to identify it

- The leaves are divided into 3–10 (or more) heart-shaped and top-notched leaflets, arranged in a palmate fashion, with all the leaflets of roughly equal size.

- Most species have three leaflets. In these species, the leaves are similar to those of some clovers. However, clover is not heart-shaped and has a white V-shaped marking on it.

- Some species exhibit rapid changes in leaf angle in response to temporary high light intensity, closing up in bright light.

- The flowers have five petals, which are usually fused at the base, and 10 stamens. The petal colour varies from white to pink, red or yellow.

- The fruit is a small capsule containing several seeds.

- The roots are often tuberous and succulent.

- The leaves and stems have a deliciously sour taste.

How to harvest

Leaves
Oxalis grows from spring to autumn, depending on the climate, and in temperate areas can grow year round. You can harvest by snipping leaves and flowers near the base with a pair of scissors so as not to disturb the roots. The whole plant is edible, but mainly the leaves, stems and flowers are used.

Flowers
Flowers can be cut at the base of the stem with scissors, as the stem and the flower can be eaten.

Nutrients

Other than being rich in vitamin C, there is limited nutritional information on this plant.

Culinary use

This delicious tart herb is great raw in salads, and can be cooked and eaten as a green vegetable. The dried leaves of common wood sorrel (*Oxalis acetosella*) may be used to make a lemony-tasting tea. The Potawatomi Native Americans cooked it with sugar to enjoy as a dessert. In India, creeping wood sorrel (*O. corniculata*) is eaten seasonally, starting in December or January.

Folk medicine

The Kiowa Native American tribe chewed wood sorrel to alleviate thirst on long trips. The Algonquian people considered it an aphrodisiac. The Cherokee ate wood sorrel to relieve mouth sores and a sore throat, while the Iroquois ate wood sorrel to help with cramps, fever and nausea.

To avoid scurvy, sailors travelling around Patagonia ate the leaves of scurvy-grass sorrel (*O. enneaphylla*) as a source of vitamin C.

The Russians make an infusion for fevers and catarrh. Around the world, it was traditionally used as a blood cleanser, for weak stomachs, to stimulate appetite, stop vomiting and remove abdominal obstructions. A juice is made as a gargle for ulcers in the mouth, to heal wounds and stop bleeding. Cloths soaked in the juice are used to reduce swelling and inflammation.

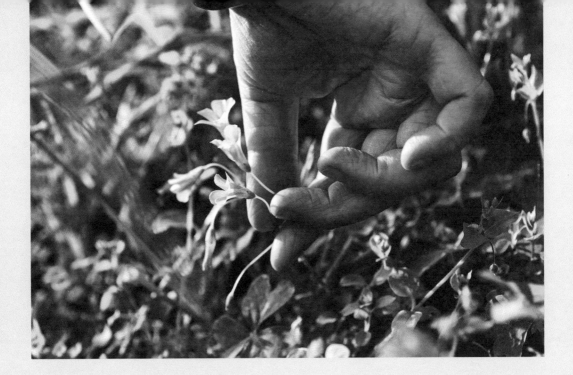

Research

Clinical trials have confirmed the use of *Oxalis corniculata* in the following areas: antioxidant,[1] antibacterial, antifungal and insecticidal.[2]

The use of *Oxalis pes-caprae* has been studied in the following areas: antioxidant and neuroprotective,[3] antibacterial[4] and antioxidant.[5]

How to use it as a medicine

It is used as a powder, an infusion, a juice, or externally as a poultice.

CAUTIONS + CONTRAINDICATIONS

People with gout, rheumatism, arthritis, hyperacidity and kidney stones should use this plant with caution due to its high oxalic acid content. Cooking or eating it with high-calcium foods, such as tahini, can reduce this issue, but caution is recommended.

Oxalis can also be used in:
- Oxalis glycetract

Oxalis lemonade

This wonderful beverage is really refreshing on hot days, and can also be made into icy poles. It's a nice gentle antibacterial drink that can help support the immune system and may be helpful with inflammation.

MAKES 2 CUPS (500 ML)
10 MINUTES

GF

1 handful of fresh oxalis leaves, stems and flowers

1 tablespoon maple syrup

2 cups (500 ml) chilled mineral water

Juice the oxalis, to give you ¼ cup (60 ml) juice. Stir in the maple syrup to make a green cordial. The cordial tastes best when used straight away, but you can make a bigger batch to store in the fridge, where it will last for up to 3 days. Due to its high oxalate content, it is best used for short periods (3–5 days at a time) then have a break for a week or more.

To use the cordial, pour into glasses and top up with the mineral water. Serve cold, garnished with a slice of fresh lemon and an oxalis flower if desired.

Oxalis & lime tarts

These tarts make a lovely party food, or a simple dessert for a dinner party. You need to use raw oxalis in the filling, to keep it deliciously tangy, as the flavour changes when cooked. Because the tart shells are chilled rather than baked, they can go soft and soggy if left out on hot days, so don't take them on summer picnics. You can also use gingernut biscuits as another base option.

Serve fresh from the fridge, garnished with fresh or dried citrus slices, berries and edible flowers.

MAKES 6 TARTS

3 HOURS SOAKING +
30 MINUTES

BISCUIT BASE

160 g (5½ oz) toasted granola

2 tablespoons coconut oil, or a stick of hard vegan butter, melted

2 teaspoons ground ginger

TART FILLING

1 cup (155 g) raw cashews, soaked in water for 3–12 hours

1 cup fresh oxalis (leaves, flowers and stems), finely chopped

juice and zest of 2 limes

½ cup (125 ml) almond milk

½ cup (125 ml) maple syrup

¼ cup (50 g) coconut oil

1 tablespoon lecithin

Put the biscuit base ingredients in a food processor and blitz for 2 minutes, or until the mixture holds together when pressed. (If using unsweetened granola, add an extra tablespoon of maple syrup.)

Line a 6-hole muffin tin with paper cases. Add 2 tablespoons of the biscuit mixture to each paper case and press it down firmly with your fingers to create a tart base.

Chill the bases in the fridge while making the filling.

Using a jug blender, or a stick blender in a jug, blend together all the filling ingredients. You need to blend for quite a while to get a smooth mixture, so keep blending for at least 5 minutes.

Pour the filling into the tart shells, then refrigerate for at least 1 hour to allow the filling to thicken. Just before serving, garnish as desired.

The tarts will keep in the fridge in an airtight container for 3–5 days.

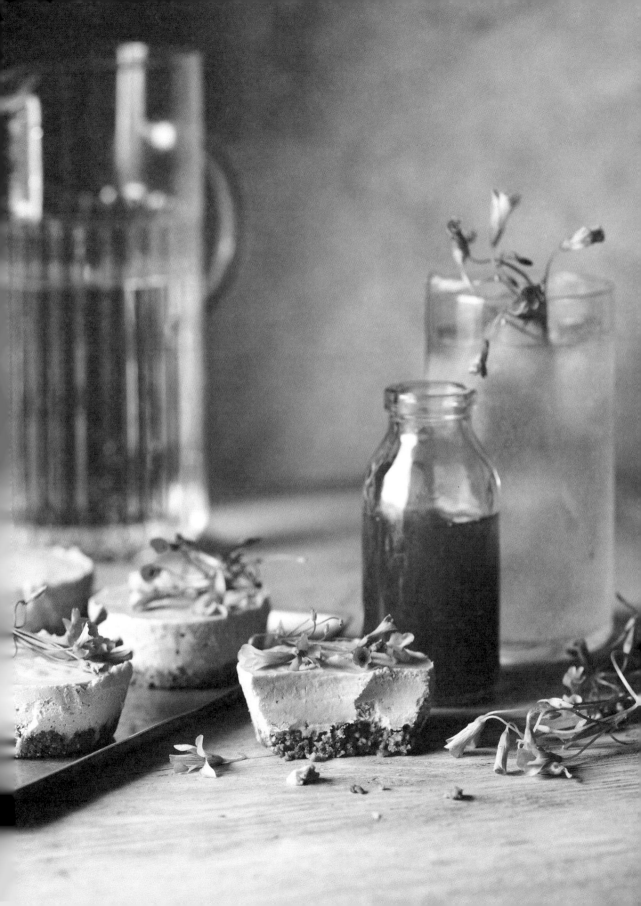

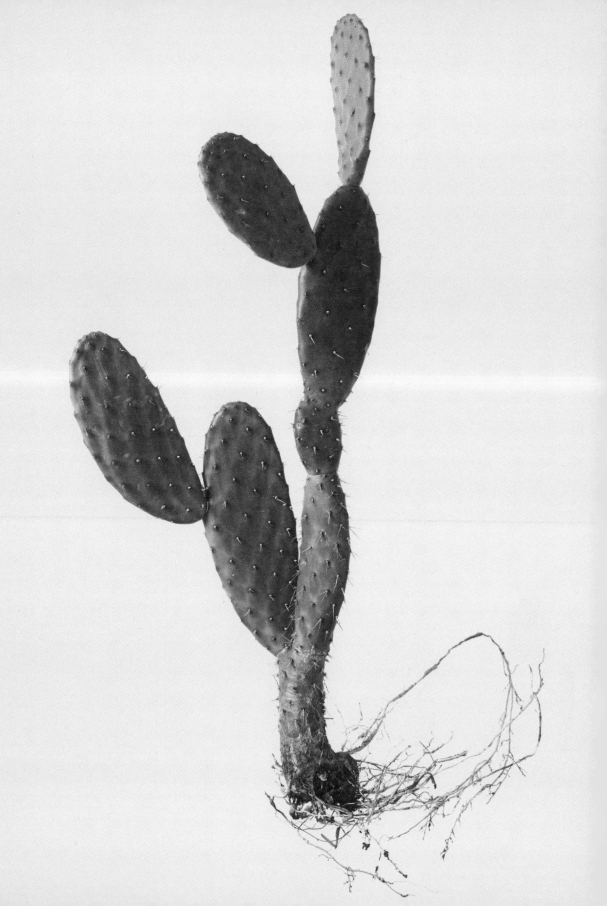

Prickly pear

COMMON NAMES:

prickly pear

SPECIES:

Opuntia stricta; may be confused with the taller, orange-flowered *Opuntia ficus-indica*, commonly called prickly pear or Indian fig.

GENUS:

Opuntia

FAMILY:

Cactaceae

DISTRIBUTION:

Thought to have originated in Mexico. Naturalised in Australia, southern Europe, Africa and southern Asia.

PLANT SPIRIT QUALITIES:

Prickly pear is good for people who like too much of a good thing, to the point where it becomes self-destructive. Parties, sex, sugar, Netflix ... in moderation, all these things provide joy and pleasure in life, but when used to excess they become destructive and addictive. If we are overindulging, binge eating or struggling with addictions, prickly pear helps us balance the impulse for work and play, fun and seriousness. The plant has prickles and a tough outer skin, but inside it has cool, soothing gel. It knows when to be tough and make a point, and when to soothe and cool down. **Key word — balance.**

How to identify it

- Prickly pear is an upright succulent cactus that grows 0.5–2 metres (1½–6½ feet) tall.
- This cactus plant has a distinctive series of flattened, succulent, oval-shaped pads, which grow to 10–35 cm (4–14 inches) long, 7–20 cm (2¾–8 inches) wide, and 1–2 cm (½–¾ inch) thick.
- The oval-shaped prickly pear pads (also called 'cladodes' or 'nopales') are green or bluish-green in colour. These are the parts that are peeled and eaten, along with the pinkish-purple fruits.
- The pads themselves are hairless, but feature small, raised circular structures (known as 'areoles'), which may each have one or two sharp spines about 2–4 cm (¾–1½ inches) long.
- The leaves are tiny cylindrical or cone-shaped structures, 4.5–6 mm (¼ inch) long, and are quickly shed from the developing stems.
- The flowers are bright yellow, but often have pinkish or reddish markings on the outer petals. They are borne singly on fleshy bases along the margins of the stems.
- The immature fruit is green, turning reddish-purple when mature.
- The succulent egg-shaped fruit is 4–8 cm (1½–3¼ inches) long and 2.5–4 cm (1–1½ inches) wide, with depressions on the ends.
- The reddish or purplish pulp in the centre of the fruit contains a large number of seeds. The seeds are 4–5 mm (¼ inch) long and 4–5 mm (¼ inch) wide, and are generally yellow or pale brown.
- The plant has shallow and horizontally spread roots.

How to harvest

Prickly pear grows year round in hot, dry and arid regions, and will produce fruit and new pads in summer.

Prickly pear pads

Harvest early in the growing season (spring), when new pads appear on the plant. The older pads have hard fibres that are unpleasant (kind of like fish bones).

To harvest the pads, wear a thick pair of gloves. Using a sharp knife, cut the pads off at the base and drop them into a bucket. Look for nice plump green pads without black, brown or white spots on them.

When you are ready to use the pads, run a very sharp knife over the front and back of the pads, and all around the edge, to completely remove all the spines. Wash the gel pads to remove any spikes that have stuck to them.

Prickly pear fruit

Wear thick gloves! Look for ripe, bright red to dark pink or purple fruit; there is also a pale green variety. Twist the fruit at the base to remove, then cut with a sharp knife into a bucket.

To remove the spikes, you can use a pair of tongs to hold the fruit over a flame to burn them off, or rub away the spikes with a stiff-bristled brush.

To use, cut off the top and bottom of each fruit using a sharp knife. Cut an incision down one side of the fruit, from top to bottom, then peel back the skin. It usually peels off easily.

The fruit can be eaten raw as is, but it is full of seeds, so you might want to push it through a sieve if using in a smoothie. If eating fresh, just spit out the seeds.

Nutrients

Sugars, fibre and vitamins A, C and E.

Culinary use

Opuntia species are a health-promoting food eaten around the world. Their sweet, edible fruits can be eaten raw or made into jams and other desserts. The young prickly pear pads are peeled and eaten as a vegetable in salads, or cooked like okra.

Folk medicine

Opuntia species have been used in traditional medicine for centuries in the management of diseases that involve oxidative stress, especially diabetes, obesity, rheumatism, asthma, high cholesterol and hypertension.

Research

Clinical trials have confirmed its use in the following areas: reduces high cholesterol and blood lipids,[1] lowers blood pressure,[2] weight loss,[3] antioxidant and anti-inflammatory,[4] scar reduction[5] and antibiotic.[6]

How to use it as a medicine

The pads and fruit are mainly consumed as a food, and medicinal effects are obtained through the diet. The inner gel can be used as a poultice.

CAUTIONS + CONTRAINDICATIONS
Caution is needed to avoid being stung by the prickles, which are painful and irritating.

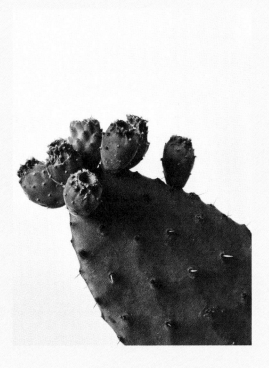

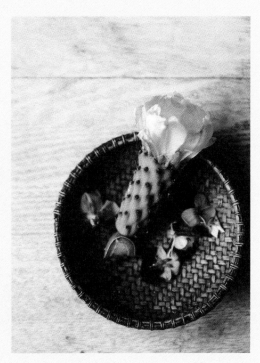

Prickly pear with tomato, onion & chilli

This traditional Mexican dish is a simple way to enjoy the health benefits of prickly pear. This is one food that can assist with weight management, so eat as much as you want! Both traditional use and current research have shown prickly pear to be helpful in reducing high cholesterol and blood lipids, lowering blood pressure and assisting with weight loss. It is also antioxidant and anti-inflammatory.

SERVES 4
45 MINUTES

GF

2 young fresh prickly pear pads

2 teaspoons salt

2 tablespoons olive oil

2 onions, finely chopped

3 garlic cloves, finely chopped

2 tomatoes, finely chopped

2 tablespoons tomato paste (concentrated purée)

1 fresh chilli, finely chopped

Harvest the prickly pear pads as per the instructions on page 258. Be sure to pick only young pads, as the older ones have hard, inedible fibres.

Cut the skin off the edges and remove the spikes by running a very sharp knife over the front and back. (If your pads are very young and fresh, you won't need to peel them.) Cut the pads into 1 cm (½ inch) cubes.

Pour 2 cups (500 ml) water into a saucepan, add the salt and bring to the boil. Add the prickly pear and simmer over medium heat for 10 minutes. The prickly pear will change colour from bright green to olive green.

Heat the olive oil in a frying pan or skillet over medium–high heat. Add the prickly pear, onion, garlic, tomatoes, tomato paste and chilli. Fry for 20–30 minutes, stirring now and then, until the slipperiness has cooked out of the prickly pear.

Remove from the heat and season with salt and pepper to taste.

You can use this dish as a filling in wraps, tacos or burritos, or as a side dish topped with guacamole, coriander (cilantro) sprigs and lime wedges. It will keep in the fridge in an airtight container for 3–5 days.

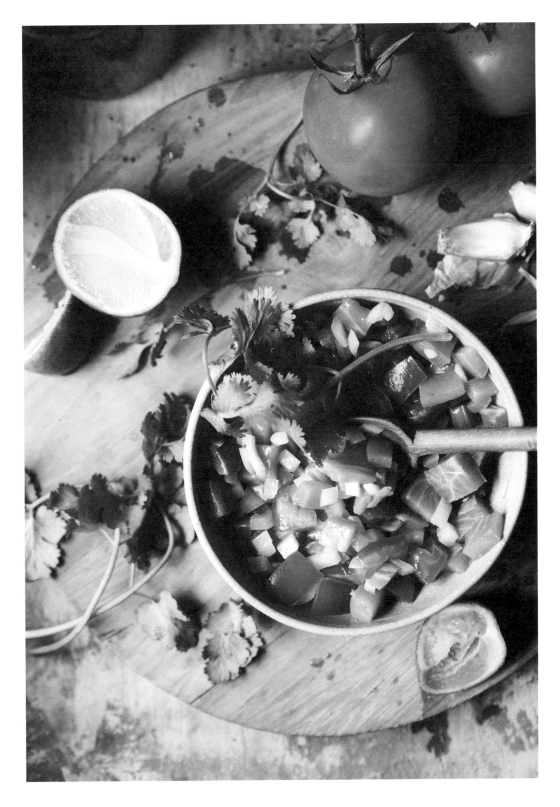

Prickly pear smoothie

Both the fruit and the pads can be used in this smoothie, which is great as part of a cleanse or detox. It is nutritious, stabilises blood sugar, has a low glycaemic index and is very low in calories, thereby assisting in weight management while still tasting delicious.

SERVES 2; MAKES 2 CUPS
10 MINUTES

GF

1 young fresh prickly pear pad

3–6 fresh prickly pear fruits

1 cup (125 g) frozen raspberries

¼ grapefruit, skin and seeds removed

ice cubes (optional)

Harvest the prickly pear pad as per the instructions on page 258. Be sure to pick only a young pad, as older ones have hard, inedible fibres. Cut the skin off the edges and remove the spikes by running a very sharp knife over the front and back. (If your pads are very young and fresh, you won't need to peel them.) Cut the pads into 4 cm (1½ inch) cubes and place in a blender.

Peel the prickly pear fruits as per the instructions on page 258. Add to the blender with the raspberries, grapefruit, ½ cup (125 ml) water, and a handful of ice cubes if you'd like your smoothie cold. Blend on high speed for 30–60 seconds.

Drink straight away, or soon after blending.

Prickly pear jam

When you come across a big crop of prickly pear fruit, this jam is one way to preserve some of it to enjoy throughout the year. It goes well with grain bread or your favourite sourdough for a delicious wild food breakfast or snack. It can also be added to muesli, porridge, smoothies and yoghurt. You can adjust the quantities, depending on how bountiful your prickly pear harvest is.

MAKES ½–¾ CUP
20 MINUTES

GF

12 fresh prickly pear fruits

2 tablespoons raw sugar

1 teaspoon lemon juice

Remove the skin from the prickly pear fruits as per the instructions on page 258. Set a sieve over a saucepan and squish the fruit through the sieve to remove the seeds. You'll want 1 cup of pulp.

Add the sugar and lemon juice to the pan. Bring to the boil, then reduce the heat and simmer for 10–15 minutes (the more fruit you're using, the longer it will take), stirring so the jam doesn't stick.

To check it's ready, dip a cold spoon into the mixture, cool for 10 seconds, then wipe your finger across the spoon. When your finger leaves a smooth clear streak across the spoon, the jam is ready.

Pour into a sterilised glass jar (see page 23) and seal with the lid. The jam will keep in the cupboard for 12 months or longer. Once opened, store in the fridge and use within 3–6 months.

Prickly pear chia pudding

SERVES 1–2
30 MINUTES

GF

12 fresh prickly pear fruits

¼ cup (20 g) chia seeds

1 tablespoon sugar or maple syrup

1 teaspoon lemon juice

This pudding has the health benefits of prickly pear and the protein, essential fatty acids and fibre of chia seeds to make an all-round nutritious meal. The colour is beautiful and feels tropical and decadent. It's a lovely breakfast served with fresh fruit.

Remove the skin from the prickly pear fruits as per the instructions on page 252. Set a sieve over a saucepan and squish the fruit through the sieve to remove the seeds.

Add the chia seeds and sugar and cook over medium heat for 5 minutes, stirring until the chia seeds start to thicken. Remove from the heat and stir in the lemon juice.

Pour into a bowl to cool, then refrigerate for 20 minutes, or until ready to serve. (The pudding will continue to thicken in the fridge, and will keep for 5–7 days in an airtight container.)

Serve with your favourite yoghurt and toppings.

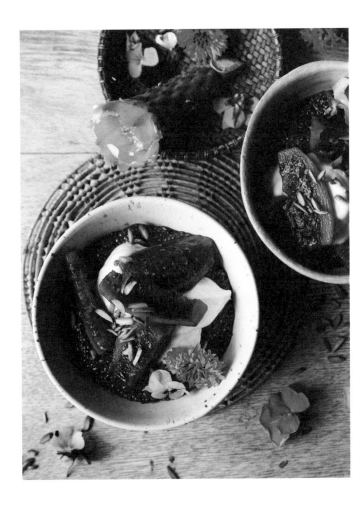

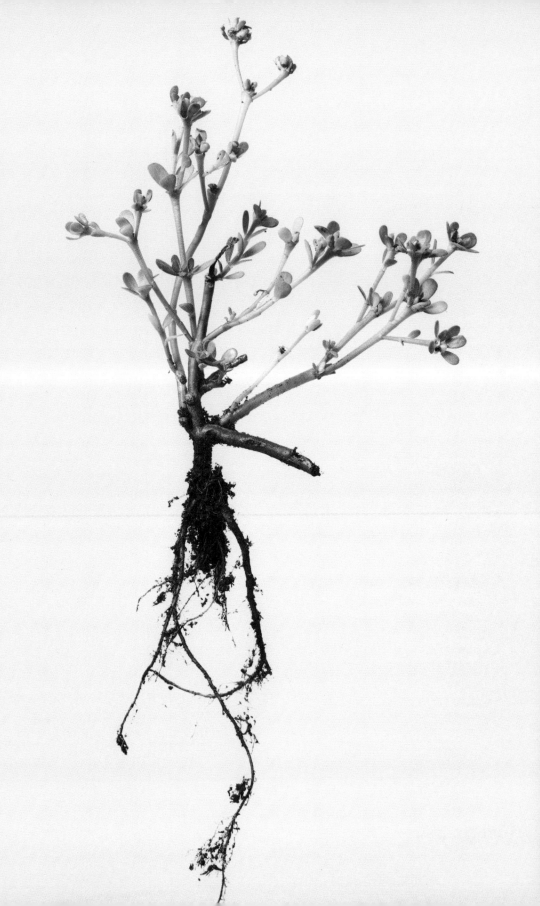

Purslane

COMMON NAMES:

purslane

SPECIES:

Portulaca oleracea

GENUS:

Portulaca

FAMILY:

Portulacaceae

DISTRIBUTION:

Origins are uncertain. Distributed throughout North Africa, the Americas and southern Europe, through the Middle East and the Indian subcontinent to Malaysia and Australasia.

PLANT SPIRIT QUALITIES:

Purslane is good for the brain, due to its high essential fatty acid content. Energetically, it also has an affinity for the brain, helping you to feel inspired by new ideas, places and adventures. (You often find purslane stretching across pathways, as though off on its own little adventure!) A good remedy for students, creatives and wannabe adventurers, and when life feels dull, as it helps you feel excited about new horizons. It fills your heart with curiosity, inspires your imagination and gives you courage for new adventures. **Key words — curiosity, knowledge, adventure, travel.**

How to identify it

- Purslane is a succulent groundcover with smooth, reddish, mostly prostrate stems.
- Its succulent green leaves may be alternate or opposite, and are clustered at the stem joints and ends.
- It has small yellow flowers, which have five regular parts and are up to 6 mm (¼ inch) wide. Depending upon rainfall, the flowers appear at any time during the year. The flowers open singly at the centre of the leaf cluster for only a few hours on sunny mornings.
- Seeds are formed in a tiny pod, opening when mature.
- Purslane has a taproot with fibrous secondary roots.

How to harvest

Purslane is an annual that grows from spring to autumn, and in temperate climates can grow all year. It is very easy to harvest as it pulls out with little effort. In order to not pull up the roots accidentally, you may want to harvest with scissors, or else gently pull up sections only, leaving enough for the patch to regenerate. The whole plant — but mainly leaves, stems and flowers — can all be eaten and used medicinally.

Nutrients

Rich in alpha-linolenic acid (ALA), omega-3 essential fatty acid (one of the highest plant sources), antioxidants, vitamin A (in some cases it has up to seven times more beta-carotene than carrots), vitamins C and E (alpha-tocopherol), iron, calcium, potassium and magnesium.

Culinary use

Purslane is a common food source around the world. The succulent leaves and young shoots are pleasantly cooling in spring salads. The older shoots are used as a cooked vegetable, and the thick stems of plants that have run to seed can be pickled in salt and vinegar to add to winter salads.

Folk medicine

Portulaca oleracea has been used around the world in the treatment of burns, headache and diseases related to the intestines, liver and stomach. It has also been used for coughs, shortness of breath, as a purgative, cardiac tonic, emollient and muscle relaxant.

As an anti-inflammatory, it has been used in arthritis, osteoporosis and psoriasis.

The World Health Organization lists it as one of the most used medicinal plants, and has described it as a 'global panacea'.

Chinese folklore considers it a vegetable for long life, and it has been used for thousands of years in traditional Chinese medicine, where its cold nature and sour taste are said to 'cool' the blood, reduce bleeding, and clear heat and toxins. It is indicated for the treatment of fever, dysentery, diarrhoea, carbuncles and eczema.

Research

Clinical trials have confirmed its use in the following areas: skin and wound healing,[1] antioxidant and anti-inflammatory,[2] ulcers,[3] ulcerative colitis,[4] inflammatory bowel disease,[5] insomnia,[6] diabetes,[7] metabolic syndrome,[8] asthma,[9] allergies,[10] neuroprotective,[11] liver protective[12] and antimicrobial.[13]

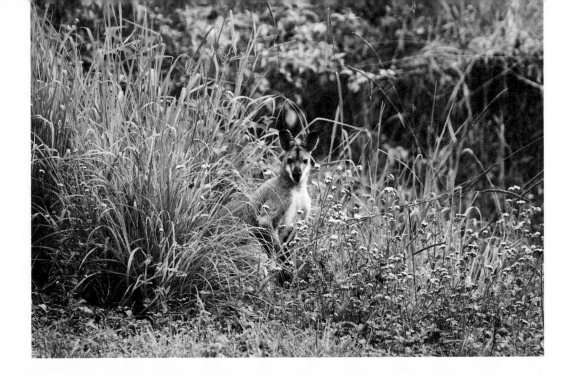

How to use it as a medicine

In traditional Chinese medicine it is used as a dried powder, with a recommended dose of 9–15 g (¼ –½ oz) of the dried aerial part. *P. oleracea* can be made into a macerate, a poultice or an infusion.

People with 'cold' underactive stomachs may like to use it heated and with warming spices such as ginger and cinnamon.

CAUTIONS + CONTRAINDICATIONS
P. oleracea is high in oxalates. Caution is recommended during pregnancy.

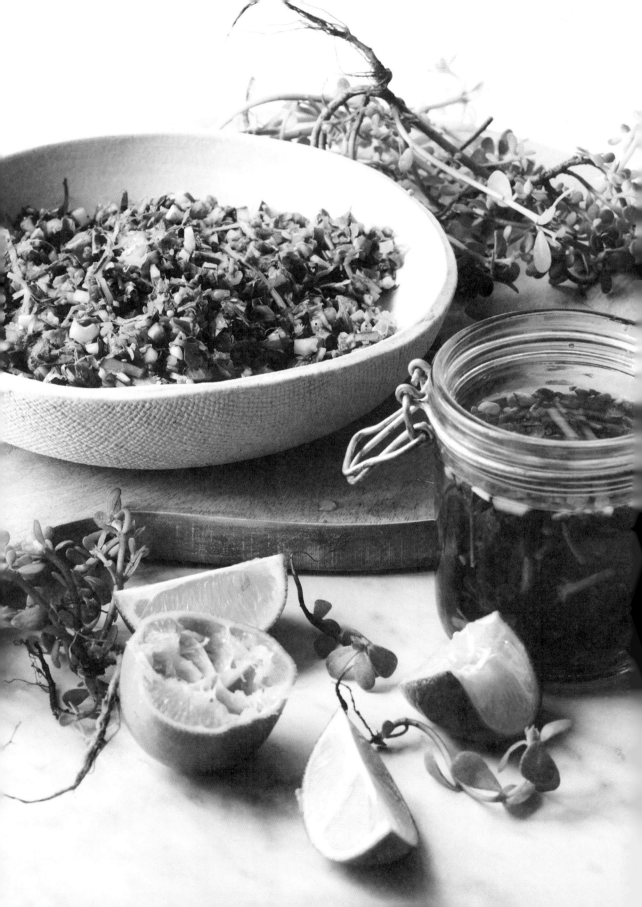

Purslane salsa verde

I could eat this green salsa all day long. It's so fresh and tangy, balanced perfectly by the heat from the jalapenos.

This recipe uses the pickled purslane from the recipe on page 270, so make that dish first.

MAKES ABOUT 1 CUP
15 MINUTES

GF

1 cup (250 ml) of pickled purslane (page 270), plus 2 tablespoons of the purslane pickle juice

1 tablespoon pickled jalapeño chillies (or to taste)

1 onion, chopped

¼ cup chopped coriander (cilantro) leaves

juice of 2 limes

1 teaspoon salt (or to taste)

Put all the ingredients in a blender and blend for 5 minutes, or until the mixture has a salsa-like consistency.

Serve with corn chips, tacos, nachos, burritos, over roast vegetables, in salad wraps, or on toast with vegan cream cheese. It's a perfect dish for a party or barbecue.

The salsa will keep in an airtight container in the fridge for 3–5 days.

Pickled purslane

MAKES ABOUT 1 CUP

15 MINUTES + 2½ WEEKS FERMENTING

GF

If you love pickles, this pickled purslane is a great addition to any meal. It's bursting with omega-3 essential fatty acids and good probiotics, and is also anti-inflammatory and healing to the gut. You can serve it as a probiotic side dish, a bit like sauerkraut.

I've given two pickling techniques below. The first is a simple vinegar pickle; the second method uses a brine and is the traditional and probiotic way to ferment vegetables.

VINEGAR PICKLES

1 handful of fresh purslane

1 cup (250 ml) apple cider vinegar

1 teaspoon salt

Cut the purslane into sections about 5–10 cm (2–4 inches) long and place in a sterilised glass jar (see page 23). Fill with the apple cider vinegar and add the salt.

If you have a metal lid, place baking paper between the lid and the jar to stop it rusting.

Cap tightly and leave to pickle for at least 2 weeks. It will then keep sealed in the fridge for up to 3 months.

LACTO-FERMENTED PICKLES

1 teaspoon salt

1 cup (250 ml) water

1 handful of fresh purslane

Combine the salt and water in a sterilised glass jar (see page 23). Add the purslane and put a lid on lightly so air can escape.

Leave on a bench or in a cupboard for 3–5 days, until bubbles appear.

Once bubbles appear, leave the jar in the fridge for 2 weeks before eating. The pickles will then keep sealed in the fridge for up to 3 months.

If bubbles appear after only a day or two on the bench, keep taste testing until the pickles are nice and sour, then store in the fridge. You may want to leave them out until day 3 or 4, even if bubbles have appeared on day 1 or 2.

Purslane gel

10 MINUTES
MAKES ½ CUP (125 ML)

1 handful of fresh purslane leaves

2 tablespoons laponite gel, or fresh aloe vera gel (see note)

12 drops of citricidal (citrus seed extract), optional

Note

To make a fresh aloe vera gel, blend 2 peeled fresh aloe vera leaves in a blender for about 10–20 seconds, and use that in this soothing gel instead.

Purslane gel can be applied to minor wounds and burns, eczema, psoriasis, and generally dry, itchy or inflamed skin. Using laponite and citricidal will make this remedy last significantly longer, but if you don't have those, just make fresh batches as needed.

Put the purslane in a blender and whiz for 10–20 seconds, until you have a smooth gel.

Mix the laponite or aloe vera gel through. If using the citricidal, stir it through to incorporate.

Transfer to a glass jar, seal with the lid, label with the ingredients and date made, and store in the fridge.

If using only the purslane and aloe vera gel, use within 3–5 days. If using both the laponite and citricidal, the expiry date is 3 months.

HOW TO USE THE GEL

Apply directly to the skin 1–4 times daily. If needed, cover with a light gauze dressing and change the dressing daily.

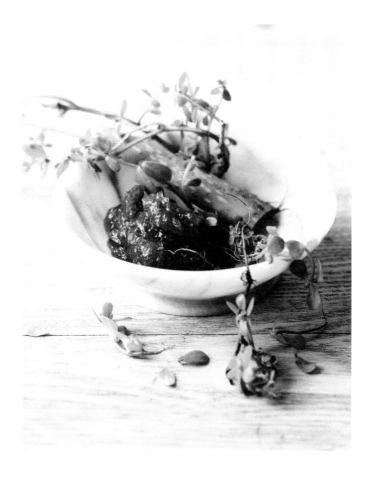

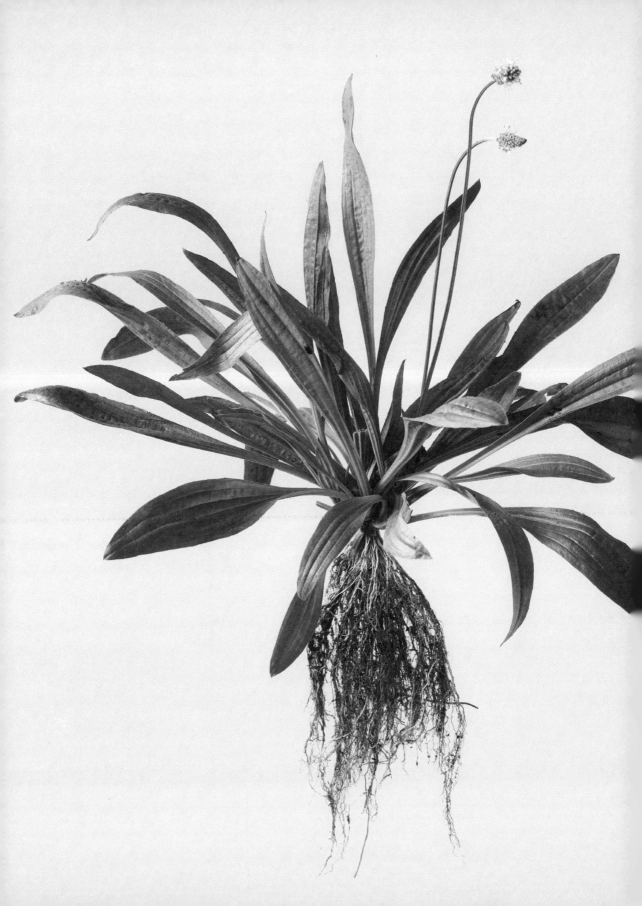

Ribwort

COMMON NAMES:

ribwort, narrow-leaf plantain

SPECIES:

Plantago lanceolata

GENUS:

Plantago

FAMILY:

Plantaginaceae

DISTRIBUTION:

Native to Europe; naturalised in the Americas, Asia and Australia.

PLANT SPIRIT QUALITIES:

Like a knight in shining armour, ribwort — 'Sir Lanceolata' — brings you the courage, strength and fortification to face your fears, to 'slay the dragons' that terrify you and keep you stuck. It is useful for anxiety, phobias and nightmares. Whenever you need courage to face a confronting or unpleasant task, call on ribwort.
Key word — courage.

How to identify it

- Ribwort is a low-growing perennial herb that forms a rosette.
- The basal leaves are lance-shaped (long, thin and pointed) and 2.5–30 cm (1–12 inches) long. They either spread outward or stand upright, and taper to a tip.
- The leaf margins are smooth or slightly toothed. The leaves are slightly hairy, with 3–7 distinct parallel veins that narrow at the tip.
- It has upright, non-branching flower stalks, with no leaves, that end in an oval inflorescence with many flowers.
- Flowers are about 4 mm (³⁄₁₆ inch) in diameter, with a green calyx and brownish corolla, and long cream-yellow stamens at the base.
- Ribwort has a well-developed root system.

How to harvest

Seeds

Ribwort will go to seed in mid to late summer. Look for the tall stalks with brown or black seeds. Cut the seed stalks at the base, leaving some plants unharvested so the colony can reproduce.

Put the heads of the seed stalk in a paper bag and give it a shake to collect the seeds, or shake the stalks over a large bowl. You can leave the stalks in the bag or bowl for a day or two to catch more seeds. If the seeds have not come off, gently massage them with your hands.

Remove the debris from the seeds by gently rubbing the seeds through your hands and blowing away the chaff.

Store the seeds in a cool, dry dark place, such as a paper bag or glass jar in a dark cupboard. Label with the name of the plant and the date harvested.

Plantain seeds from the ribwort species *Plantago ovata* are also known as psyllium, which is often used for treating constipation.

Leaves

The leaves can be harvested all year. The best time to harvest them is in the morning, when they are fresh and full of moisture.

Use a sharp pair of scissors or gently use your fingers to cut the leaves just above the base of the plant. Generally, it's best to pick leaves from the bottom if you want to continue to harvest from the same plant.

Rinse the leaves in water to remove any dirt or debris, then shake them in a colander or pat dry with a towel.

Use fresh, or freeze or dry the leaves for later use.

Nutrients

Zinc and potassium. The seeds are a good source of protein.

Culinary use

Young leaves can be eaten cooked or raw. They are rather bitter and fibrous, but when young can be used as a pot herb. The fibres can be removed prior to eating. The seeds can be used as a sago-like porridge, or ground into bread, but preparation can be laborious. For simple use, add a leaf or two to a green smoothie.

Folk medicine

The *Plantago* species appear in texts by the Greek physician Dioscorides (c. 40–90 AD), the Anglo–Saxons, and in the folklore of Indigenous peoples in Australia, New Zealand and the United States.

Ribwort is used by herbalists for coughs, wounds, inflamed skin and insect bites, where it is applied topically. In the upper respiratory tract, it is used as a mucous membrane tonic, as the mucilage covers the mucosa with a protective layer, soothing irritation. In the lower respiratory tract it is used as an expectorant. In the genitourinary system, it has historically been used for haemorrhoids and minor bladder infections.

Research

Clinical trials have confirmed its use in the following areas: respiratory tract infections,[1] antiviral,[2] antimicrobial,[3] anti-inflammatory,[4] antioxidant,[5] wound healing,[6] weight gain,[7] antipeptic ulcer activity[8] and antiparasitic.[9]

How to use it as a medicine

It is used as a tincture, an infusion, a glycetract and a poultice.

Ribwort can also be used in:
- Ribwort glycetract
- Ribwort tea
- Ribwort poultice
- Ribwort infused oil
- Wild wilted greens
- Wild greens powder

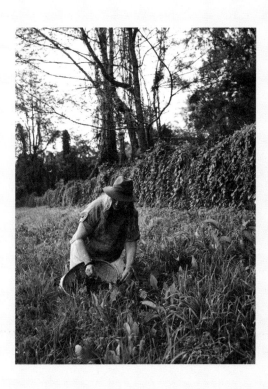

Crispy fried ribwort with tempeh & greens on greens

The challenge with eating ribwort is the stringy nature of the leaves. By making a green glaze out of the leaves and removing the stringy fibres, you get the health benefits of the antioxidants and anti-inflammatory effects of ribwort — no strings attached! Also, by frying the leaves until crispy, you get to enjoy ribwort in a whole new way that goes beyond just another steamed or stir-fried vegetable. This dish is jumping with flavour and texture, with wild ribwort as the star.

SERVES 4
30 MINUTES

GF

2 teaspoons sesame oil

1 thumb-sized piece of fresh ginger, finely chopped

4 garlic cloves, finely chopped

300 g (10½ oz) block of tempeh, thinly sliced

½ head of broccoli, cut into florets

10 green beans, trimmed

6–10 asparagus spears, chopped

1 handful of snow peas (mangetout)

1 handful of fresh ribwort leaves, finely chopped

¼ cup (40 g) salted, roasted cashews

RIBWORT GLAZE

1 handful of fresh ribwort leaves, finely chopped

2 tablespoons white miso paste

2 tablespoons rice wine vinegar

2 tablespoons coconut sugar

CRISPY FRIED RIBWORT LEAVES

5–10 fresh ribwort leaves

2 tablespoons rice bran oil

pinch of salt

To make the ribwort glaze, bring 2 cups (500 ml) water to the boil in a saucepan. Add the ribwort and blanch for 1–2 minutes.

Strain the ribwort through a sieve. Set the sieve over a bowl, then press on the ribwort with the back of a spoon to squeeze the water out.

Tip the blanched ribwort into a blender (or into a jug, if using a stick blender). Add the miso, vinegar, sugar and 1 tablespoon water. Blend for 2 minutes, then strain through a sieve, composting the pulp. Set aside.

Warm the sesame oil in a heavy-based frying pan over medium heat. Fry the ginger and garlic for 1–2 minutes, until lightly browned.

Add the tempeh slices and brown them on both sides, then add the broccoli and beans and fry for 3 minutes.

Toss in the asparagus, snow peas and ribwort and fry for another 1–2 minutes. Drizzle with the ribwort glaze and cook for a further minute, mixing it through.

Transfer to a serving bowl and top with the cashews.

For the crispy fried ribwort, heat the rice bran oil in the pan over high heat. Standing back from the pan in case the oil starts spitting, throw the ribwort leaves in and cook for 1–2 minutes, until crisp. Using tongs, quickly remove from the pan and drain on paper towel to absorb the oil, giving the leaves a gentle pat.

Sprinkle with the salt, scatter them over the glazed vegetables and serve straight away, before the crispy leaves go soggy.

This dish is lovely served with steamed rice.

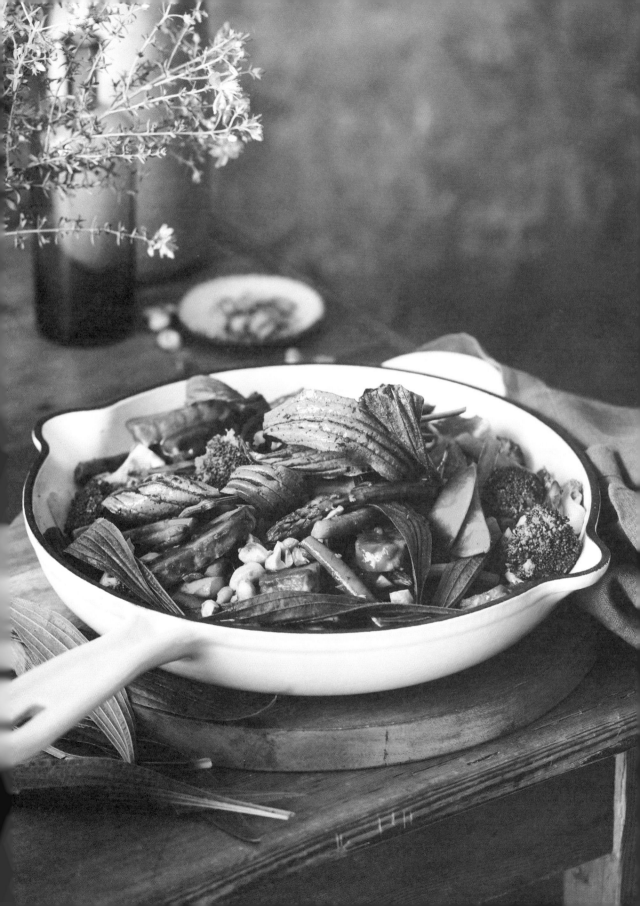

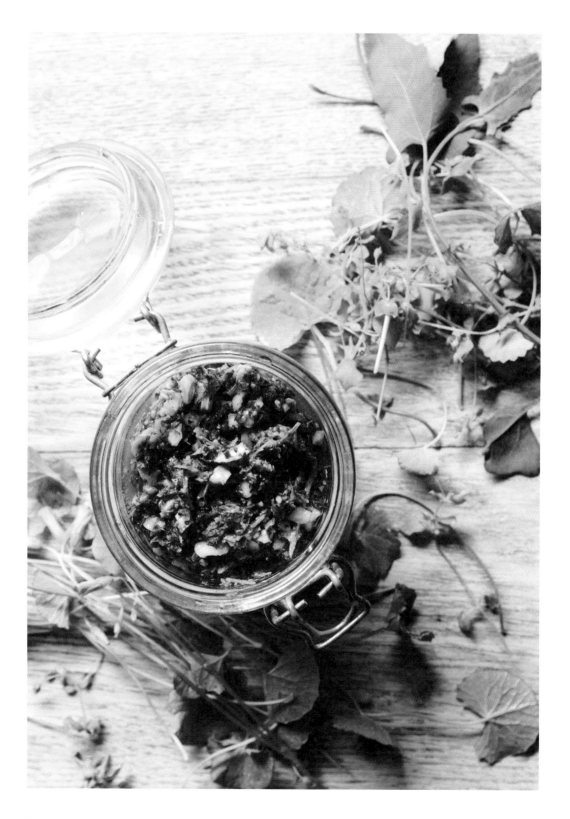

Wild weed pesto

MAKES ABOUT 1 CUP
15 MINUTES

A wild weed pesto is a great way to pack lots of wild plants into a single dish that is loaded with nutrition and healing benefits. I use all or any of the following wild greens in my pesto: nettle, nasturtium, purslane, cobbler's pegs, nodding top, plantain, oxalis, chickweed, amaranth leaves, blackberry nightshade leaves, fat hen, cleavers, wild garlic, dandelion and bush basil/tulsi.

Feel free to add anything edible you have growing abundantly. Remember to balance the flavour with more of the palatable herbs and less of the bitter ones. Unless you want a bitter pesto — then go for bitter, my friend. I'm all for it.

This pesto can be eaten as a dip with raw chopped vegetables or crackers, or slathered on pizza, pasta or bread.

---

3 handfuls of fresh wild greens

2 tablespoons lemon juice

2 tablespoons extra virgin olive oil

2 garlic cloves, peeled

¼ cup (40 g) raw cashews or macadamia nuts

1 tablespoon nutritional yeast

1 tablespoon maple syrup

¼ teaspoon salt

Wash and coarsely chop all your greens.

Put all the ingredients in a blender or food processor and blitz until your pesto is as smooth or chunky as you'd like it to be. I recommend stopping after 1 minute of blending and scraping down the sides to have a taste, then adding anything to balance the flavour and deciding if you want to keep blitzing for a smoother texture.

Your pesto will keep in an airtight container in the fridge for 3–5 days.

Ribwort & horseradish syrup

MAKES 200 ML (7 FL OZ)
15 MINUTES

1 small handful of fresh ribwort leaves

1 tablespoon horseradish paste (store-bought is fine)

1 tablespoon lemon juice

1 tablespoon maple syrup or honey

1–2 garlic cloves, peeled

Ribwort is a mucous membrane tonic because the mucilage covers the mucosa with a protective layer, soothing irritation, and helping the tissues of the sinuses to heal. Horseradish clears and unblocks mucus from the sinuses. Garlic is a potent antibiotic, helping clear infection.

This is a very hot syrup due to the horseradish and garlic, so it's not ideal for children or people who can't handle heat. The combination is intensely powerful, but clears the head quickly. The recipe is flexible, though, so feel free to adjust the amount of garlic, horseradish or maple syrup to taste.

Put all the ingredients in a blender and whiz until smooth. If you like a thick, pulpy syrup, leave as is. If you find it too fibrous, strain through a sieve lined with muslin (cheesecloth).

Pour into a sterilised jar (see page 23). Seal with the lid, then label with the ingredients and date made.

The syrup will keep for 3–4 days in the fridge, or up to 3 months in the freezer.

HOW TO USE THE SYRUP
Take 1–2 teaspoons 3–4 times daily.

Ribwort ointment

MAKES ¼ CUP (60 ML)
20 MINUTES

50 ml (1¾ fl oz) ribwort infused oil, made using the slow method (2 weeks) on page 30, or the fast method (1–2 days) on page 31

5 g (⅛ oz) shea butter

5 g (⅛ oz) sunflower wax

5–10 drops of tea tree oil

Ribwort has antiseptic, antihistamine, anti-inflammatory and soothing qualities, making it perfect to use on insect bites and stings, and small cuts and scrapes.

In a Pyrex or heatproof glass jug, combine the ribwort infused oil, shea butter and sunflower wax. Place the jug in a saucepan, then pour about 5 cm (2 inches) water into the pan to make a water bath.

Bring the water to a slow boil. Stir the mixture in the jug until all the ingredients have melted, about 8–10 minutes.

Remove from the heat. Add 5 drops of tea tree essential oil and mix until incorporated. Smell the ointment and put a little on your skin to see how it feels. If you think that's enough tea tree, add no more. If you think it needs more, add it drop by drop, testing as you go.

Pour into a sterilised amber glass jar (see page 23) and allow to set.

Seal with the lid, then label with the ingredients, date made, and an expiry date of 12 months. If making multiple batches, add a batch number. Store in a dark, cool cupboard or drawer.

Apply to insect bites, stings and small cuts and scrapes as needed.

Head & chest tonic for excess mucus

This glycetract is good when there is lots of mucus in the head from a head cold or sinus infection, or you are hacking up lots of mucus from the lungs. The ribwort is drying and helps expel mucus, while also soothing inflammation in the sinuses and lungs. The echinacea helps boost the immune system to fight the infection, and the ginger and orange peel warm the body and improve circulation. It's a good tonic to have in the house over winter.

MAKES 1 CUP (250 ML)

15 MINUTES + 2 WEEKS INFUSING

1 small handful of dried ribwort leaves

¼ cup (12 g) dried echinacea purpurea root

2 teaspoons dried ginger root or powder

2 teaspoons dried orange peel

150 ml (5 fl oz) vegetable glycerine

100 ml (3½ fl oz) distilled water

Sterilise a 2 cup (500 ml) glass jar (or even slightly bigger) in the dishwasher, or in a pot of boiling water for 10 minutes (see page 23).

Place all the ingredients in the sterilised jar. Shake the jar vigorously to mix the herbs into the water and glycerine. You may want to stir it a bit with a spoon.

Label with the ingredients, date made and the date it will be ready, which is 2 weeks from the day of making. Leave the jar on the bench for 2 weeks, shaking it once a day.

If, after 3–5 days, the herbs are becoming a dry clump, add 75 ml (2½ fl oz) more glycerine and 50 ml (1¾ fl oz) more distilled water and give it another good stir. Check the consistency to make sure that, when you shake it, the herbs are moving freely in the jar.

After 2 weeks, strain the herb mixture into a bowl through a large sieve lined with muslin (cheesecloth). It will be thick and slippery. Set the sieve aside and, holding the ball of muslin tightly between both hands, squeeze more of the herbal liquid into the bowl.

When strained, pour the mixture into the sterilised jar and label with the ingredients and date made.

Store the mixture in the fridge, where it will last up to 3 months.

If the cough has passed, you can store it in the freezer, where it will last up to 12 months.

HOW TO USE THE TONIC

Take 2 teaspoons 3–4 times daily.

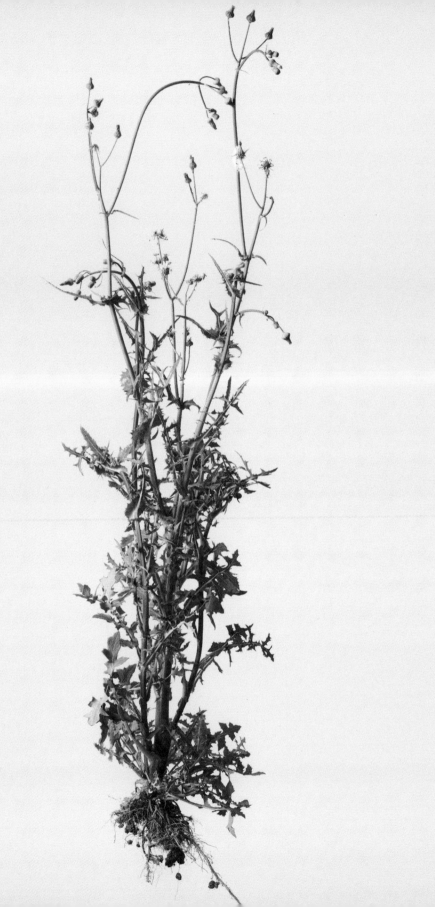

Sow thistle

COMMON NAMES:

Sow thistle, hare thistle, milk thistle

SPECIES:

Sonchus oleraceus

GENUS:

Sonchus

FAMILY:

Asteraceae

DISTRIBUTION:

Native to Europe and Western Asia. Found in almost every corner of the earth, including Alaska and the Arctic Circle.

PLANT SPIRIT QUALITIES:

Aggression and passivity are sides of the same coin. Sow thistle helps you balance these two forces within yourself and your life. If you have been overly passive, allowing others to take advantage of you or hurt you, or if you have weak boundaries, sow thistle can help you strengthen your sense of self, defend your boundaries and stand up for yourself. On the other hand, if you have been overly aggressive, abusive or dominating, sow thistle helps you to soften, mellow and be more open and vulnerable. Sow thistle brings balance to your strengths and weaknesses, and helps you to stand in your true power. **Key words — aggression, passivity.**

How to identify it

- This is an erect, hairless, branched annual or biennial herb about 1 metre (3 feet) tall.
- It has hollow stems, which have a milky sap.
- The basal leaves are up to 30 cm (12 inches) long and form a rosette.
- The leaves are soft and lobed or toothed, similar to dandelion leaves, except they grow up the central stalk.
- The stem leaves are somewhat smaller, and wrapping around the stem.
- The stems and leaves can be green or purplish in colour.
- The yellow dandelion-like flower heads are clustered, each about 2 cm (¾ inch) in diameter, with all the florets having a radiating petal-like blade.
- These 'flowers' are at the ends of branches.
- The tiny fruits are short and flattened, topped by a tuft of fine, soft bristles.

How to harvest

The best time to harvest sow thistle is when the leaves are young and tender, rather than bitter and spiky — usually in spring or early summer.

Leaves, stems and young flowers
Avoid picking plants near roadsides or areas where pesticides or chemicals may have been used.

Wear gloves to protect your hands from the prickly edges of the plant. Use scissors or secateurs to cut off the leaves near the base — or you can harvest the whole plant above ground and use the leaves, stems and young flowers.

Rinse them thoroughly under running water to remove any dirt or debris and wash the bitter sap from the stems.

Seeds
When the flowers turn into fluffy seed heads, collect them in a paper bag. Store the seeds in a cool, dry place until you're ready to sow them.

You can replant the seeds by sowing them in well-draining soil, about 5 mm to 1 cm (¼–½ inch) deep. Water the area gently to keep the soil moist, but not waterlogged. Germination should occur within a couple of weeks, and you can thin the seedlings as they grow.

Nutrients

Protein, calcium, phosphorus, iron, vitamin A, thiamine (B2), riboflavin (B2), niacin (B3) and vitamin C.

Culinary use

Young leaves can be eaten raw or cooked. Sow thistle has a mild flavour, especially in spring. It can be added to salads, cooked like spinach or used in soups and stews. You may want to remove the prickles on the stems. Stems can be cooked like asparagus or rhubarb, and are best if the outer skin is removed first.

Folk medicine

In the Philippines, *Sonchus oleraceus* is used as a cathartic laxative, with strong effects on the liver, duodenum and colon. It is also used to treat fluid in the lungs and abdomen. It is administered with manna, aniseed and carbonate of magnesia, or with stimulants and aromatics.

In Bengal, an infusion of leaves and roots is given as a tonic and febrifuge (fever reducer). In Indochina, stems are used as a sedative and tonic.

In Italy it is used as a laxative and diuretic, with the juice of the plant given for cleaning and healing ulcers.

In Brazilian folk medicine it is used as a general tonic, and also to treat headaches, pain, hepatitis, infections, inflammation and rheumatism.

In India, the juice of fresh leaves is taken orally for its liver protective effects.

More generally, an infusion of the leaves is used for delayed menstruation and to boost milk production. Latex in the sap is used for warts, and the leaves are applied as a poultice on inflammatory swellings. An infusion of the leaves and roots has been used to treat fevers.

The Maori people of New Zealand have used it as a chewing gum, as it contains 0.14% rubber.

Research

Clinical trials have confirmed its use in the following areas: pain relief,[1] antidepressant and anti-anxiety,[2] diabetes,[3] obesity,[4] prebiotic,[5] wound healing,[6] ulcers,[7] anti-inflammatory,[8] antifungal[9] and kidney protection.[10]

How to use it as a medicine

The juice is traditionally used as a gum, an infusion, or externally as a sap or poultice.

CAUTIONS + CONTRAINDICATIONS
None known, but it can have a strong laxative effect. Due to its constituents and use for delayed menstruation, it should be avoided during pregnancy.

Sow thistle can also be used in:
- Anti-inflammatory gel
- Wild weed pesto
- Sow thistle glycetract

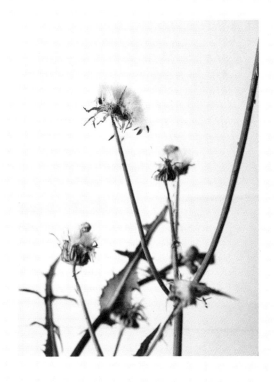

Sow thistle & jackfruit

SERVES 4
1 HOUR

GF

1 tablespoon olive oil,
plus extra for drizzling

1 brown onion, finely chopped

3 garlic cloves, crushed

1 teaspoon dried Italian herbs

1 teaspoon smoked paprika

2 bay leaves

2 tablespoons tamari

400 g (14 oz) tin of young
jackfruit, strained

4 cups (1 litre) water with
1 stock cube added, or 4 cups
(1 litre) vegetable stock

400 g (14 oz) tin of chopped
tomatoes

1 carrot, cut into chunks

2 potatoes, peeled and
cut into chunks

1 sweet potato, cut into chunks

2 handfuls of fresh sow thistle
leaves, finely chopped

1 small handful of chopped
parsley

This is a veganised version of a traditional Maori dish that is normally made with *puha* (sow thistle) and pork. You'll be amazed how the sow thistle and jackfruit soak up the marvellous flavour of this stew to give a vegan slow-cooked pork vibe. It's a real keeper, as any leftovers can be saved for lunch or dinner the next day — and it is especially nourishing during winter when you crave those hot, hearty meals.

Sow thistle is an antioxidant and anti-inflammatory, and helps maintain healthy metabolism and hormonal balance, while jackfruit is rich in minerals including calcium and magnesium, which help protect bone density and relieve arthritis.

Heat the olive oil in a large heavy-based saucepan. Add the onion and garlic and sauté for 5 minutes until translucent.

Stir in the herbs, paprika, bay leaves and tamari. Break the jackfruit up a bit with your hands, then sauté with the onion mixture for a couple of minutes.

Pour in the stock and tomatoes. Add the remaining vegetables and sow thistle. Bring to the boil, then reduce the heat and simmer for 40 minutes, or until the potato is tender.

Using a potato masher, mash some of the potatoes to thicken the stew to your desired thickness. (I like to leave some potato still in chunks.)

Season with salt and pepper to taste. Serve garnished with the parsley and a drizzle of olive oil.

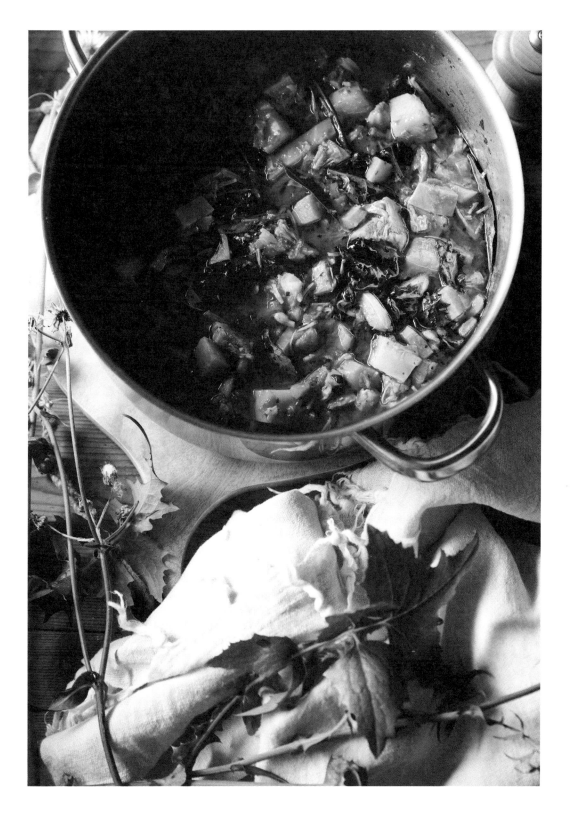

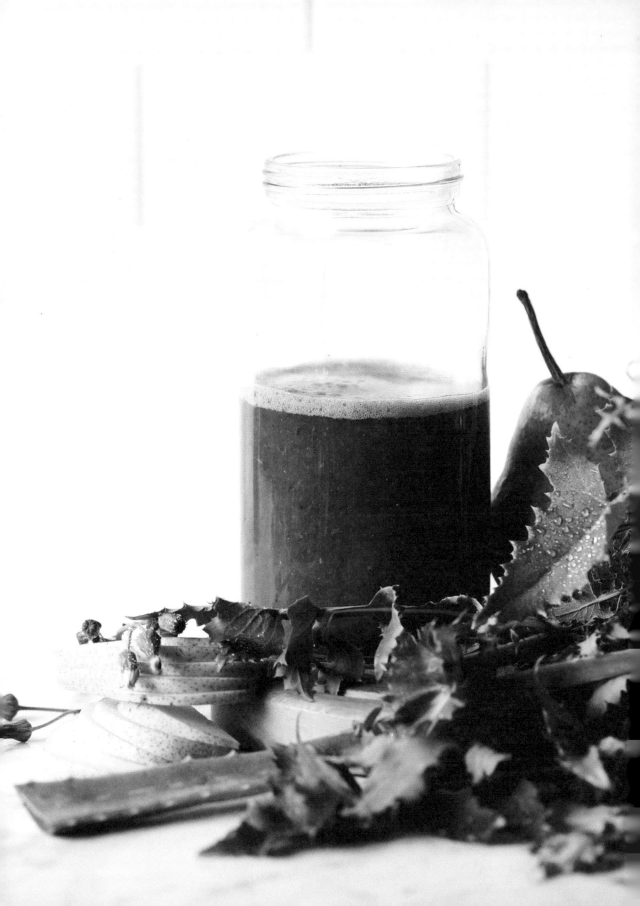

Sow thistle, aloe & pear juice for constipation

Around the world, sow thistle is used as a laxative with strong effects on the liver, duodenum and colon. It is anti-inflammatory and cleansing for the gut and intestinal tract. If you have long-term constipation, it is good to explore the reason with a health practitioner who can help you understand why. This recipe can be used short term when needed to get things moving, or for a longer time for general gut health.

MAKES 1½ CUPS (375 ML)
15 MINUTES

GF

1 medium-sized fresh aloe vera leaf, about 20 cm (8 inches) long and 5 cm (2 inches) wide (see note)

2 handfuls of fresh sow thistle leaves, coarsely chopped

1 cup (250 ml) pear juice

Peel the aloe vera by cutting the spines from the sides, then using a sharp knife to slice the skin off the front and back.

Cut the aloe gel into cubes and place in a jug. Add the sow thistle and pear juice and blitz using a stick blender for 1–2 minutes. (You can also use a jug blender, but you may need to add a tiny bit of water to blend properly.)

Strain the juice through a sieve lined with muslin (cheesecloth), into a jar with a lid.

The juice will keep in the fridge for 2–3 days. If you want to keep it longer, freeze the juice in ice cube trays and thaw as needed. The juice will last up to 3 months frozen.

HOW TO USE THE JUICE

Drink 1 cup (250 ml) before bed to help stimulate a bowel movement. People's sensitivity to this recipe varies greatly, so you may want to start with ¼ (60 ml) or ½ cup (125 ml) to see how you respond.

Note
You'll need enough aloe vera to give ¼ cup (60 ml) fresh gel when peeled and cut into 2 cm (¾ inch) cubes.

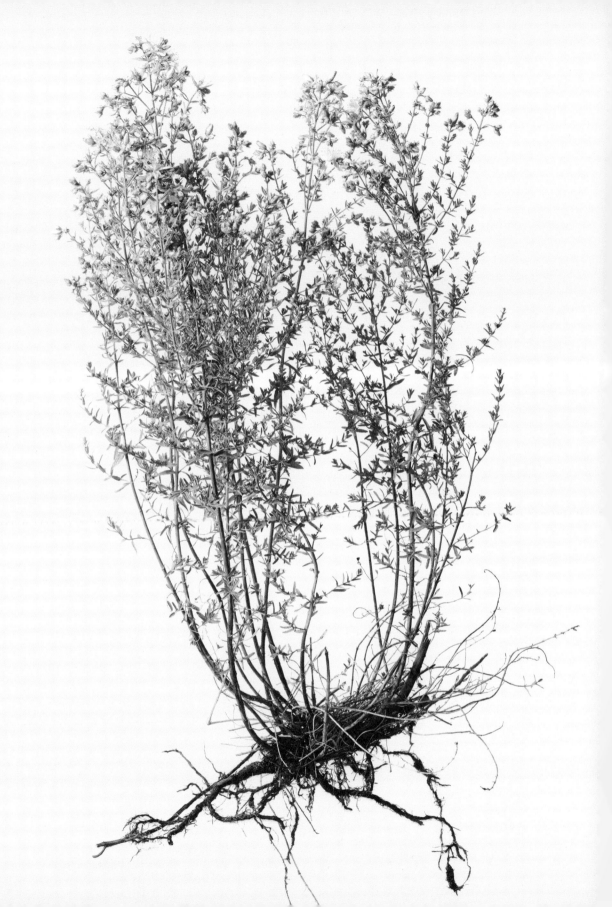

St John's wort

COMMON NAMES:

St John's wort

SPECIES:

Hypericum perforatum; there are over 370 *Hypericum* species

GENUS:

Hypericum

FAMILY:

Hypericaceae

DISTRIBUTION:

Native to Europe and Asia, but has spread to temperate regions worldwide. Listed as a noxious weed in more than 20 countries, with introduced populations in South America, North America, India, New Zealand, Australia and South Africa.

PLANT SPIRIT QUALITIES:

St John's wort is a classic remedy for depression. Energetically, it helps bring satisfaction, light and happiness back into your life. St John's wort has hundreds of tiny 'holes' in its leaves, allowing the light through. It's when you feel the most cracked, the most broken, that you are most open to the light. It helps clear patterns of depression, allowing you to move into a new frequency of light and happiness. **Key words — satisfaction, light, happiness.**

How to identify it

- St John's wort has a five-petalled, bright yellow flower about 22 mm (¾ inch) in diameter.
- If you look closely at the flowers, or use a magnifying glass, you will see small black dots that, when rubbed on your fingers, leave a red oil. The red pigment in the oil contains hypericin, which is responsible for many of the plant's beneficial effects.
- The fruit has a sticky capsule that splits open in summer, to release seeds the following autumn and winter.
- The tiny seed is cylindrical, only 0.5–1 mm long, and can be pale to dark brown or black, with a pitted seed coat.
- Held up to light, the leaves appear to have a number of tiny 'holes', which are actually oil glands. These 'perforations' led to the species name *perforatum*.
- It has erect, woody, flowering stems, which are cylindrical and sometimes have a reddish tinge.
- Stems branch near the top and have two opposing longitudinal ribs or ridges.
- Leaves and branches are always opposite one another on the stem.
- The plant grows to a height of about 60–90 cm (2–3 feet).
- St John's wort has one set of roots that grow vertically to about 1 metre (3 feet) deep into the soil, and another set that grow horizontally and produce buds that form into new plants.
- Deep soils favour the development of vertical roots. In shallow soils, roots generally grow laterally and sucker more readily than vertical roots.

How to harvest flowers

The best time to harvest St John's wort is when it is in full bloom. This usually occurs in midsummer, when the flowers are bright yellow and the plant is most potent.

When harvesting the flowers, use a pair of scissors or secateurs (and wearing gloves can be good to protect your hands from the red-staining hypericin). Snip off the top 10–15 cm (4–6 inches) of the plant, just above a leaf node (the point where the leaf joins the stem). This encourages the plant to continue growing and producing more flowers.

Harvest only a small portion of the plant to ensure it can continue to grow sustainably.

Fresh flowers can be added to oil to make an infused oil.

If you want to dry them, spread the flowers and leaves in a single layer on a clean, dry surface, such as a drying rack or a cloth. Leave in a warm, well-ventilated area away from direct sunlight to dry completely for 1–2 weeks, or until the flowers and leaves crumble easily when touched.

When dry, store in an airtight glass jar in a cool, dark place. Label with the name of the plant and the date harvested.

Nutrients

Protein, fats, vitamins A and C, carotenoids, rutin and pectin.

Culinary use

St John's wort is not a common food source, but flowers and fresh leaves can be used in salads, and the dried plant enjoyed as a tea. It has also been used as an ingredient in the distillation of vodka, as a dye and as an infused oil.

Folk medicine

Many famous ancient physicians, including Dioscorides, Pliny the Elder and Hippocrates, have described using St John's wort as a topical treatment for wounds and burns, and internally for kidney, stomach and lung ailments, but it was Nicholas Culpeper who first suggested it as a remedy for melancholy and madness in 1652.

In Christian Europe, the plant came into flower around St John's Day, 24 June, which is how it acquired its common name. The red pigment is also said to symbolise the blood of Saint John.

Hypericum perforatum has been used orally and topically by traditional herbalists all around the world, as a sedative, analgesic, anti-inflammatory, diuretic and antimalarial, and to heal wounds, burns, rheumatism, haemorrhoids, ulcers, neuralgia, myalgia, gastroenteritis, contusions, sprains, diarrhoea, menorrhagia, trauma, hysteria, bedwetting and depression.

Research

Clinical trials have confirmed its use in the following areas: depression in adults and children,[1] menopausal symptoms and depression,[2] anxiety,[3] obsessive-compulsive disorder (OCD),[4] drug and alcohol dependence,[5] premenstrual syndrome,[6] antibacterial,[7] antiviral,[8] potential treatment for Covid-19,[9] wound healing,[10] pain relief,[11] neuralgia[12] and obesity.[13]

How to use it as a medicine

H. perforatum is used in an extensive number of preparations as a tablet, fluid extract, powder, tincture, infusion, infused oil and poultice.

CAUTIONS + CONTRAINDICATIONS

St John's wort has been found to affect the metabolism and actions of many medications, including warfarin, the oral contraceptive pill, digoxin, indinavir, cyclosporine, phenprocoumon, HIV protease inhibitors, theophylline, triptans, alprazolam, amitriptyline, fexofenadine, irinotecan, methadone, nevirapine, simvastatin and tacrolimus.

When used with SSRIs (serotonin reuptake inhibitor antidepressants, such as sertraline, paroxetine, nefazodone) or buspirone, St John's wort can cause serotonergic syndrome — a cluster of symptoms including high body temperature, agitation, increased reflexes, tremor, sweating, dilated pupils and diarrhoea.

Other side effects caused by simultaneous use with SSRIs include nausea, rash, fatigue, restlessness, photosensitivity, acute neuropathy and episodes of mania.

Always check interactions with medications, or ask your pharmacist to do this for you.

Some internal-use preparations of St John's wort, particularly at high doses, have been associated with increased photosensitivity, resulting in higher risk of sunburn — a risk that is less common at the lower oral doses used for treating depression.

With topical applications, the risk of photo-sensitisation is extremely minimal and unlikely, unless use is long-term or at a high dose, or the skin is very fair or damaged.

It is not recommended after organ transplants.

St John's wort can also be used in:
- Blackberry nightshade ointment
- St John's wort tea
- St John's wort glycetract
- Capsules

St John's wort infused oil

---

2 WEEKS

MAKES AS MUCH OIL AS YOU HAVE FLOWERS

enough fresh St John's wort flowers to fill a jar of your choosing

olive oil, to fill your jar

This is a beautiful rich red oil made from the fresh flowers of St John's wort. It can be used on its own or in creams, balms and ointments to help with inflammation, pain (especially nerve pain from nerve damage, cold sores, genital herpes and shingles), as well as wounds, burns, rheumatism, haemorrhoids, ulcers, bruises and sprains. Make sure you read the Cautions + Contraindications information on page 293 before using this oil.

Use fresh flowers straight off the plant, or let them wilt for an hour or so to remove some of the moisture, but don't let them dry out. Once the flowers are dry, the oil in them will thicken, and won't infuse into the olive oil.

Snip or crush the flowers a bit with either the blade or handle end of your scissors. This will help release their oil.

Fill a sterilised glass jar (see page 23) with the flowers; some leaves and stems from the tips of the plants can be added as well. Fill the jar with olive oil, completely covering the flowers.

Seal with the lid, then label with the ingredients, date made, and the date it will be ready, which is 2 weeks from the day of making.

Leave to infuse in sunlight, or on a shelf, for 2 weeks. The oil will take on a rich dark red colour during that time.

After 2 weeks, strain the oil through muslin (cheesecloth). There is often a sediment or residue at the bottom of the jar. Pour the oil slowly through the cheesecloth to avoid using this residue. For a purer oil, strain it through a coffee filter — it can take a day to go through, so be patient. This more refined straining method is usually only necessary for commercial production.

Store your oil in a cool dark place, and label with the ingredients and date made. The oil should keep for up to 12 months; after that time, smell the oil to check it hasn't gone rancid.

HOW TO USE THE OIL

Use this oil in creams and ointments, or apply directly to the skin for nerve pain and healing of minor wounds.

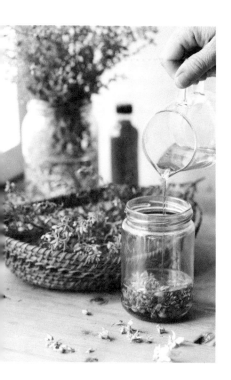

St John's wort pain ointment

Recent clinical trials have confirmed the use of St John's wort for pain, especially nerve pain. This ointment is good where there is nerve and muscular pain or arthritis. Simply apply directly to the sore area and massage into the skin.

MAKES ¼ CUP (60 ML)
20 MINUTES

50 ml (1¾ fl oz) St John's wort infused oil (see note)

5 g (⅛ oz) cayenne pepper

5 g (⅛ oz) shea butter

5 g (⅛ oz) sunflower wax

5–10 drops of wintergreen essential oil

Note
Make your infused St John's wort oil from fresh flowers, either by the slow method (2 weeks) on page 30, or by the fast method for fresh herbs on page 31. The slow method will produce a richer, redder oil.

In a Pyrex or other heatproof glass jug, combine the St John's wort infused oil, cayenne pepper, shea butter and sunflower wax. Place the jug in a saucepan, then pour about 5 cm (2 inches) water into the pan to make a water bath.

Bring the water to a slow boil. Stir the mixture in the jug until all the ingredients have melted, about 8–10 minutes.

Remove from the heat. Strain through a sieve lined with muslin (cheesecloth) set over a bowl, to remove the cayenne pepper.

Mix in the wintergreen essential oil, drop by drop, testing on your inner wrist to see how heating it feels and how strong it smells, before adding more if desired.

Pour into a sterilised amber glass jar (see page 23) and allow to set.

Seal with the lid, then label with the ingredients, date made, and an expiry date of 12 months. If making multiple batches, add a batch number. Store in a dark, cool cupboard or drawer.

CAUTION!
This oil has a heating sensation. Patch test on a small area before using, and wait 15 minutes for the heat to build. Avoid the face and eyes and wash your hands immediately after use. Also read the Cautions + Contraindications information on page 293 before using this oil.

Natural vegan sun lotion

MAKES 150 ML (5 FL OZ)

45 MINUTES + 30 MINUTES INFUSING

2 tablespoons dried calendula and/or dried St John's wort flowers

2 tablespoons infused calendula oil (see notes)

2 tablespoons St John's wort oil (see notes)

1 teaspoon red raspberry seed oil (available online)

1 teaspoon carrot seed oil

2 tablespoons olivem 1000

2 tablespoons shea butter

1 tablespoon vegetable glycerine

1 tablespoon zinc oxide powder (be careful not to inhale the powder)

12 drops of citricidal (citrus seed extract)

When hot sun exposure is unavoidable and you need some protection, a natural sun lotion like this one may come in handy. While this lotion shouldn't be relied on to offer complete sun protection, it may be helpful in nourishing the skin and countering some of the damaging effects of sun exposure.

Generally, though, also try to minimise sun exposure between 11 am and 2 pm. During the middle of the day, stay in the shade, and if swimming, wear a rashie (long-sleeved protective clothing).

The strength of your ingredients and batches will vary considerably, so always test each batch you make.

Do a patch test on yourself by rubbing some cream on certain parts of your skin and not on others, then spend a short amount of time in the morning or late afternoon sun. Observing any change in skin colour of the creamed/uncreamed skin will give you a sense of how much sun protection your cream offers.

Infuse the calendula or St John's wort flowers in ½ cup (125 ml) water overnight, or for a minimum of 30 minutes.

Strain and compost the water-infused flowers. Pour the infused liquid into a small saucepan, but leave it off the heat.

Pop some ice cubes in a large bowl half filled with water, to have an ice bath ready for when you are mixing your cream. (You can leave the ice bath in the fridge or freezer until needed.)

In a Pyrex or other heatproof glass jug, combine the calendula oil, St John's wort oil, raspberry seed oil, carrot seed oil, olivem 1000, shea butter and glycerine. Place the jug in another saucepan, then pour about 5 cm (2 inches) water into the pan to make a water bath. Bring the water to the boil, then reduce the heat to a slow boil. Stir the mixture in the jug until all the ingredients have melted, about 8–10 minutes. Take off the heat.

Add the zinc oxide to the jug and mix to incorporate, being careful not to breathe in the powder. Add the citricidal.

Reheat the oil mixture in the jug, as well as the infused flower water in the other pan, until close to boiling point — but take them off the heat as soon as bubbles start to form.

The oil mixture and the infusion need to be as close as possible to the same temperature to incorporate smoothly and avoid a gritty cream, so as soon as the oils have melted and the infusion is near boiling, pour the jug mixture into the flower infusion, place the saucepan in the ice bath (this will help the mixture thicken much more quickly) and start mixing with a fork or whisk. (If making a large batch, a stick blender will be much faster.)

Stop mixing when the mixture forms nice stiff peaks, like whipped cream.

Spoon into sterilised amber glass jars (see page 23). Seal with the lid, then label with the ingredients, date made, and an expiry date of 3 months.

Best stored in a dark, cool cupboard or drawer, or in the fridge.

Notes

Make your infused St John's wort oil from fresh flowers, either by the slow method (2 weeks) on page 30, or by the fast method for fresh herbs on page 31. The slow method will produce a richer, redder oil.

You also need infused calendula oil, which is best made from dried flowers via the slow method on page 30.

For best results, read the section on creams in Herbal Medicine-making Fundamentals on page 34 before making your cream.

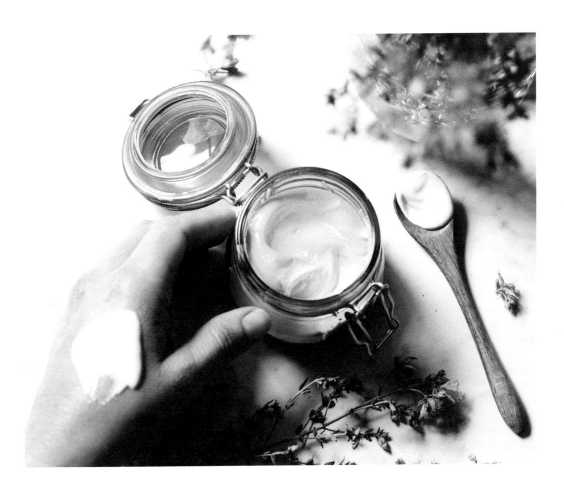

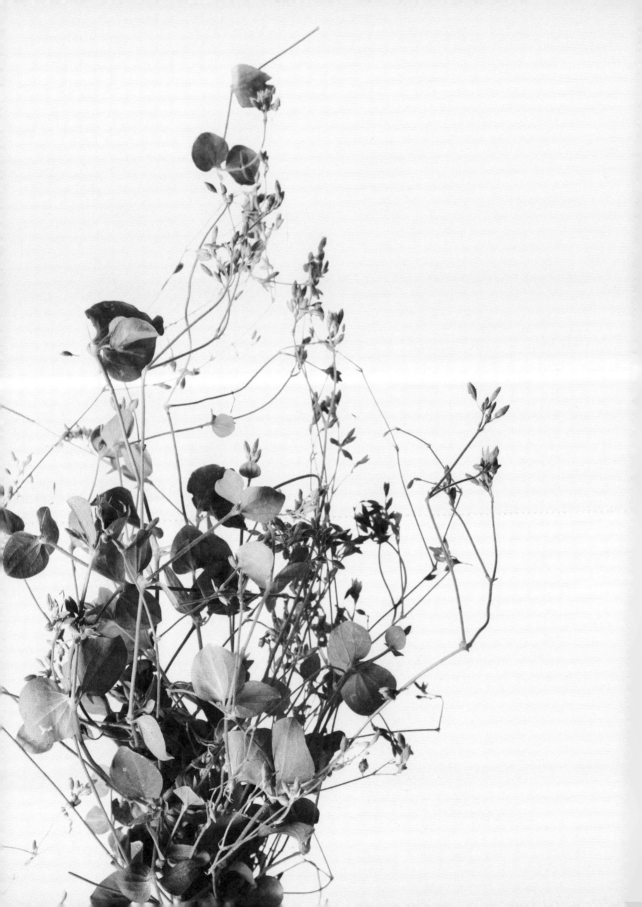

Tropical chickweed

COMMON NAMES:

tropical chickweed

SPECIES:

Drymaria cordata

GENUS:

Drymaria

FAMILY:

Caryophyllaceae

DISTRIBUTION:

Native to Mexico and Central and South America, as well as central and southern Africa. Also naturalised in the Caribbean region, the southern United States, Asia, India and throughout Oceania.

PLANT SPIRIT QUALITIES:

Tropical chickweed helps you stay committed to the things and people that help you stay healthy and happy. It can strengthen your dedication to your spiritual or creative practice, your exercise regime, a healthy diet or relationships with your loved ones. Tropical chickweed is like a life coach that encourages you to keep committed when enthusiasm starts to fade, and boredom, restlessness and laziness creep in. It can help inspire you stay on track and keep doing those day-to-day things that serve your highest good.
Key word — commitment.

How to identify it

- Tropical chickweed is slender, with smooth, hairless stems — unlike European chickweed, which has a hairy stem.

- It grows to about 30 cm (12 inches) long, frequently rooting at the nodes.

- Leaves are roughly heart-shaped, opposite each other and attached to stems.

- Veins are clearly seen on the underside of the leaves, radiating outwards from the bottom end of the leaf.

- The small flowers are loosely clustered towards the tips of the branches, and are borne on stalks (pedicels) some 2–15 mm ($\frac{1}{16}$–$\frac{5}{8}$ inch) long.

- The flowers have five narrow green sepals, 3–5 mm ($\frac{1}{8}$–$\frac{1}{4}$ inch) long, that are covered with sticky (glandular) hairs. They also have five white petals about 2–3 mm ($\frac{1}{16}$–$\frac{1}{8}$ inch) long, plus two or three stamens, and an ovary topped with three styles.

- The five white petals are usually deeply two-lobed, and may be easily mistaken for 10 petals at first glance. Flowering occurs throughout most of the year.

- Tropical chickweed does **not** have milky sap. If you have a plant that you think is chickweed and it has milky sap, you have the wrong plant (most likely, petty spurge).

How to harvest

In tropical climates, this plant grows all year except midsummer, when it gets too hot. It is very easy to harvest as it pulls out with little effort. In order to not pull up the roots accidentally, you may want to harvest with scissors or else gently pull up sections only, leaving enough for the patch to regenerate.

The whole plant (but mainly the leaves and stems) can all be eaten and used medicinally. You can use the plant fresh, or dry it for later use.

Nutrients

Vitamin C, vitamin A, B vitamins, potassium, calcium and phosphorus.

Folk medicine

A traditional medicine in Africa, India, Nepal and the Americas, *Drymaria cordata* has been used topically for snakebite, wounds, burns, eczema, dermatitis, tumours and leprosy. In Africa and India it is also used for sore joints, eye infections, fevers, coughs and bronchitis. It is also used as a laxative and diuretic, and to increase appetite.

In Nigeria, *D. cordata* (commonly called 'Calabar woman's eye') is used to treat convulsions, fever conditions and sleeping disorders in children.

Local tribespeople from the Garo and Khasi hills of Meghalaya, India, wrap this herb in big leaves, which are folded, tied and placed over a fire. When the plant is heated, the vapour is inhaled as a treatment for cough and sinusitis, or an acute cold.

Research

Clinical trials have confirmed its use in the following areas: pain and fever,[1] cough suppressant,[2] antibacterial,[3] antioxidant,[4] diabetes,[5] epilepsy[6] and anti-anxiety.[7]

How to use it as a medicine

As an infusion, a tincture, an inhalation and topically as a poultice.

CAUTIONS + CONTRAINDICATIONS
May potentially cause skin sensitivity in some people, but this is rare.

Tropical chickweed can also be used in:

- Wild weed pesto
- Anti-inflammatory gel
- Tropical chickweed glycetract
- Tropical chickweed tea

Tropical chickweed anti-inflammatory juice

I tend to think of tropical chickweed as nature's ibuprofen because of its powerful anti-inflammatory effects. It has traditionally been used for coughs, colds and flus, as well as inflammation in the joints caused by arthritis. Drink this juice as part of a treatment protocol that targets your specific condition to help reduce pain and inflammation.

MAKES 2 CUPS (500 ML)
10 MINUTES

GF

3 handfuls of fresh tropical chickweed

1 handful of mint sprigs

½ pineapple, peeled and chopped into chunks

2 Lebanese (short) cucumbers, chopped into chunks (or 1 thick-skinned cucumber, peeled)

Place all the ingredients in a juicer and juice them.

Add ½ cup (125 ml) water to dilute the mixture a little.

Serve with or without ice.

HOW TO USE THE JUICE

Drink 3–4 cups (750 ml–1 litre) a day for pain and inflammation.

You can make a double batch in the morning to drink throughout the day.

Tropical chickweed healing cream

MAKES 12 ML (½ FL OZ)

30 MINUTES + 30 MINUTES INFUSING

2 tablespoons dried tropical chickweed, or 1 handful of fresh tropical chickweed leaves

3 tablespoons infused tropical chickweed oil (see note)

1½ tablespoons olivem 1000

1 teaspoon vegetable glycerine

12 drops of citricidal (citrus seed extract)

Note

Make your infused tropical chickweed oil by the fast method for fresh herbs on page 31.

Due to its ibuprofen-like anti-inflammatory effects, this cream can be used for pain and inflammation in the joints and muscles caused by injury or arthritis. Use it regularly throughout the day to manage pain and increase mobility.

For best results, read the section on creams in Herbal Medicine-making Fundamentals on page 34 before making your cream.

Infuse the dried or fresh tropical chickweed in ½ cup (125 ml) hot boiled water overnight, or for at least 30 minutes.

Strain and compost the herbs. Add the liquid infusion to a small saucepan, but leave it off the heat.

Pop some ice cubes in a large bowl half filled with water, to have an ice bath ready for when you are mixing your cream. (You can leave the ice bath in the fridge or freezer until needed.)

In a Pyrex or other heatproof glass jug, combine the tropical chickweed infused oil, olivem 1000 and glycerine. Place the jug in another saucepan, then pour about 5 cm (2 inches) water into the pan to make a water bath. Bring the water to the boil, then reduce the heat to a slow boil. Stir frequently until the ingredients have melted, about 8–10 minutes.

Add the citricidal to your tropical chickweed infusion in the other pan. Heat the infusion until close to boiling point — but take it off the heat as soon as bubbles form.

The oil mixture and the infusion need to be as close as possible to the same temperature to incorporate smoothly and avoid a gritty cream, so as soon as the wax has melted and the infusion is near boiling, pour the melted oil mixture into the infusion, place the saucepan in the ice bath (this will help the mixture thicken much more quickly) and start mixing with a fork or whisk. (If making a large batch, a stick blender will be much faster.)

Stop mixing when it forms nice stiff peaks like whipped cream.

Spoon into sterilised amber glass jars (see page 23). Seal with the lid, then label with the ingredients, date made, and an expiry date of 3 months. Store in the fridge.

HOW TO USE THE CREAM

Apply the cream every 3–4 hours to affected areas.

Tropical chickweed inhalation

**MAKES ENOUGH FOR
1 INHALATION**

15 MINUTES

1 handful of fresh tropical chickweed

1 cup (250 ml) boiling water

This is a classic steam inhalation traditionally used for spasmodic coughs, bronchitis, whooping cough, asthma, sinusitis and eye inflammation – in conjunction with appropriate medical care. It needs to be repeated three times daily for 3 days, but can be used for a week or more, depending on the severity of the symptoms.

Traditionally the chickweed is wrapped in a banana leaf and steamed in a pot of hot boiled water, then a straw is fed through a hole in the leaf and the steam is inhaled into the nose for sinus problems, or opened and inhaled for lung problems.

Coarsely chop the tropical chickweed.

Pour the boiling water into a heatproof bowl and add the chickweed.

Cover your head and shoulders with a towel, so that the rising steam is collected under the towel, and place your head over the bowl, about 20 cm (8 inches) away.

Inhale deeply for bout 10–15 minutes, until the water cools and the steam disappears.

CAUTION!
While inhaling, be careful not to scald your nose or face.

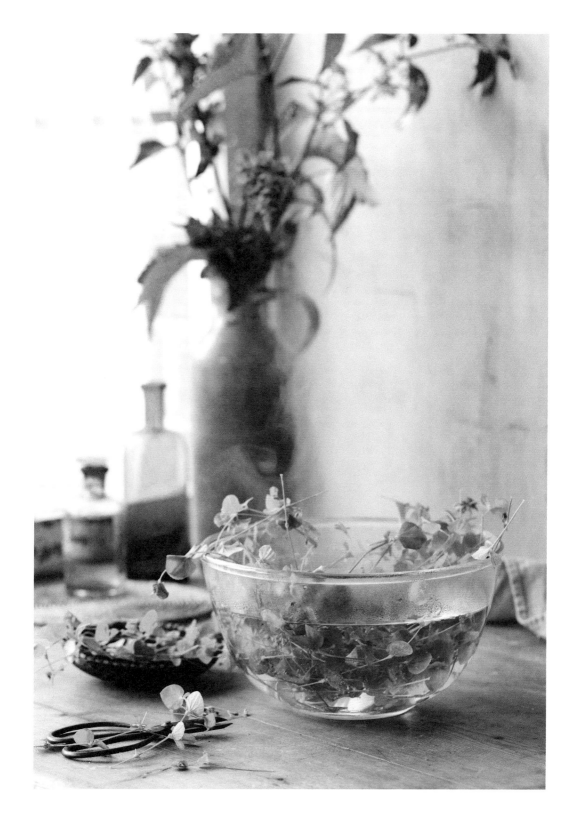

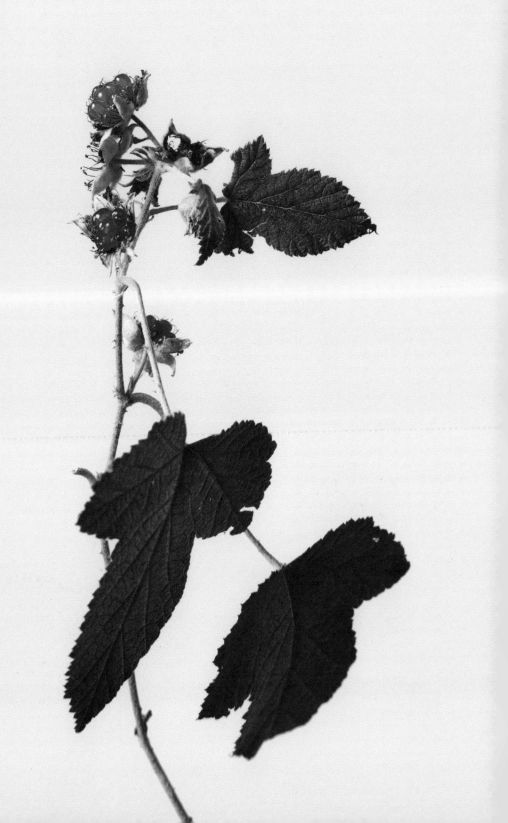

Wild raspberry

COMMON NAMES:

Wild raspberry

SPECIES:

Rubus spp. Pictured is *Rubus moluccanus*.
There are 250–700 *Rubus* species.

GENUS:

Rubus

FAMILY:

Rosaceae

DISTRIBUTION:

Native to Europe. Naturalised in Australia,
New Zealand, North America and South
America.

PLANT SPIRIT QUALITIES:

Wild raspberry helps you find the balance
between high and low standards. If you
are overly fussy and nitpicky, expecting
everything to always be perfect, wild
raspberry encourages you to relax. When
you are lazy and sloppy, it will inspire
you to raise your standards and do a
better job. It can smooth friction caused
by extreme behaviour, thoughts, actions
and expectations, by helping us find the
right balance of freedom and discipline
so that life becomes smoother and more
harmonious. **Key word — perfectionism.**

How to identify it

Rubus rosifolius

- The plant has pale to dark green compound leaves, ending with two leaves on either side, with a single leaf at the very end.
- The leaves have toothed margins, with glandular hairs on both sides of the leaflets.
- Leaves stay green all year.
- Stems are covered in sharp prickles.
- Flowers are white, either in panicles or solitary.
- Red, edible aggregate fruits are 2 cm (¾ inch) long, and ripen in late summer to early autumn in eastern Australia.
- Roots form runners, which give rise to multiple plants, facilitating wide spreading of plants.

Rubus moluccanus

- *Rubus moluccanus* is a tall shrub that can form thickets up to 10 metres (30 feet) across.
- The stems have stiff prickles.
- The oval to heart-shaped leaves can be up to 25 cm (10 inches) in diameter, in contrast to the thin lance-shaped leaves of *R. rosifolius*. The leaves are also a darker shade of green than those of *R. rosifolius*.
- The leaf margins are finely toothed.
- *R. moluccanus* has white or pink flowers in spring and summer.
- The bright red fruit ripens in late summer to early autumn and is 1–3 cm (½–1¼ inches) in diameter.
- *R. moluccanus* is quite variable, with five taxonomic varieties recognised.

How to harvest

Leaves

Raspberry leaves are best harvested in early summer, when they have a nice flush of new growth. Wearing gloves and using secateurs, cut the leaves off the prickly stems, or cut stems below the lowest leaf, letting them fall into a basket or bag. Leaves can be used fresh or dried.

Berries

Berries can be picked by hand during fruiting in late summer to early autumn. They can be eaten fresh or frozen for later use.

Nutrients

The fruit of wild raspberries is a great source of antioxidants, carbohydrates, vitamins A, B, C, E and folate, and is rich in minerals, especially manganese, calcium, magnesium, selenium and phosphorus. It also contains ferric citrate (a form of iron), which makes it useful in anaemia.

Culinary uses

The fruit is eaten raw or cooked in all manner of desserts, jams and sauces. It can be used daily on breakfast cereal, in fruit salads and smoothies, or eaten on its own as a snack. Raspberry cordial also has antibacterial effects.

Folk medicine

The most common *Rubus* species used in medicine is *R. idaeus,* or *R. strigosus,* which used to be considered a subspecies of *R. idaeus.*

Midwives and herbalists around the world have used raspberry leaf for women during their childbearing years, as it is thought to nourish both mother and child, facilitate an easier labour, ease after-birth pains and stimulate breast milk production. It has also been used for nausea in morning sickness, and for heavy menstrual bleeding and period pain.

While it is mainly thought of as a herb for the female reproductive system, it has also been used to treat diarrhoea and constipation. It can also be used for sore throats, mouths and eyes, particularly where there is inflammation, pain and a discharge of either pus or mucus.

Research

Clinical trials on *Rubus* species — in particular *Rubus idaeus* — have confirmed their use in the following areas: antioxidant,[1] antibacterial and anti-diarrhoea[2] and diabetes.[3]

Clinical trials on *Rubus rosifolius* have confirmed its use in the following areas: antioxidant[4] and diabetes.[5]

How to use it as a medicine

Drink an infusion of 2–4 teaspoons of dried leaves or 3–6 chopped fresh leaves per cup (250 ml) of hot boiled water, three times per day. (For a stronger medicinal drink, you can let it stand overnight and drink it the next day. It can be diluted with water until palatable.)

CAUTIONS + CONTRAINDICATIONS

In the first trimester of pregnancy, it should not be used without the supervision of your medical practitioner. It is typically only recommended from 18–20 weeks of pregnancy until birth or afterwards, especially if needed for breast milk production.

Avoid in instances of constipation due to dehydration and tightness in the bowel. However, in constipation caused by a lack of tone, it can be beneficial.

Use the leaves with caution if you have low iron, as their high tannin content can reduce the absorption of nutrients. This is rarely an issue if taken at least 2 hours away from meals. The fruit, on the other hand, can be beneficial for low iron levels, being high in ferric citrate and vitamin C.

Wild raspberry can also be used in:
- Wild greens powder
- Wild raspberry glycetract

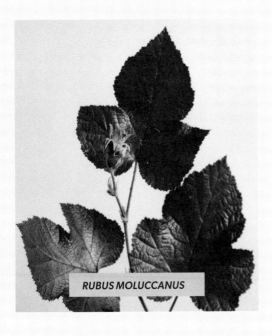

RUBUS MOLUCCANUS

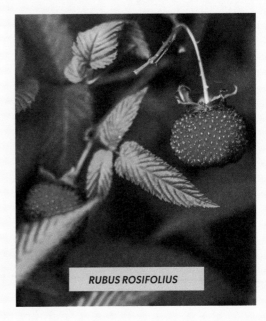

RUBUS ROSIFOLIUS

Wild raspberry muffins

Light in texture and full of fruit, these vegan muffins are a great way to use wild raspberries. The raspberry and yogurt combination is fresh and tangy and creates a very moist muffin — and we all know how disappointing a dry muffin can be!

MAKES 12 REGULAR OR 6 LARGE MUFFINS

45 MINUTES

1 medium banana

¾ cup (185 g) vegan yoghurt

¼ cup (60 ml) rice bran oil

1 teaspoon pure vanilla extract

1½ cups (210 g) plain (all-purpose) spelt flour, or gluten-free all-purpose flour

1 cup (130 g) coconut or rapadura sugar

2 teaspoons baking powder

½ teaspoon bicarbonate of soda (baking soda)

a pinch of salt

1½ cups (185 g) fresh wild raspberries

Preheat the oven to 180°C (350°F) and grease a 12-hole muffin tin, or two 6-hole muffin tins.

Lightly mash the banana in a bowl, then add the yoghurt, oil and vanilla and mix into a paste.

In another bowl, mix together the flour, coconut sugar, baking powder, bicarbonate of soda and salt.

Add the wet ingredients and gently stir in a figure-eight motion until combined. Don't overmix, as you want the batter to have air bubbles, to ensure lighter muffins.

Set aside 12 of the best raspberries to garnish the muffins. Cut the remaining raspberries in half, then very gently fold them through the batter. (It's best to cut them up so they cook better in the batter.)

Spoon the batter into the muffin holes, filling each one only halfway, to give the muffins space to rise. Top each muffin with a raspberry.

Bake for 20–30 minutes, or until a skewer poked in the centre comes out clean.

Remove from the oven, then let the muffins cool in the tin before turning out onto a wire rack or wooden chopping board.

There is A LOT of moisture in these muffins, so they might become soggy after a day or two. Store them in an airtight container with paper towel under and over them and they will keep on the bench for 2–3 days, or in the fridge for up to 1 week.

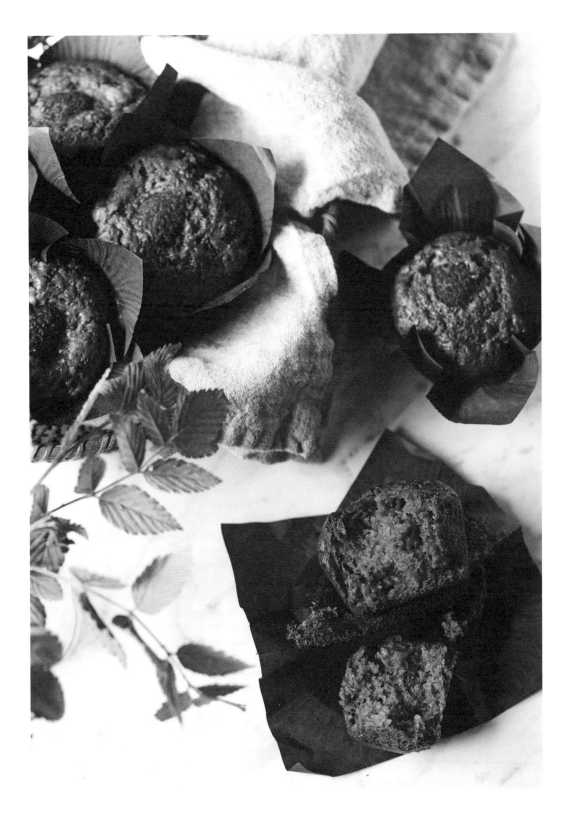

Wild raspberry leaf fermented tea

Fermenting berry leaves brings out a rich, fruity flavour that is much more aromatic than just the dried leaves on their own. Fermentation also produces beneficial probiotics and anti-inflammatory effects. Raspberry tones and strengthens the blood vessels and is beneficial to the gut microbiome.

**MAKES 10 SERVES
(10 TEASPOONS)**

**30 MINUTES +
7 DAYS FERMENTING
AND DEHYDRATING**

GF

4 handfuls of fresh wild raspberry leaves (pulled off the stems wearing a pair of gloves)

Using a sharp knife, scrape the back of each raspberry leaf to remove the tops of the spiky spines. Fold each leaf in half or into quarters, with the spiky side facing inwards. Roll each leaf into a ball and place in a sterilised glass jar (see page 23).

Store the jar in a cupboard for 5–7 days for the leaves to ferment. During this time, they will turn brown.

After a week, dry the leaves by putting them in a dehydrator at a low setting for 12 hours, or in the oven at the lowest setting with the door ajar for 4 hours, or laid flat in a cardboard box in a car in the sun for a day or two. When dry, the leaves should be crunchy.

They are now tea leaves and can be steeped into a tea by adding 1 teaspoon dried leaves to 1 cup (250 ml) hot boiled water.

Store the tea leaves in an airtight container. They will keep in a cool, dark cupboard for up to a year.

Wild raspberry cordial

This sweet, tart cordial has a strong raspberry taste and can be good for diarrhoea, improving the gut microbiome and reducing parasites. You can make it without the sugar (although it won't last as long in the fridge), or sweeten it with ½ cup (125 ml) honey or maple syrup instead.

Serve diluted with chilled still or sparkling water and ice. It's also delicious as a sauce drizzled over ice cream, yoghurt or pancakes.

**MAKES 2 CUPS (500 ML)
30 MINUTES**

GF

2 cups (250 g) wild raspberries

1 cup (185 g) golden caster (superfine) sugar

zest and juice of 1 lemon

Combine all the ingredients in a saucepan with 300 ml (10½ fl oz) water. Bring to a slow rolling boil until the sugar dissolves, then reduce the heat and simmer for 5 minutes. Remove from the heat and allow to cool for 15 minutes.

Stir in the lemon juice, then pour through a sieve set over a bowl, pressing the liquid and pulp through with the back of a spoon.

Pour into a sterilised bottle (see page 23) and seal with the lid. The cordial will keep in the fridge for about 1 month.

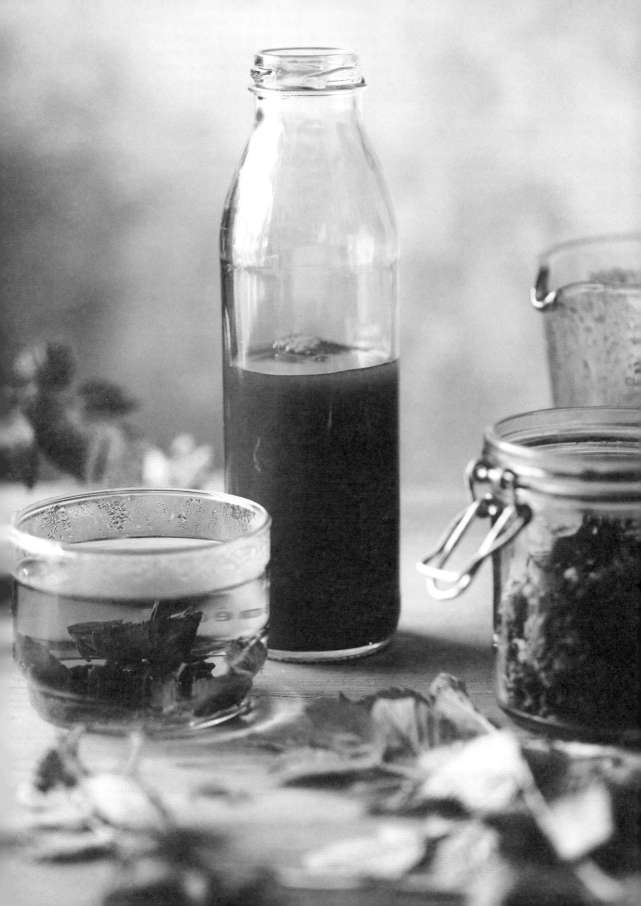

References

SOURCES FOR NUTRITION TABLE, PAGE 14

1. Self Nutrition Data (common vegetables in table 1, all raw), 2018, nutritiondata.self.com

2. Weise V, *Cooking Weeds*. Devon: Prospect Books, 2004.

3. Kallas J, *Edible Wild Plants*. Utah: Gibbs Smith, 2010.

4. Muchuweti M *et al*. Assessment of the nutritional value of wild leafy vegetables consumed in the Buhera district of Zimbabwe: A preliminary study. *Acta Hortic* 2009; 806: 323–30.

5. Plants for a Future, 2019, *Bidens pilosa*, pfaf.org/user/Plant.aspx?LatinName=bidens+pilosa

6. Nutrition and You, *Purslane nutrition facts*, 2019, nutrition-and-you.com/purslane.html

7. Adjatin A *et al*. Proximate, mineral and vitamin C composition of vegetable Gbolo [*Crassocephalum rubens* (Juss. ex Jacq.) S. Moore and *C. crepidioides* (Benth.) S. Moore] in Benin. *Int J Biol Chem Sci* 2013; 710: 319–31.

8. Bomkazi GM *et al*. Nutritional assessment of *Chenopodium album* L. (Imbikicane) young shoots and mature plant-leaves consumed in the Eastern Cape Province of South Africa. *2nd International Conference on Nutrition and Food Sciences IPCBEE* 2013; 53: 97–102.

9. Nutritionvalue.org, 2019, *Amaranth leaves raw*, nutritionvalue.org/Amaranth_leaves%2C_raw_nutritional_value.html

10. Narzary H *et al*. Proximate and vitamin-C analysis of wild edible plants consumed by Bodos of Assam, India. *J Mol Pathophysiol* 2015; 4: 11–16.

AMARANTH

1. Yong YY *et al*. Biofilm inhibiting activity of betacyanins from red pitahaya (*Hylocereus olyrhizus*) and red spinach (*Amaranthus dubius*) against *Staphylococcus aureus* and *Pseudomonas aeruginosa* biofilms. *J Appl Microbiol* 2018; 126(1): 68–78.

2. Sabbione AV *et al*. Amaranth peptides decreased the activity and expression of cellular tissue factor on LPS activated THP-1 human monocytes. *Food Funct* 2018; 17(7): 3823–34.

3. Nardo AE *et al*. Amaranth as a source of antihypertensive peptides. *Front Plant Sci* 2020; 11: 578631.

4. Baraniak J *et al*. The dual nature of amaranth-functional food and potential medicine. *Foods* 2022; 11(4): 618.

5. Valenzuela Z *et al*. Amaranth, quinoa and chia bioactive peptides: a comprehensive review on three ancient grains and their potential role in management and prevention of type 2 diabetes. *Crit Rev Food Sci Nutr* 2022; 62(10): 2707–21.

ASTHMA WEED

1. Sharma N *et al*. Evaluation of the antioxidant, anti-inflammatory, and anticancer activities of *Euphorbia hirta* ethanolic extract. *Molecules* 2014; 19(9): 14567–81.

Balasubramanian B *et al*. Protective effect of *Euphorbia thymifolia* and *Euphorbia hirta* against carbon tetrachloride-induced hepatotoxicity in Wistar rats. *Drug Dev Ind Pharm* 2022; 48(8): 406–16.

Xia M *et al*. Anti-inflammatory and anxiolytic activities of *Euphorbia hirta* extract in neonatal asthmatic rats. *AMB Express* 2018; 8(1): 179.

2. Ibid.

Ahmad SF *et al*. Anti-inflammatory effect of *Euphorbia hirta* in an adjuvant-induced arthritic murine model. *Immunol Invest* 2014; 43(3): 197–211.

3. Singh GD *et al*. Inhibition of early and late phase allergic reactions by *Euphorbia hirta* L. *Phytother Res* 2006; 20(4): 316–21.

Gil TY *et al*. *Euphorbia hirta* leaf ethanol extract suppresses TNF-alpha/IFN-gamma-induced inflammatory response via down-regulating JNK or STAT1/3 pathways in human keratinocytes. *Life* (Basel) 2022; 12(4): 589.

Youssouf MS *et al*. Anti-anaphylactic effect of *Euphorbia hirta*. *Fitoterapia* 2007; 78(7–8): 535–9.

4. Ahmad SF *et al*. Anti-inflammatory effect of *Euphorbia hirta* in an adjuvant-induced arthritic murine model. *Immunol Invest* 2014; 43(3): 197–211.

Chen J *et al*. In vitro anti-inflammatory activity of fractionated *Euphorbia hirta* aqueous extract on rabbit synovial fibroblasts. *Biomed J* 2015; 38(4): 301–6.

Lee KH *et al*. The effect of water extracts of *Euphorbia hirta* on cartilage degeneration in arthritic rats. *Malays J Pathol* 2008; 30(2): 95–102.

5. Gyuris A *et al*. Antiviral activities of extracts of *Euphorbia hirta* L. against HIV-1, HIV-2 and SIVmac251. *In Vivo* 2009; 23(3): 429–32.

6. Perumal S *et al*. Chemical analysis, inhibition of biofilm formation and biofilm eradication potential of *Euphorbia hirta* L. against clinical isolates and standard strains. *BMC Complement Altern Med* 2013; 13: 346.

Perumal S *et al*. Anti-infective potential of caffeic acid and epicatechin 3-gallate isolated from methanol extract of *Euphorbia hirta* (L.) against *Pseudomonas aeruginosa*. *Nat Prod Res* 2015; 29(18): 1766–9.

7. Kumar S *et al*. *Euphorbia hirta*: its chemistry, traditional and medicinal uses, and pharmacological activities. *Pharmacogn Rev* 2010; 4(7): 58–61.

BLACKBERRY NIGHTSHADE

1. Javed T *et al*. In-vitro antiviral activity of *Solanum nigrum* against hepatitis C virus. *Virology J* 2011; 19(8): 26.

Sharma D *et al*. *Solanum nigrum* L. in COVID-19 and post-COVID complications: a propitious candidate. *Mol Cell Biochem* 2023; 1: 20.

2. Zakaria ZA *et al*. Antinociceptive, anti-inflammatory and antipyretic effects of *Solanum nigrum* aqueous extract in animal models. *Methods Find Exp Clin Pharmacol* 2009; 31 (2): 81–8.

3. Campisi A *et al*. Antioxidant activities of *Solanum nigrum* L. leaf extracts determined in in vitro cellular models. *Foods* 2019; 8(2): 63.

Akula US *et al*. In vitro 5-lipoxygenase inhibition of polyphenolic antioxidants from undomesticated plants of South Africa. *J Med Plants Res* 2008; 2: 207–12.

Ravi V *et al*. Anti-inflammatory effect of methanolic extract of *Solanum nigrum* Linn. berries. *Int J Appl Res Nat Prod* 2009; 2: 33–6.

Chen X *et al*. *Solanum nigrum* Linn.: an insight into current research on traditional uses, phytochemistry, and pharmacology. *Front Pharmacol* 2022; 13: 918071.

4. Wannang NN *et al*. Anti-seizure activity of the aqueous leaf extract of *Solanum nigrum* linn. (Solanaceae) in experimental animals. *Afr Health Sci* 2008; 8: 74–9.

5. Lin HM *et al*. Hepatoprotective effects of *Solanum nigrum* Linn. extract against CCl(4)-induced oxidative damage in rats. *Chem Biol Interact J* 2008; 171: 283–93.

6. Chen X *et al*. *Solanum nigrum* Linn.: an insight into current research on traditional uses, phytochemistry, and pharmacology. *Front Pharmacol* 2022; 13: 918071.

BLUE TOP

1. Durodola JJ. Antibacterial property of crude extracts from herbal wound healing remedy – *Ageratum conyzoides*. *Planta Med* 1977; 32(8): 388–90.

Almagboul AZ *et al*. Antimicrobial activity of certain Sudanese plants in folkloric medicine: screening for antibacterial activity. *Part II Fitoterapia* 1985; 56: 103–9.

Nogueira J *et al*. *Ageratum conyzoides* essential oil as aflatoxin suppressor of *Aspergillus flavus*. *Int J Food Microbiol* 2010; 137(1): 55–60.

Abena JAA *et al*. Analgesic effects of a raw extract of *Ageratum conyzoides* in the rat. *Encephale* 1993; 19(4): 329–32.

Marques Neto JF *et al*. Effects of *Ageratum conyzoides* L. in the treatment of osteoarthritis. *Revista Brasil Reumatol* 1988; 28(4): 109–14.

2. Chahal R *et al*. *Ageratum conyzoides* L. and its secondary metabolites in the management of different fungal pathogens. *Molecules* 2021; 26(10): 2933.

3. Abena JAA *et al*. Analgesic effects of a raw extract of *Ageratum conyzoides* in the rat. *Encephale* 1993; 19(4): 329–32.

Hossain H *et al*. Antinociceptive and anti-oxidant potential of the crude ethanol extract of the leaves of *Ageratum conyzoides* grown in Bangladesh. *Pharma Biol* 2013; 51(7): 893–8.

4. Detering M *et al*. *Ageratum conyzoides* L. inhibits 5-alpha-reductase gene expression in human prostate cells and reduces symptoms of benign prostatic hypertrophy in otherwise healthy men in a double blind randomized placebo controlled clinical study. *BioFactors* 2017; 43(6): 789–800.

5. Adelakun SA *et al*. Therapeutic effects of aqueous extract of bioactive active component of *Ageratum conyzoides* on the ovarian-uterine and hypophysis-gonadal axis in rat with polycystic ovary syndrome: Histomorphometric evaluation and biochemical assessment. *Metabol Open* 2022; 15: 100201.

6. Durodola JJ. Antibacterial property of crude extracts from herbal wound healing remedy – *Ageratum conyzoides*. *Planta Med* 1977; 32(8): 388–90.

   Chah KF *et al*. Antibacterial and wound healing properties of methanolic extracts of some Nigerian medicinal plants. *J Ethnopharmacol* 2006; 104(1): 164–7.

7. Hossain H *et al*. Antinociceptive and antioxidant potential of the crude ethanol extract of the leaves of *Ageratum conyzoides* grown in Bangladesh. *Pharmaceut Biol* 2013; 51(7): 893–8.

   Adebayo AH *et al*. Anticancer and antiradical scavenging activity of *Ageratum conyzoides* L. (Asteraceae). *Pharmacognosy* 2010; 6(21): 62.

   Yadav N *et al*. Phytochemical constituents and ethnopharmacological properties of *Ageratum conyzoides* L. *Phytother Res* 2019; 33(9): 2163–78.

8. Agunbiade OS *et al*. Hypoglycaemic activity of *Commelina africana* and *Ageratum conyzoides* in relation to their mineral composition. *Afr Health Sci* 2012; 12(2): 198–203.

   Nyunaï N *et al*. Hypoglycaemic and antihyperglycaemic activity of *Ageratum conyzoides* L. in rats. *Afr J Tradit Complement Altern Med* 2009; 6(2): 123–30.

9. Singh, SB *et al*. Ethnobotany, phytochemistry and pharmacology of *Ageratum conyzoides* Linn (Asteraceae). *J Med Plants Res* 2013; 7(8): 371–85.

BROADLEAF PLANTAIN

1. Cardoso FCI *et al*. A protocol for systematic review of *Plantago major* L. effectiveness in accelerating wound-healing in animal models. *Syst Rev* 2019; 8(1): 337.

   Ashkani-Esfahani S *et al*. The healing effect of *Plantago major* and *Aloe vera* mixture in excisional full thickness skin wounds: stereological study. *World J Plast Surg* 2019; 8(1): 51–7.

   Zubair M *et al*. Promotion of wound healing by *Plantago major* L. leaf extracts: ex-vivo experiments confirm experiences from traditional medicine. *Nat Prod Res* 2016; 30(5): 622–4.

   Thomé RG *et al*. Evaluation of healing wound and genotoxicity potentials from extracts hydroalcoholic of *Plantago major* and *Siparuna guianensis*. *Exp Biol Med* (Maywood) 2012; 237(12): 1379–86.

   Anaya-Mancipe JM *et al*. Electrospun nanofibers loaded with *Plantago major* L. extract for potential use in cutaneous wound healing. *Pharmaceutics* 2023; 15(4): 1047.

2. Chiang LC *et al*. In vitro cytotoxic, antiviral and immunomodulatory effects of *Plantago major* and *Plantago asiatica*. *Am J Chinese Med* 2003; 31(2): 225–34.

3. Hetland G *et al*. Protective effect of *Plantago major* L. pectin polysaccharide against systemic *Streptococcus pneumoniae* infection in mice. *Scand J Immunol* 2000; 52(4): 348–55.

   Chiang LC *et al*. Antiviral activity of *Plantago major* extracts and related compounds in vitro. *Antiviral Res* 2002; 55(1): 53–62.

4. Oto G *et al*. *Plantago major* protective effects on antioxidant status after administration of 7,12-Dimethylbenz(a)anthracene in rats. *Asian Pacific J Cancer Prev* 2011; 12(2): 531 5.

   Türel I *et al*. Hepatoprotective and anti-inflammatory activities of *Plantago major* L. *Indian J Pharm* 2009; 41(3): 20–4.

5. Boskabadi J *et al*. The relaxant effect of *Plantago major* on rat tracheal smooth muscles and its possible mechanisms. *Iran J Allergy Asthma Immunol* 2020; 19(4): 386–96.

   Farokhi F *et al*. Histopathologic changes of lung in asthmatic male rats treated with hydro-alcoholic extract of *Plantago major* and theophylline. *Avicenna J Phytomed* 2013; 3(2): 143–51.

CAT'S EAR

1. Senguttuvan J *et al*. Phytochemical analysis and evaluation of leaf and root parts of the medicinal herb, *Hypochaeris radicata* L. for in vitro antioxidant activities. *Asian Pac J Trop Biomed* 2014; 4: S359–67.

2. Jamuna S *et al*. In-vitro antibacterial activity of leaf and root extracts of *Hypochaeris radicata* L. (Asteraceae) – a medicinal plant species inhabiting the high hills of Nilgiris, the Western Ghats. *Int J Pharm Pharmaceut Sci* 2013; 5(1): 175–8.

3. Senguttuvan J *et al*. In vitro antifungal activity of leaf and root extracts of the medicinal plant, *Hypochaeris radicata* L. *Int J Pharm Pharmaceut Sci* 2013; 5: 758–61.

CHICKWEED

1. Rani N *et al*. Quality assessment and anti-obesity activity of *Stellaria media* (Linn.) Vill. *BMC Complement Altern Med* 2012; 12(1): 106.

   Chidrawar V *et al*. Antiobesity effect of *Stellaria media* against drug induced obesity in Swiss albino mice. *AYU* (*Int Quarterly J Res Ayurveda*), 2011; 32(4): 576.

2. Shan Y *et al*. Purification and characterization of a novel anti-HSV-2 protein with antiproliferative and peroxidase activities from *Stellaria media*. *Acta Biochimica et Biophysica Sinica* 2013; 45(8): 649–55.

   Ma L *et al*. Anti-hepatitis B virus activity of chickweed [*Stellaria media* (L.) Vill.] extracts in hepG2.2.15 cells. *Molecules* 2012; 17(7): 8633–46.

3. Rogozhin EA *et al*. A novel antifungal peptide from leaves of the weed *Stellaria media* L. *Biochimie* 2015; 116: 125–32.

4. Gorina YV *et al*. Evaluation of hepatoprotective activity of water-soluble polysaccharide fraction of *Stellaria media* L. *Bull Exp Biol Med* 2013; 154(5): 645–8.

CHINESE MUGWORT

1. Wang M *et al*. Sesquiterpene lactones from *Artemisia verlotiorum* and their anti-inflammatory activities. *Fitoterapia* 2023; 169: 105560.

2. de Lima TC *et al*. Evaluation of the central properties of *Artemisia verlotiorum*. *Planta Med* 1993; 59(4): 326–9.

3. Calderone V *et al*. Vascular effects of aqueous crude extracts of *Artemisia verlotiorum* Lamotte (Compositae): in vivo and in vitro pharmacological studies in rats. *Phytother Res* 1999; 13(8): 645–8.

4. Cafarchia C *et al*. Antifungal activity of essential oils from leaves and flowers of *Inula viscosa* (Asteraceae) by Apulian region. *Parassitologia* 2002; 44(3–4): 153–6.

CLEAVERS

1. Ilina T *et al*. Phytochemical profiles and in vitro immunomodulatory activity of ethanolic extracts from *Galium aparine* L. *Plants* (Basel) 2019; 8(12): 541.

2. Sharifi-Rad M *et al*. Anti-methicillin-resistant *Staphylococcus aureus* (MRSA) activity of Rubiaceae, Fabaceae and Poaceae plants: a search for new sources of useful alternative antibacterials against MRSA infections. *J Cell Molec Biol* (Noisy le Grand) 2016; 62(9): 39–45.

3. Laanet PR *et al*. Phytochemical screening and antioxidant activity of selected Estonian *Galium* species. *Molecules* 2023; 28(6): 2867.

5. Quinlan FJ. *Galium aparine* as a remedy for chronic ulcers. *BMJ* 1883; 1(1172): 1173–4.

CLOVER, WHITE

1. Ahmad S *et al*. Phytochemical profile and pharmacological properties of *Trifolium repens*. [published online ahead of print] *J Basic Clin Physiol Pharmacol* 2020, Aug 10: /j/jbcpp.ahead-of-print/jbcpp-2020-0015/ jbcpp-2020-0015.xml

2. Tundis R *et al*. *Trifolium repens* and *T. repens* (Leguminosae): edible flower extracts as functional ingredients. *Foods* 2015; (3): 338–48.

COBBLER'S PEGS

1. Yan Z *et al*. Bioactive polyacetylenes from *Bidens pilosa* L and their anti-inflammatory activity. *Nat Prod Res* 2022; 36(24): 6353–8.

   Pereira RL *et al*. Immunosuppressive and anti-inflammatory effects of methanolic extract and the polyacetylene isolated from *Bidens pilosa* L. *Immunopharmacology* 1999; 43(1): 31–7.

2. Bartolome AP *et al*. *Bidens pilosa* L. (Asteraceae): botanical properties, traditional uses, phytochemistry, and pharmacology. *Evid Based Complement Altern Med* 2013; 2013: 340215.

   Chang SL *et al*. Polyacetylenic compounds and butanol fractions from *Bidens pilosa* can modulate the differentiation of helper T cells and prevent autoimmune diabetes in non-obese diabetic mice. *Planta Med* 2004; 70(11): 1045–51.

   Ubillas RP *et al*. Antihyperglycemic acetylenic glucosides from *Bidens pilosa*. *Planta Med* 2000; 66(1): 82–3.

   Hsu YJ *et al*. Anti-hyperglycemic effects and mechanism of *Bidens pilosa* water extract. *J Ethnopharmacol* 2009; 122(2): 379–83.

3. Yoshida N *et al*. *Bidens pilosa* supresses interleukin-1beta-induced cyclooxygenase-2 expression through inhibition of mitogen activated protein kinases phosphorylation in normal human dermal fibroblasts. *J Pharmacol Exp Therapeut* 2006; 318(1): 181–7.

   Seyama MH *et al*. Improvement of the anti-inflammatory and antiallergic activity of *Bidens pilosa* L var. *radiata* SCHERFF treated with enzyme (Cellulosine). *J Health* 2008; 54(3): 294–301.

4. Xagorari A *et al*. Luteolin inhibits an endotoxin-stimulated phosphorylation cascade and proinflammatory cytokine production in macrophages. *J Pharmacol Exp Therapeut* 2001; 296(1): 181–7.

   Chiang YM *et al*. Cytopiloyne, a novel polyacetylenic glucoside from *Bidens pilosa*, functions as a T helper cell modulator. *J Ethnopharmacol* 2007; 110(3): 532–8.

   Xuan TD *et al*. Chemistry and pharmacology of *Bidens pilosa*: an overview. *J Pharm Investig* 2016; 46(2): 91–132.

Chang SL et al. Flavonoids, centaurein and centaureidin, from *Bidens pilosa*, stimulate IFN-β expression. *J Ethnopharmacol* 2007; 112(2): 232–6.

Chang CLT et al. The distinct effects of a butanol fraction of *Bidens pilosa* plant extract on the development of TH1-mediated diabetes and Th2-mediated airway inflammation in mice. *J Biomed Sci* 2005; 12(1): 79–89.

5. Chiang YM et al. Metabolite profiling and chemopreventive bioactivity of plant extracts from *Bidens pilosa*. *J Ethnopharmacol* 2004; 95(2–3): 409–19.

Muchuweti M et al. Screening of antioxidant and radical scavenging activity of *Vigna ungiculata*, *Bidens pilosa* and *Cleome gynandra*. *Am J Food Technol* 2007; 2(3): 161–8.

Yoshida N et al. *Bidens pilosa* supresses interleukin-1beta-induced cyclooxygenase-2 expression through inhibition of mitogen activated protein kinases phosphorylation in normal human dermal fibroblasts. *J Pharmacol Exp Therapeut* 2006; 296(1): 181–7.

Deba F et al. Chemical composition and antioxidant, antibacterial and antifungal activities of the essential oils from *Bidens pilosa* Linn. var. *Radiata*. *Food Control* 2008; 19(4): 346–52.

6. Bartolome AP et al. *Bidens pilosa* L. (Asteraceae): botanical properties, traditional uses, phytochemistry, and pharmacology. *Evid Based Complement Altern Med* 2013.

7. Shandukani PD et al. Antibacterial activity and in situ efficacy of *Bidens pilosa* Linn and *Dichrostachys cinerea* Wight et Arn extracts against common diarrhoea-causing waterborne bacteria. *BMC Complement Altern Med* 2018; 18(1): 171.

Chiang YM et al. Cytopiloyne, a novel polyacetylenic glucoside from *Bidens pilosa*, functions as a T helper cell modulator. *J Ethnopharmacol* 2007; 110(3): 532–8.

Deba F et al. Chemical composition and antioxidant, antibacterial and antifungal activities of the essential oils from *Bidens pilosa* Linn. var. *Radiata*. *Food Control* 2008; 19(4): 346–52.

Afolayan AO. Screening the root extracts from *Bidens pilosa* L. var. *Radiata* (Asteraceae) for antimicrobial potentials. *J Med Plant Res* 2009; 3(8): 568–72.

Tobinaga S et al. Isolation and identification of a potent antimalarial and antibacterial polyacetylene from *Bidens pilosa*. *Planta Med* 2009; 75(6): 624–8.

8. Gomez AA et al. Antifungal and antimycotoxigenic metabolites from native plants of northwest Argentina: isolation, identification and potential for control of *Aspergillus* species. *Nat Prod Res* 2020; 34(22): 3299–302.

Deba F et al. Chemical composition and antioxidant, antibacterial and antifungal activities of the essential oils from *Bidens pilosa* Linn. var. *Radiata*. *Food Control* 2008; 19(4): 346–52.

Deba F et al. Herbicidal and fungicidal activities and identification of potential phytotoxins from *Bidens pilosa* L var. *radiata* Scherff. *Weed Biol Manag* 2007; 7(2): 77–83.

Afolayan AO. Screening the root extracts from *Bidens pilosa* L. var. *Radiata* (Asteraceae) for antimicrobial potentials. *J Med Plant Res* 2009; 3(8): 568–72.

9. Dimo T et al. Possible mechanisms of action of the neutral extract from *Bidens pilosa* L. leaves on the cardiovascular system of anaesthetized rats. *Phytother Res* 2003; 17(10): 1135–9.

Dimo T et al. Hypotensive effects of methanol extract from *Bidens pilosa* and *Ocimum suave*. *Afr J Pharm Pharmacol* 2011; 5(2): 132–6.

Nguelefack TB et al. Relaxant effects of the neutral extract of the leaves of *Bidens pilosa* Linn on isolated rat vascular smooth muscle. *Phytother Res* 2005; 19(3): 207–10.

10. Kyakulaga HA et al. Wound healing potential of the ethanolic extracts of *Bidens pilosa* and *Ocimum suave*. *Afr J Pharm Pharmacol* 2011; 5(2): 132–6.

11. Tan PV et al. Effects of methanol, cyclohexane and methylene chloride extracts of *Bidens pilosa* on various gastric ulcer models in rats. *J Ethnopharmacol* 2000; 73(3): 415–21.

Yamamoto K et al. Gastric cytoprotective anti-ulcerogenic actions of hydroxychalcones in rats. *Planta Med* 1992; 58(5): 389–93.

DANDELION

1. Kamal FZ et al. Chemical composition, antioxidant and antiproliferative activities of *Taraxacum officinale* essential oil. *Molecules* 2022; 27(19): 6477.

2. Newell CA et al. *Herbal Medicines: A Guide for Health-Care Professionals*. London: The Pharmaceutical Press, 1996.

3. Pfingstgraf IO et al. Protective effects of *Taraxacum officinale* L. (dandelion) root extract in experimental acute chronic liver failure. *Antioxidants* (Basel) 2021; 10(4): 504.

Xu L et al. Protective effects of taraxasterol against ethanol-induced liver injury by regulating CYP2E1/Nrf2/HO-1 and NF-kB signaling pathways in mice. *Oxid Med Cell Longev* 2018; 8284107.

Hfaiedh M et al. Hepatoprotective effect of *Taraxacum officinale* leaf extract on sodium dichromate-induced liver injury in rats. *Environ Toxicol* 2016; 31(3): 339–49.

Maliakal PP et al. Effect of herbal teas on hepatic drug metabolizing enzymes in rats. *J Pharmaceutics Pharmacol* 2001; 53(10): 1323–9.

4. Li W et al. Anti-inflammatory effects and mechanisms of dandelion in RAW264.7 macrophages and zebrafish larvae. *Front Pharmacol* 2022; 13: 906927.

Tita B. *Taraxacum officinale* W: pharmacological effect of ethanol extract. *Pharmacol Res* 1993; 27(1): 23–4.

Newell CA et al. *Herbal Medicines: A Guide for Health-Care Professionals*. London: The Pharmaceutical Press, 1996.

Cho S. Alternation of hepatic antioxidant enzyme activities and lipid profile in streptozotocin induced diabetic rats by supplementation of dandelion water extract. *Clinica Chimica Acta* 2002; 317(1–2): 109–17.

5. Wirngo FE et al. The physiological effects of dandelion (*Taraxacum officinale*) in type 2 diabetes. *Rev Diabet Stud* 2016; 13(2–3): 113–31.

6. Kania-Dobrowolska M et al. Dandelion (*Taraxacum officinale* L.) as a source of biologically active compounds supporting the therapy of co-existing diseases in metabolic syndrome. *Foods* 2022; 11(18): 2858.

DOCK

1. Lee KH et al. Antimalarial activity of nepodin isolated from *Rumex crispus*. *Arch Pharmacol Res* 2013; 36(4): 430–5.

2. Pelzer CV et al. More than just a weed: an exploration of the antimicrobial activity of *Rumex crispus* using a multivariate data analysis approach. *Planta Med* 2022; 88(9–10): 753–61.

3. Shiwani S et al. Carbohydrase inhibition and anti-cancerous and free radical scavenging properties along with DNA and protein protection ability of methanolic root extracts of *Rumex crispus*. *Nutr Res Pract* 2012; 6(5): 389–95.

4. Maksimović Z et al. Antioxidant activity of yellow dock (*Rumex crispus* L. Polygonaceae) fruit extract. *Phytother Res* 2011; 25(1): 10–15.

5. Park ES et al. *Rumex crispus* and *Cordyceps militaris* mixture ameliorates production of pro-inflammatory cytokines induced by lipo-polysaccharide in C57BL/6 mice splenocytes. *Prev Nutr Food Sci* 2018; 23(4): 374–81.

6. Süntar I et al. Preventive effect of *Rumex crispus* L. on surgically induced intra-abdominal adhesion model in rats. *Daru* 2021; 29(1): 101–15.

FAT HEN

1. Amodeo V et al. *Chenopodium album* L. and *Sisymbrium officinale* (L.) Scop.: phytochemical content and in vitro antioxidant and anti-inflammatory potential. *Plants* (Basel) 2019; 8(11): 505.

Adedapo A et al. Comparison of the nutritive value and biological activities of the acetone, methanol and water extracts of the leaves of *Bidens pilosa* and *Chenopodium album*. *Acta Poloniae Pharmaceutica* 2011; 68(1): 83–92.

Kaur C et al. Anti-oxidant activity and total phenolic content of some Asian vegetables. *Int J Food Sci Technol* 2002; 37: 153–61.

Elif Korcan S et al. Evaluation of antibacterial, antioxidant and DNA protective capacity of *Chenopodium album*'s ethanolic leaf extract. *Chemosphere* 2013; 90(2): 374–9.

2. Chamkhi I et al. Genetic diversity, antimicrobial, nutritional, and phytochemical properties of *Chenopodium album*: a comprehensive review. *Food Res Int* 2022; 154: 110979.

3. Singh PK et al. Evaluation of antibacterial activities of *Chenopodium album* L. *Int J Appl Biol Pharmaceut Technol* 2011; 2(3): 398–401.

Nayak DP et al. Antimicrobial and anthelmintic evaluation of *Chenopodium album*. *Int J Pharma World Res* 2010; 1(4): 1–15.

Elif Korcan S et al. Evaluation of antibacterial, antioxidant and DNA protective capacity of *Chenopodium album*'s ethanolic leaf extract. *Chemosphere* 2013; 90(2): 374–9.

Kaur C et al. Anti-oxidant activity and total phenolic content of some Asian vegetables. *Int J Food Sci Technol* 2002; 37: 153–61.

4. Dutt S et al. Possible mechanism of action of antiviral proteins from the leaves of *Chenopodium album* L. *Indian J Biochem Biophys* 2004; 41(1): 29–33.

5. Amjad L et al. Antibacterial activity of the *Chenopodium album* leaves and flowers extract. *World Acad Sci Engineer Technol* 2012; 61: 903–6.

Jabbar A *et al*. Anthelmintic activity of *Chenopodium album* (L) and *Caesalpinia crista* (L) against trichostrongylid nematodes of sheep. *J Ethnopharmacol* 2007; 114(1): 86–91.

Sharma P *et al*. Phytoextract-induced developmental deformities in malaria vector. *Bioresource Technol* 2006; 97(14): 1599–604.

Russo S *et al*. Effect of extracts of *Chenopodium album* L. on the larval and adult states of *Oryzaephilus surinamensis* L. (Coleoptera: Silvanidae). *IDESIA* 2011; 29(1): 51–7.

6. CABI, 2019. Invasive species compendium, *Chenopodium album* (Fat Hen), www.cabi. org/isc/datasheet/12648#830a2108-328a-4d27-880b-90bc720be91c>

Ahmad, M *et al*. Evaluation of spasmolytic and anlgesic activity of ethanolic extract of *Chenopodium album* Linn and its fractions. *J Med Plants Res* 2012; 6(31): 4691–7.

7. Hussain S *et al*. *Chenopodium album* extract ameliorates carbon tetrachloride induced hepatotoxicity in rat model. *Saudi J Biol Sci* 2022; 29(5): 3408–13.

Nigam V *et al*. Hepatoprotective activity of *Chenopodium album* Linn against paracetamol induced liver damage. *Pharmacol Online* 2011; 3: 312–28.

Pal A *et al*. Hepatoprotective activity of *Chenopodium album* linn. plant against paracetamol induced hepatic injury in rats. *Int J Pharm Pharmaceut Sci* 2013; 3: 55–7.

8. Pande M *et al*. Sexual function improving effect of *Chenopodium albumm* (Bathua sag) in normal male mice. *Biomed Pharmacol J* 2008; 1: 325–32.

Baldi A *et al*. Effect of *Chenopodium album* on sexual behaviour and sperm count in male rats. *Acta Horticulturae* 2013; 972: 22.

Kumar S *et al*. *Chenopodium album* seed extract-induced sperm cell death: exploration of a plausible pathway. *Contraception* 2008; 77(6): 456–62.

Kumar S *et al*. *Chenopodium album* seed extract: a potent sperm-immobilizing agent both in vitro and in vivo. *Contraception* 2007; 75(1): 71–8.

9. Poonia A *et al*. *Chenopodium album* Linn: review of nutritive value and biological properties. *J Food Sci Technol* 2015; 52(7): 3977–85.

FENNEL

1. Domínguez-Vigil IG *et al*. Antigiardial activity of *Foeniculum vulgare* hexane extract and some of its constituents. *Plants* (Basel) 2022; 11(17): 2212.

Rather MA *et al*. *Foeniculum vulgare*: a comprehensive review of its traditional use, phytochemistry, pharmacology, and safety. *Arab J Chem* 2016; 9: S1574–83.

2. Ibid.

3. Ibid.

4. Tognolini M *et al*. Protective effect of *Foeniculum vulgare* essential oil and anethole in an experimental model of thrombosis. *Pharmacol Res* 2007; 56: 254–60.

5. Choi EM *et al*. Anti-inflammatory, analgesic and antioxidant activities of the fruit of *Foeniculum vulgare*. *Fitoterapia* 2004; 75: 557–65.

6. Albert-Puleo M. Fennel and anise as estrogen agents. *J Ethnopharmacol* 1980; 2: 337–44.

7. Mahboubi M. *Foeniculum vulgare* as valuable plant in management of women's health. *J Menopausal Med* 2019; 25(1): 1–14.

Ostad SN *et al*. Effect of fennel essential oil on uterine contraction as a model for dysmenorrhea, pharmacology and toxicology study. *J Ethnopharmacol* 2001; 76: 299–304.

Pattanittum P *et al*. Dietary supplements for dysmenorrhoea. *Cochrane Database Syst Rev* 2016; 3(3): CD002124.

8. Lee HW *et al*. Fennel (*Foeniculum vulgare* Miller) for the management of menopausal women's health: A systematic review and meta-analysis. *Complement Ther Clin Pract* 2021; 43: 101360.

Kargozar R *et al*. A review of effective herbal medicines in controlling menopausal symptoms. *Electron Physician* 2017; 9(11): 5826–33.

9. Ozbek H *et al*. Effect of *Foeniculum vulgare* essential oil. *Fitoterapia* 2003; 74: 317–19.

10. El-Soud NA *et al*. Activities of *Foeniculum vulgare* Mill. essential oil in streptozotocin induced diabetic rats. *Maced J Med Sci* 2011; 4(2): 139–46.

GOTU KOLA

1. Sun B *et al*. Therapeutic potential of *Centella asiatica* and its triterpenes: a review. *Front Pharmacol* 2020; 11: 568032.

Chandrika UG *et al*. Gotu kola (Centella asiatica): nutritional properties and plausible health benefits. *Adv Food Nutr Res* 2015; 76: 125–57.

Ratz-Łyko A *et al*. Moisturizing and anti-inflammatory properties of cosmetic formulations containing *Centella asiatica* extract. *Indian J Pharm Sci* 2016; 78(1): 27–33.

Torbati FA *et al*. Ethnobotany, phytochemistry and pharmacological features of *Centella asiatica*: a comprehensive review. *Adv Exp Med Biol* 2021; 1308: 451–99.

2. Park KS. Pharmacological effects of *Centella asiatica* on skin diseases: evidence and possible mechanisms. *Evid Based Complement Alternat Med* 2021; 2021: 5462633.

Bylka W *et al*. *Centella asiatica* in dermatology: an overview. *Phytother Res* 2014; 28(8): 1117–24.

Gohil K *et al*. Pharmacological review on *Centella asiatica*: a potential herbal cure-all. *Indian J Pharm Sci* 2010; 72(5): 546.

3. Lee Y *et al*. Inhibitory effect of *Centella asiatica* extract on DNCB-induced atopic dermatitis in HaCaT cells and BALB/c mice. *Nutrients* 2020; 12(2): 411.

4. Gohil K *et al*. Pharmacological review on *Centella asiatica*: a potential herbal cure-all. *Indian J Pharm Sci* 2010; 72(5): 546.

5. Cotellese R *et al*. *Centella asiatica* (Centellicum®) facilitates the regular healing of surgical scars in subjects at high risk of keloids. *Minerva Chirurgica* 2018; 73(2): 151–6.

6. Ganie IB *et al*. Biotechnological intervention and secondary metabolite production in *Centella asiatica* L. *Plants* (Basel) 2022; 11(21): 2928.

Puttarak P *et al*. Effects of Centella asiatica (L.) Urb. on cognitive function and mood related outcomes: a systematic review and meta-analysis. *Sci Rep* 2017; 7(1): 10646.

Wong JH *et al*. Mitoprotective effects of *Centella asiatica* (L.) Urb.: anti-Inflammatory and neuroprotective opportunities in

neurodegenerative disease. *Front Pharmacol* 2021; 12: 687935.

Wattanathorn J *et al*. Positive modulation of cognition and mood in the healthy elderly volunteer following the administration of *Centella asiatica*. *J Ethnopharmacol* 2008; 116(2): 325–32.

7. Puttarak P *et al*. Effects of *Centella asiatica* (L.) Urb. on cognitive function and mood related outcomes: a systematic review and meta-analysis. *Sci Rep* 2017; 7(1): 10646.

Wattanathorn J *et al*. Positive modulation of cognition and mood in the healthy elderly volunteer following the administration of *Centella asiatica*. *J Ethnopharmacol* 2008; 116(2): 325–32.

8. Gohil K *et al*. Pharmacological review on *Centella asiatica*: a potential herbal cure-all. *Ind J Pharm Sci* 2010; 72(5): 546.

9. Bradwejn J *et al*. A double-blind, placebo-controlled study on the effects of Gotu kola (*Centella asiatica*) on acoustic startle response in healthy subjects. *J Clin Psychopharmacol* 2000; 20(6): 680–4.

10. Razali NNM *et al*. Cardiovascular protective effects of *Centella asiatica* and its triterpenes: a review. *Planta Med* 2019; 85(16): 1203–15.

HERB ROBERT

1. Swiatek L *et al*. Herb robert's gift against human diseases: anticancer and antimicrobial activity of *Geranium robertianum* L. *Pharmaceutics* 2023; 15(5): 1561.

Graca VC *et al*. Chemical characterization and bioactive properties of aqueous and organic extracts of *Geranium robertianum* L. *Food Funct* 2016; 7(9): 3807–14.

Gebarowska E *et al*. Chemical composition and antimicrobial activity of *Geranium robertianum* L. essential oil. *Acta Pol Pharm* 2017; 74(2): 699–70.

2. Bawish BM *et al*. Promising effect of *Geranium robertianum* L. leaves and aloe vera gel powder on Aspirin®-induced gastric ulcers in Wistar rats: anxiolytic behavioural effect, antioxidant activity, and protective pathways. *Inflammopharmacol* 2023; 31(6): 3183–201.

Graca VC *et al*. Chemical characterization and bioactive properties of aqueous and organic extracts of *Geranium robertianum* L. *Food Funct* 2016; 7(9): 3807–14.

Ben Jemia M *et al*. Antioxidant activity of Tunisian Geranium robertianum L. (Geraniaceae). *Nat Prod Res* 2013; 2(22): 2076–83.

3. Catarino MD *et al*. Antioxidant and anti-inflammatory activities of *Geranium robertianum* L. decoctions. *Food Funct* 2017; 8(9): 3355–65.

4. Paun G *et al*. Evaluation of *Geranium* spp., *Helleborus* spp. and *Hyssopus* spp. polyphenolic extracts inhibitory activity against urease and alpha-chymotrypsin. *J Enzyme Inhib Med Chem* 2014; 29(1): 28–34.

5. Panahi Y *et al*. Investigation of the effectiveness of *Syzygium aromaticum*, *Lavandula angustifolia* and *Geranium robertianum* essential oils in the treatment of acute external otitis: a comparative trial with ciprofloxacin. *J Microbiol Immunol Infect* 2014; 47(3): 211–16.

6. Ferreira FM *et al*. 'MitoTea': *Geranium robertianum* L. decoctions decrease blood glucose levels and improve liver mitochondrial oxidative phosphorylation in diabetic Goto-

Kakizaki rats. *Acta Biochimica Polonica* 2010; 57(4): 399–402.

7. Corina P *et al*. Treatment with acyclovir combined with a new Romanian product from plants. *Oftalmologia*. [Article in Romanian.] 1999; 46(1): 55–7.

8. Bawish BM *et al*. Promising effect of *Geranium robertianum* L. leaves and aloe vera gel powder on Aspirin®-induced gastric ulcers in Wistar rats: anxiolytic behavioural effect, antioxidant activity, and protective pathways. *Inflammopharmacol* 2023; 10.1007/s10787-023-01205-0.

9. Ibid.

LANTANA

1. Carstairs S *et al*. Ingestion of *Lantana camara* is not associated with significant effects in children. *Pediatrics* 2010; 127(2): e1585–8.

2. Kurade N *et al*. Chemical composition and antibacterial activity of essential oils of *Lantana camara*, *Ageratum houstonianum* and *Eupatorium adenophorum*. *Pharm Biol* 2010; 48(5): 539–44.

   Costa J *et al*. Chemical composition and resistance-modifying effect of the essential oil of *Lantana camara* Linn. *Pharmacogn Mag* 2010; 6(22): 79.

3. Badakhshan M *et al*. A comparative study: antimicrobial activity of methanol extracts of *Lantana camara* various parts. *Pharmacogn Res* 2009; 1(6): 348–51.

4. Udappusamy V *et al*. Lantana camara L. essential oil mediated nano-emulsion formulation for biocontrol application: anti-mosquitocidal, anti-microbial and antioxidant assay. *Arch Microbiol* 2022; 204(7): 388.

   Huy Hung N *et al*. *Lantana camara* essential oils from Vietnam: chemical composition, molluscicidal, and mosquito larvicidal activity. *Chem Biodivers* 2021; 18(5): e2100145.

   Murugesan S *et al*. Chemical constituents and toxicity assessment of the leaf oil of *Lantana camara* Linn. from Tamil Nadu regions. *Asian J Plant Sci Res* 2016; 6(3): 32–42.

   Moyo B *et al*. An in-vivo study of the efficacy and safety of ethno-veterinary remedies used to control cattle ticks by rural farmers in the Eastern Cape Province of South Africa. *Trop Anim Health Prod* 2009; 41(7): 1569–76.

   Kandeda AK *et al*. An aqueous extract of Lantana camara attenuates seizures, memory impairment, and anxiety in kainate-treated mice: evidence of GABA level, oxidative stress, immune and neuronal loss modulation. *Epilepsy Behav* 2022; 129: 108611.

5. Udappusamy V *et al*. Lantana camara L. essential oil mediated nano-emulsion formulation for biocontrol application: anti-mosquitocidal, anti-microbial and antioxidant assay. *Arch Microbiol* 2022; 204(7): 388.

   El-Din MIG *et al*. Comparative LC-LTQ-MS-MS analysis of the leaf extracts of *Lantana camara* and *Lantana montevidensis* growing in Egypt with insights into their antioxidant, anti-inflammatory, and cytotoxic activities. *Plants* (Basel) 2022; 11(13): 1699.

6. Kandeda AK *et al*. An aqueous extract of *Lantana camara* attenuates seizures, memory impairment, and anxiety in kainate-treated mice: evidence of GABA level, oxidative stress, immune and neuronal loss modulation. *Epilepsy Behav* 2022; 129: 108611.

MALLOW

1. Barros L *et al*. Leaves, flowers, immature fruits and leafy flowered stems of *Malva sylvestris*: a comparative study of the nutraceutical potential and composition. *Food Chem Toxicol* 2010; 48(6): 1466–72.

2. Mousavi SM *et al*. A review on health benefits of *Malva sylvestris* L. nutritional compounds for metabolites, antioxidants, and anti-inflammatory, anticancer, and antimicrobial applications. *Evid Based Complement Alternat Med* 2021; 2021: 5548404.

   Martins CAF *et al*. Anti-inflammatory effect of *Malva sylvestris*, *Sida cordifolia*, and *Pelargonium graveolens* is related to inhibition of prostanoid production. *Molecules* 2017; 22(11): 1883.

   Benso B *et al*. *Malva sylvestris* inhibits inflammatory response in oral human cells. An in vitro infection model. *PLoS One* 2015; 10(10): e0140331.

   Benso B *et al*. Anti-inflammatory, anti-osteoclastogenic and antioxidant effects of *Malva sylvestris* extract and fractions: in vitro and in vivo studies. *PLoS One* 2016; 11(9).

   Qin H *et al*. *Malva sylvestris* attenuates cognitive deficits in a repetitive mild traumatic brain injury rat model by reducing neuronal degeneration and astrocytosis in the hippocampus. *Med Sci Monit* 2017; 23: 6099–106.

3. Watanabe E *et al*. Determination of the maximum inhibitory dilution of cetylpyridinium chloride-based mouthwashes against *Staphylococcus aureus*: an in vitro study. *J Appl Oral Sci* 2008; 16: 275–9.

   Bonjar S. Evaluation of antibacterial properties of some medicinal plants used in Iran. *J Ethnopharmacol* 2004; 94: 301–5.

   Mousavi SM *et al*. A review on health benefits of *Malva sylvestris* L. nutritional compounds for metabolites, antioxidants, and anti-inflammatory, anticancer, and antimicrobial applications. *Evid Based Complement Alternat Med* 2021; 2021: 5548404.

4. Nasiri E *et al*. Effect of *Malva sylvestris* cream on burn injury and wounds in rats. *Avicenna J Phytomed* 2015; 5(4): 341–54.

   Prudente AS *et al*. Pre-clinical efficacy assessment of *Malva sylvestris* on chronic skin inflammation. *Biomed Pharmacother* 2017; 93: 852–60.

5. Hamedi A *et al*. Effects of *Malva sylvestris* and its isolated polysaccharide on experimental ulcerative colitis in rats. *Evid Based Complement Altern Med* 2016; 21(1): 14–22.

6. Mohamadi Z *et al*. Amelioration of renal and hepatic function, oxidative stress, inflammation and histopathologic damages by *Malva sylvestris* extract in gentamicin induced renal toxicity. *Biomed Pharmacother* 2019; 112: 108635.

   Ben Saad A *et al*. *Malva sylvestris* extract protects upon lithium carbonate-induced kidney damages in male rat. *Biomed Pharmacother* 2016; 84: 1099–107.

   Azmoonfar R *et al*. Radioprotective effect of *Malva sylvestris* L. against radiation-induced liver, kidney and intestine damages in rat: a histopathological study. *Biochem Biophys Rep* 2023; 34: 101455.

   Batiha GE *et al*. The phytochemical profiling, pharmacological activities, and safety of *Malva sylvestris*: a review. *Naunyn Schmiedebergs Arch Pharmacol* 2023; 396(3): 421–40.

7. Benso B *et al*. *Malva sylvestris* inhibits inflammatory response in oral human cells. An in vitro infection model. *PLoS One* 2015;10(10): e0140331.

NASTURTIUM

1. Gasparotto A *et al*. Natriuretic and diuretic effects of *Tropaeolum majus* (Tropaelaceae) in rats. *J Ethnopharmacol* 2009; 122: 517–22.

2. Traka M *et al*. Glucosinolates, isothiocyanates and human health. *Phytochem Rev* 2009; 8: 269–82.

   Kleinwächter M *et al*. The glucosinolate-myrosinase system in nasturtium (*Tropaeolum majus* l.): variability of biochemical parameters and screening for clones feasible for pharmaceutical utilization. *J Agric Food Chem* 2008; 56: 11165–70.

3. Jakubczyk K *et al*. Garden nasturtium (*Tropaeolum majus* L.): a source of mineral elements and bioactive compounds. *Rocz Panstw Zakl Hig* 2018; 69(2): 119–26.

4. Gasparotto A *et al*. Antihypertensive effect of isoquercitrin and extracts from *Tropaeolum majus* L: evidence for the inhibition of angiotensin converting enzyme. *J Ethnopharmacol* 2011; 134: 363–74.

5. Albrecht U *et al*. A combination of *Tropaeolum majus* herb and *Armoracia rusticana* root for the treatment of acute bronchitis. *Phytomedicine* 2023; 116: 154838.

6. Jurca T *et al*. The effect of *Tropaeolum majus* L. on bacterial infections and in vitro efficacy on apoptosis and DNA lesions in hyperosmotic stress. *J Physiol Pharmacol* 2018; 69(3).

   Kaiser SJ *et al*. Natural isothiocyanates express antimicrobial activity against developing and mature biofilms of *Pseudomonas aeruginosa*. *Fitoterapia* 2017; 119: 57–63.

   Jurca T *et al*. A phytocomplex consisting of *Tropaeolum majus* L. and *Salvia officinalis* L. extracts alleviates the inflammatory response of dermal fibroblasts to bacterial lipopolysaccharides. *Oxid Med Cell Longev* 2020; 8516153.

   Jurca T *et al*. The effect of *Tropaeolum majus* L. on bacterial infections and in vitro efficacy on apoptosis and DNA lesions in hyperosmotic stress. *J Physiol Pharmacol* 2018; 69(3).

7. Jakubczyk K *et al*. Garden nasturtium (*Tropaeolum majus* L.) – a source of mineral elements and bioactive compounds. *Rocz Panstw Zakl Hig* 2018; 69(2): 119–26.

NETTLE

1. Mohammadi A *et al*. The *Urtica dioica* extract enhances sensitivity of paclitaxel drug to MDA-MB-468 breast cancer cells. *Biomed Pharmacother* 2016; 83: 835–42.

   Mohammadi A *et al*. Urtica dioica dichloromethane extract induce apoptosis from intrinsic pathway on human prostate cancer cells (PC3). *Cell Mol Biol* (Noisy le Grand) 2016; 62(3): 78–83.

   Konrad L *et al*. Antiproliferative effect on human prostate cancer cells by a stinging nettle root (*Urtica dioica*) extract. *Planta Med* 2000; 66(1): 44–7.

2. Qujeq D *et al*. Effect of *Urtica dioica* leaf alcoholic and aqueous extracts on the number and the diameter of the islets in diabetic rats. *Int J Mol Cell Med* 2013; 2(1): 21–6.

   Patel SS *et al*. Antidepressant and anxiolytic like effects of *Urtica dioica* leaves in streptozotocin induced diabetic mice. *Metab Brain Dis* 2018; 33(4): 1281–92.

Amiri-Behzadi *et al.* Effects of *Urtica dioica* supplementation on blood lipids, hepatic enzymes and nitric oxide levels in type 2 diabetic patients: a double blind, randomized clinical trial. *Avicenna J Phytomed* 2016; 6(6): 686–95.

Kianbakht S *et al.* Improved glycemic control in patients with advanced type 2 diabetes mellitus taking *Urtica dioica* leaf extract: a randomized double-blind placebo-controlled clinical trial. *Clin Lab* 2013; 59(9–10): 1071–6.

3. Sökeland J *et al.* Combination of Sabal and *Urtica* extract vs. finasteride in benign prostatic hyperplasia (Aiken stages I to II): comparison of therapeutic effectiveness in a one year double-blind study. [Article in German.] *Der Urologe* 1997; 36(4): 327–33.

Safarinejad MR. *Urtica dioica* for treatment of benign prostatic hyperplasia: prospective, randomized, double-blind, placebo-controlled, crossover study. *J Herb Pharmacother* 2005; 5: 1–11.

4. Mittman P. Randomized, double-blind study of freeze-dried *Urtica dioica* in the treatment of allergic rhinitis. *Planta Med* 1990; 56(1): 44–7.

NODDING TOP

1. Aniya Y *et al.* Free radical scavenging and hepatoprotective actions of the medicinal herb, *Crassocephalum crepidioides* from the Okinawa islands. *Biol Pharm Bull* 2005; 28(1): 19–23.

2. Ibid.

3. Galba Jean B *et al.* Neuroprotective effects of the ethanolic leaf extract of *Crassocephalum crepidioides* (Asteraceae) on diazepam-induced amnesia in mice. *Adv Pharmacol Pharm Sci* 2022: 1919469, Sep 28.

4. Ayodele OO *et al.* In vitro anticoagulant effect of *Crassocephalum crepidioides* leaf methanol extract and fractions on human blood. *J Exp Pharmacol* 2019; 11: 99–107.

Ayodele OO *et al.* Modulation of blood coagulation and hematological parameters by *Crassocephalum crepidioides* leaf methanol extract and fractions in STZ-induced diabetes in the rat. *Sci World J* 2020; 2020: 1036364.

5. Bahar E *et al.* Beta-cell protection and antidiabetic activities of *Crassocephalum crepidioides* (Asteraceae) Benth. S. Moore extract against alloxan-induced oxidative stress via regulation of apoptosis and reactive oxygen species (ROS). *BMC Complement Altern Med* 2017; 17(1): 179.

6. Can NM *et al.* Wound healing activity of *Crassocephalum crepidioide* (Benth.) S. Moore. leaf hydroethanolic extract. *Oxid Med Cell Longev* 2020; 2020: 2483187.

OXALIS

1. Handique JG *et al.* Antioxidant activities and total phenolic and flavonoid contents in three indigenous medicinal vegetables of north-east India. *Nat Prod Commun* 2012; 7(8): 1021–3.

Romojaro A *et al.* Nutritional and antioxidant properties of wild edible plants and their use as potential ingredients in the modern diet. *Int J Food Sci Nutr* 2013; 64(8): 944–52.

Ahmad B *et al.* Amelioration of carbon tetrachloride-induced pulmonary toxicity with *Oxalis corniculata*. *Toxicol Ind Health* 2015; 31(12): 1243–51.

2. Rehman A *et al.* Antibacterial, antifungal, and insecticidal potentials of *Oxalis corniculata* and

its isolated compounds. *Int J Anal Chem* 2015; 2015: 842468.

3. Gaspar MC *et al.* Polyphenolic characterisation and bioactivity of an *Oxalis pes-caprae* L. leaf extract. *Nat Prod Res* 2018; 32(6): 732–8.

4. Gul F *et al.* Phytochemistry, biological activities and in silico molecular docking studies of *Oxalis pes-caprae* L. compounds against SARS-CoV-2. *J King Saudi Univ Sci* 2022; 34(6): 102136.

5. Güçlütürk I *et al.* Evaluation of anti-oxidant activity and identification of major polyphenolics of the invasive weed *Oxalis pes-caprae*. *Phytochem Anal* 2012; 23(6): 642–6.

PRICKLY PEAR

1. Harrabi B *et al.* Polysaccharides extraction from *Opuntia stricta* and their protective effect against HepG2 cell death and hypolipidaemic effects on hyperlipidaemia rats induced by high-fat diet. *Arch Physiol Biochem* 2017; 123(4): 225–37.

Garoby-Salom S *et al.* Dietary cladode powder from wild type and domesticated *Opuntia* species reduces atherogenesis in apoE knock-out mice. *J Physiol Biochem* 2016; 72(1): 9–70.

Rahimi P *et al.* Effects of betalains on atherogenic risk factors in patients with atherosclerotic cardiovascular disease. *Food Funct* 2019; 10(12): 8286–97.

2. Rahimi P *et al.* Effects of betalains on atherogenic risk factors in patients with atherosclerotic cardiovascular disease. *Food Funct* 2019; 10(12): 8286–97.

3. Chong Pee-Win. A review of the efficacy and safety of litramine IQP-G-002AS, an *Opuntia ficus-indica* derived fiber for weight management. *Evid Based Complement Altern Med* 2014; 2014: 943713.

Uebelhack R *et al.* Effects of cactus fiber on the excretion of dietary fat in healthy subjects: a double blind, randomized, placebo-controlled, crossover clinical investigation. *Curr Ther Res Clin Exp* 2014; 76: 39–44.

4. Izuegbuna O *et al.* Chemical composition, antioxidant, anti-inflammatory, and cytotoxic activities of *Opuntia stricta* cladodes. *PLoS One* 2019; 14(1): e0209682.

Zhu X *et al.* HPLC analysis and the antioxidant and preventive actions of *Opuntia stricta* juice extract against hepato-nephrotoxicity and testicular injury induced by cadmium exposure. *Molecules* 2022; 27(15): 4972.

Kharrat N *et al.* Synergistic effect of polysaccharides, betalain pigment and phenolic compounds of red prickly pear (*Opuntia stricta*) in the stabilization of salami. *Int J Biol Macromol* 2018; 111: 561–8.

Koubaa M *et al.* Seed oil extraction from red prickly pear using hexane and supercritical CO_2: assessment of phenolic compound composition, antioxidant and antibacterial activities. *J Sci Food Agric* 2017; 97(2): 613–20.

Yeddes N *et al.* Comparative study of antioxidant power, polyphenols, flavonoids and betacyanins of the peel and pulp of three Tunisian *Opuntia* forms. *Antioxidants (Basel)* 2013; 19(2): 37–51.

5. Fang Q *et al.* *Opuntia* extract reduces scar formation in rabbit ear model: a randomized controlled study. *Int J Low Extrem Wounds* 2015; 14(4): 343–52.

6. Koubaa M *et al.* Seed oil extraction from red prickly pear using hexane and supercritical CO_2: assessment of phenolic compound composition, antioxidant and antibacterial activities. *J Sci Food Agric* 2017; 97(2): 613–20.

PURSLANE

1. Lv WJ *et al.* *Portulaca oleracea* L. extracts alleviate 2,4-dinitrochlorobenzene-induced atopic dermatitis in mice. *Front Nutr* 2022; 9: 986943.

Barros ASA *et al.* Study of the non-clinical healing activities of the extract and gel of *Portulaca capilosa* L. in skin wounds in Wistar rats: a preliminary study. *Biomed Pharmacother* 2017; 96: 182–90.

Rashed A. Simple evaluation of the wound healing activity of a crude extract of *Portulaca oleracea* L. (growing in Jordan) in *Mus musculus* JVI-1. *J Ethnopharmacol* 2003; 88(2–3): 131–6.

Zhao H *et al.* *Portulaca oleracea* L. aids calcipotriol in reversing keratinocyte differentiation and skin barrier dysfunction in psoriasis through inhibition of the nuclear factor kB signaling pathway. *Exp Ther Med* 2014; 9(2): 303–10.

2. Baradaran Rahimi V *et al.* Anti-inflammatory and anti-oxidant activity of *Portulaca oleracea* extract on LPS-induced rat lung injury. *Molecules* (Basel) 2019; 24(1): 139.

Zhou YX *et al.* *Portulaca oleracea* L: a review of phytochemistry and pharmacological effects. *Bio Med Res Int* 2015; 2015: 925631.

3. Karimi G *et al.* Evaluation of the gastric antiulcerogenic effects of *Portulaca oleracea* L. extracts in mice. *Phytother Res* 2004; 18(6): 484–7.

4. Yang X *et al.* Protective effects of ethanol extract from *Portulaca oleracea* L on dextran sulphate sodium-induced mice ulcerative colitis involving anti-inflammatory and antioxidant. *Am J Transl Res* 2016; 8(5): 2138–48.

Yang Y *et al.* Network pharmacology-based research into the effect and potential mechanism of *Portulaca oleracea* L. polysaccharide against ulcerative colitis. *Comput Biol Med* 2023; 161: 106999.

5. Kim Y *et al.* *Portulaca oleracea* extracts and their active compounds ameliorate inflammatory bowel diseases in vitro and in vivo by modulating TNF-β, IL-6 and IL-1β signaling. *Food Res Int* 2018; 106: 335.

Kong R *et al.* *Portulaca* extract attenuates development of dextran sulfate sodium induced colitis in mice through activation of PPARγ. *PPAR Res* 2018; 2018: ID 6079101.

6. Kim Y *et al.* Ibid.

Kong R *et al.* Ibid.

Hamedi S *et al.* Hypnotic effect of *Portulaca oleracea* L on pentobarbital-induced sleep in mice. *Curr Drug Discov Technol* 2019; 16(2): 198–203.

7. Zheng G *et al.* *Portulaca oleracea* L. alleviates liver injury in streptozotocin-induced diabetic mice. *Drug Des Devel Ther* 2017; 12: 47.

Hu Q *et al.* Effects of polysaccharide from *Portulaca oleracea* L. on voltage-gated Na channel of INS-1 cells. *Biomed Pharmacother* 2018; 101: 572–8.

8. Ebrahimian Z *et al.* Effects of *Portulaca oleracea* L. (purslane) on the metabolic syndrome: a review. *Iran J Basic Med Sci* 2022; 25(11): 1275–85.

Jalali J *et al.* Ameliorative effects of *Portulaca oleracea* L. (purslane) on the metabolic syndrome: a review. *J Ethnopharmacol* 2022; 299: 115672.

9. Khazdair MR *et al.* Anti-asthmatic effects of *Portulaca oleracea* and its constituents: a review. *J Pharmacopunct* 2019; 22(3): 122–30.

10. Khazdair MR et al. Experimental and clinical studies on the effects of Portulaca oleracea L. and its constituents on respiratory, allergic, and immunologic disorders, a review. Phytother Res 2021; 35(12): 6813–42.

11. Martins WB et al. Neuroprotective effect of Portulaca oleracea extracts against 6-hydroxydopamine-induced lesion of dopaminergic neurons. Anais da Acad Brasil de Ciencias 2016; 88(3): 1439–50.

    Abdel Moneim AE. The neuroprotective effects of purslane (Portulaca oleracea) on rotenone-induced biochemical changes and apoptosis in brain of rat. CNS Neurol Disord Drug Targets 2013; 12(6): 830–41.

12. Farkhondeh T et al. The hepato-protective effects of Portulaca oleracea L. extract: review. Curr Drug Discov Technol 2019; 16(2): 122–6.

    Farkhondeh T et al. The therapeutic effects of Portulaca oleracea L. in hepatogastric disorders. Gastroenterol Hepatol 2019; 42(2): 127–32.

    Dar MA et al. Amelioration of experimental hepatotoxicity in rats by Portulaca oleraceaLinn. from Kashmir Himalaya. Comb Chem High Throughput Screen 2022; 25(6): 1072–81.

13. Tleubayeva MI et al. Component composition and antimicrobial activity of CO_2 extract of Portulaca oleracea growing in the Territory of Kazakhstan. Sci World J 2021; 2021: 5434525.

    Liu Y et al. Antiviral activity of Portulaca oleracea L. extracts against porcine epidemic diarrhea virus by partial suppression on myd88/NF-κb activation in vitro. Microb Pathogen 2021; 154: 104832.

    Li YH et al. Antiviral activity of Portulaca oleracea L. against influenza A viruses. J Ethnopharmacol 2019; 241: 112013.

RIBWORT

1. Wegener T et al. Plantain (Plantago lanceolata L.), anti inflammatory action In upper respiratory tract infections. [Article in German.] Wiener Medizinische Wochenschrift 1999; 149(8–10): 211–6.

   Kraft K. Therapeutic profile in a ribwort herb fluid extract in acute respiratory illness in children and adults. In: Loew D, Rietbrock N (eds). Phytopharmaceuticals III. Research and Clinical Application, Darmstadt: Steinkopff Verlag, 1997, 199–209.

2. Bajrai LH et al. Identification of antiviral compounds against monkeypox virus profilin-like protein A42R from Plantago lanceolata. Molecules (Basel) 2022; 27(22): 7718.

   Abdin M. Possible role for Plantago lanceolata in the treatment of HIV infection. Townsend Letter 2006; 275: 92–3.

3. Rahamouz-Haghighi S et al. In vitro evaluation of cytotoxicity and antibacterial activities of ribwort plantain (Plantago lanceolata L.) root fractions and phytochemical analysis by gas chromatography-mass spectrometry. Arch Razi Institute 2022; 77(6): 2131–43.

   Ferrazzano GF et al. Determination of the in vitro and in vivo antimicrobial activity on salivary streptococci and lactobacilli and chemical characterisation of the phenolic content of a Plantago lanceolata infusion. Biomed Res Int 2015; article ID 286817.

   Rahamooz-Haghighi S et al. Establishment and elicitation of transgenic root culture

of Plantago lanceolata and evaluation of its anti-bacterial and cytotoxicity activity. Prep Biochem Biotech 2021; 51(3): 207–24.

4. Kalantari A et al. Self-nanoemulsifying drug delivery systems containing Plantago lanceolata — an assessment of their antioxidant and anti-inflammatory effects. Molecules (Basel) 2017; 22(10): 1773.

   Vigo E et al. In-vitro anti-inflammatory activity of Pinus sylvestris and Plantago lanceolata extracts: effect on inducible NOS, COX-1, COX-2 and their products in J774A.1 murine macrophages. J Pharm Pharmacol 2005; 57(3): 383–91.

   Herold A et al. Hydroalcoholic plant extracts with anti-inflammatory activity. Roumanian Arch Microbiol Immunol 2003; 62(1–2): 117–29.

   Marchesan M et al. Investigation of the anti-inflammatory activity of liquid extracts of Plantago lanceolata L. Phytother Res 1998; 12: S33–34.

5. Sanna F et al. Antioxidant contents in a Mediterranean population of Plantago lanceolata L. exploited for quarry reclamation interventions. Plants 2022; 11(6): 791.

   Kalantari A et al. Self-nanoemulsifying drug delivery systems containing Plantago lanceolata — an assessment of their antioxidant and anti-inflammatory effects. Molecules (Basel) 2017; 22(10): 1773.

   Vigo E et al. In-vitro anti-inflammatory activity of Pinus sylvestris and Plantago lanceolata extracts: effect on inducible NOS, COX-1, COX-2 and their products in J774A.1 murine macrophages. J Pharm Pharmacol 2005; 57(3): 383–91.

   Herold A et al. Hydroalcoholic plant extracts with anti-inflammatory activity. Roumanian Arch Microbiol Immunol 2003; 62(1–2): 117–29.

   Marchesan M et al. Investigation of the anti-inflammatory activity of liquid extracts of Plantago lanceolata L. Phytother Res 1998; 12: S33–34.

6. Kurt B et al. Effects of Plantago lanceolata L. extract on full-thickness excisional wound healing in a mouse model. Biotechnic Histochem 2018; 93(4): 249–57.

   Kovac I et al. Plantago lanceolata L. water extract induces transition of fibroblasts into myofibroblasts and increases tensile strength of healing skin wounds. J Pharm Pharmacol 2015; 67(1): 117–25.

7. Yoshida T et al. Plantago lanceolata L. leaves prevent obesity in C57BL/6 J mice fed a high-fat diet. Nat Prod Res 2013; 27(11): 982–7.

8. Melese E et al. Evaluation of the antipeptic ulcer activity of the leaf extract of Plantago lanceolata L. in rodents. Phytother Res 2011; 25(8): 1174–80.

9. Kozan E et al. Evaluation of some plants used in Turkish folk medicine against parasitic infections for their in vivo anthelmintic activity. J Ethnopharmacol 2006; 108: 211–16.

SOW THISTLE

1. Vilela FC et al. Evaluation of the antinociceptive activity of extracts of Sonchus oleraceus L. in mice. J Ethnopharmacol 2009; 124(2): 306–10.

2. Vilela FC et al. Antidepressant-like activity of Sonchus oleraceus in mouse models of immobility tests. J Med Food, 2010; 13(1): 219–22.

   Vilela FC et al. Anxiolytic-like effect of Sonchus oleraceus L. in mice. J Ethnopharmacol 2009; 124(2): 325–7.

3. Chen L et al. Sonchus oleraceus Linn extract enhanced glucose homeostasis through the AMPK/Akt/ GSK-3β signalling pathway in diabetic liver and HepG2 cell culture. Food Chemical Toxicol 2020; 136: 111072.

   Chen L et al. Anti-inflammatory effect of self-emulsifying delivery system containing Sonchus oleraceus Linn extract on streptozotocin-induced diabetic rats. Food Chemical Toxicol 2020; 135: 110953.

   Chen L. Chlorogenic acid and caffeic acid from Sonchus oleraceus Linn synergistically attenuate insulin resistance and modulate glucose uptake in HepG2 cells. Food Chem Toxicol 2019; 127: 182–87.

4. Chen CY et al. Lipid extract from a vegetable (Sonchus oleraceus) attenuates adipogenesis and high fat diet-induced obesity associated with AMPK activation. Front Nutrit 2021; 8, 624283.

5. Kassim MA. Dietary modulation of the human colonic microbiota through plant-derived prebiotic compounds. Masters thesis, Department of Biotechnology, Durban University of Technology, 2007.

6. Prichoa FC et al. Tissue injuries of Wistar rats treated with hydroalcoholic extract of Sonchus oleraceus. Braz J Pharm Sci 2011; 47(3): 605–13.

7. Vecchia CAD et al. Sonchus oleraceus L. promotes gastroprotection in rodents via antioxidant, anti-inflammatory, and anti-secretory activities. Evid Based Complement Altern Med: eCAM 2022; 2022: 7413231.

   Alothman EA et al. Evaluation of anti-ulcer and ulcerative colitis of Sonchus oleraceus L. Saudi Pharm J 2018; 26(7): 956–9.

8. Chen L et al. Sonchus oleraceus Linn protects against LPS-induced sepsis and inhibits inflammatory responses in RAW264.7 cells. J Ethnopharmacol 2019; 236: 63–9.

9. El-Desouky TA. Evaluation of effectiveness of aqueous extract for some leaves of wild edible plants in Egypt as anti-fungal and anti-toxigenic. Heliyon 2021; 7(2): e06209

10. Torres-González L et al. Nephroprotective effect of Sonchus oleraceusextract against kidney injury induced by ischemia-reperfusion in Wistar rats. Oxid Med Cell Longev 2018; 9572803.

ST JOHN'S WORT

1. Kenda M et al. Medicinal plants used for anxiety, depression, or stress treatment: an update. Molecules 2022; 27(18): 6021.

   Moragrega I et al. Medicinal plants in the treatment of depression: evidence from pre-clinical studies. Planta Med 2021; 87(9): 656–5.

   Lind K et al. St John's Wort for depression. Cochrane Database Syst Rev 2005; 18(2): April.

   Lind K et al. St John's Wort for treating depression. Cochrane Database Syst Rev 2008; 8(4): CD000448.

   Greeson JM et al. St John's wort (Hypericum perforatum): a review of the current pharmacological, toxicological, and clinical literature. Psychopharmacol 2001; 153(4): 402–14.

   Hübner WD et al. Experience with St John's Wort (Hypericum perforatum) in children under 12 years with symptoms of depression and psychovegetative disturbances. Phytother Res 2001; 15(4): 367–70.

2. Eatemadnia A et al. The effect of Hypericum perforatum on postmenopausal symptoms

and depression: A randomized controlled trial. *Complement Ther Med* 2019; 45: 109–13.

3. Khan A et al. Anti-anxiety properties of selected medicinal plants. *Curr Pharm Biotechnol* 2022; 23(8): 1041–60.

4. Taylor LH et al. An open-label trial of St John's wort (*Hypericum perforatum*) in obsessive-compulsive disorder. *J Clin Psychiatry* 2000; 61(8): 575–8.

5. Uzbay TI. *Hypericum perforatum* and substance dependence: a review. *Phytother Res* 2008; 22(5): 578–82.

   Subhan F et al. Adulterant profile of illicit street heroin and reduction of its precipitated physical dependence withdrawal syndrome by extracts of St John's wort (*Hypericum perforatum*). *Phytother Res* 2009; 23(4): 564–71.

6. Canning M et al. The efficacy of *Hypericum perforatum* (St John's wort) for the treatment of premenstrual syndrome: a randomized, double-blind, placebo-controlled trial. *CNS Drugs* 2010; 24(3): 207–25.

   Huang KL et al. St John's wort (*Hypericum perforatum*) as a treatment for premenstrual dysphoric disorder: case report. *Int J Psychiatry* 2003; 33(3): 295–7.

7. Delcanale P et al. Photodynamic action of *Hypericum perforatum* hydrophilic extract against *Staphylococcus aureus*. *Photochem Photobiol Sci* 2020; 19(3): 324–31.

   Nazlı O et al. Antimicrobial and antibiofilm activity of polyurethane/*Hypericum perforatum* extract (PHPE) composite. *Bioorg Chem* 2019; 82: 224–8.

   Heydarian M et al. Characterization of *Hypericum perforatum* polysaccharides with antioxidant and antimicrobial activities: Optimization based statistical modelling. *Int J Biol Macromol* 2017; 104(Pt A): 287–93.

   Okmen G et al. The biological activities of *Hypericum perforatum* L. *Afr J Trad Complement Altern Med* 2016; 14(1): 213–18.

8. Mohamed FF et al. *Hypericum perforatum* and its ingredients hypericin and pseudo-hypericin demonstrate an antiviral activity against SARS-CoV-2. *Pharmaceuticals* (Basel) 2022; 15(5): 530.

   Bajrai LH et al. In vitro screening of anti-viral and virucidal effects against SARS-CoV-2 by *Hypericum perforatum* and *Echinacea*. *Sci Rep* 2022; 12(1): 21723.

   Pang R et al. In vitro anti-hepatitis B virus effect of *Hypericum perforatum* L. *J Huazhong Univ Sci Tech* 2010; 30(1): 98–102.

   Maury W et al. Identification of light-independent inhibition of human immunodeficiency virus-1 infection through bioguided fractionation of *Hypericum perforatum*. *Virol J* 2009; 13(6): 101.

9. Nawrot J et al. Medicinal herbs in the relief of neurological, cardiovascular, and respiratory symptoms after COVID-19 infection: a literature review. *Cells* 2022; 11(12): 1897.

   Yalçın S et al. Determination of potential drug candidate molecules of the *Hypericum perforatum* for COVID-19 treatment. *Curr Pharmacol Rep* 2021; 7(2): 42–8.

   Masiello P et al. Can *Hypericum perforatum* (SJW) prevent cytokine storm in COVID-19 patients? *Phytother Res* 2020; 34(7): 1471–3.

10. Sotirova Y et al. Bigel formulations of nanoencapsulated St John's wort extract — an approach for enhanced wound healing. *Gels* 2023; 9(5): 360.

Yalçınkaya E et al. Efficiency of *Hypericum perforatum*, povidone iodine, tincture benzoin and tretinoin on wound healing. *Food Chem Toxicol* 2022; 166: 113209.

Uzunhisarcikli E et al. Role of *Hypericum perforatum* oil and pomegranate seed oil in wound healing: an in vitro study. *Z Naturforsch C J Biosci* 2021; 77(5–6): 189–95.

Altiparmak M et al. Comparison of systemic and topical *Hypericum perforatum* on diabetic surgical wounds. *J Invest Surg* 2018; 31(1): 29–37.

Süntar IP et al. Investigations on the in vivo wound healing potential of *Hypericum perforatum* L. *J Ethnopharmacol* 2010; 127(2): 468–77.

11. Galeotti N. *Hypericum perforatum* (St. John's Wort) beyond depression: a therapeutic perspective for pain conditions. *J Ethnopharmacol* 2017; 200: 136–46.

12. Goel R et al. Nanoencapsulation and characterisation of *Hypericum perforatum* for the treatment of neuropathic pain. *J Microencapsul* 2023; 40(6): 402–11.

   Assiri K et al. *Hypericum perforatum* (St John's wort) as a possible therapeutic alternative for the management of trigeminal neuralgia (TN) — a case report. *Complement Ther Med* 2017; 30: 36–9.

13. Chen S et al. The phytochemical hyperforin triggers thermogenesis in adipose tissue via a Dlat-AMPK signaling axis to curb obesity. *Cell Metab* 2021; 33(3): 565–80.

   Tokgöz H et al. *Hypericum perforatum* L.: a medicinal plant with potential as a curative agent against obesity-associated complications. *Mol Biol Rep* 2020; 47(11): 8679–86.

TROPICAL CHICKWEED

1. Ambu G et al. Traditional uses of medicinal plants by ethnic people in the Kavrepalanchok District, Central Nepal. *Plants* (Basel) 2020; 9(6): 759.

   Barua C et al. Analgesic and anti-nociceptive activity of hydroethanolic extract of *Drymaria cordata* Willd. *Ind J Pharmacol* 2011; 43(2): 121.

   Akindele A et al. Analgesic and antipyretic activities of *Drymaria cordata* (Linn.) Willd (Caryophyllaceae) extract. *Afr J Trad Complement Altern Med* 2011; 9(1): 25–35.

2. Mukherjee PK et al. Studies on antitussive activity of *Drymaria cordata* Willd. (Caryophyllaceae). *J Ethnopharmacol* 1997; 56(1): 77–80.

3. Mukherjee PK et al. Antibacterial evaluation of *Drymaria cordata* Willd (Fam. Caryophyllaceae) extract. *Phytother Res* 1997; 11: 249–50.

4. Nono RN et al. Antioxidant C-glycosylflavones of *Drymaria cordata* (Linn.) Willd. *Arch Pharmacol Res* 2015; 39(1): 43–50.

5. Patra S et al. Antidiabetic effect of *Drymaria cordata* leaf against streptozotocin-nicotinamide-induced diabetic albino rats. *J Adv Pharm Technol Res* 2020; 11(1): 44–52.

6. Picard G et al. Assessment of in vitro pharmacological effect of neotropical Piperaceae in GABAergic bioassays in relation to plants traditionally used for folk illness by the Yanesha (Peru). *J Ethnopharmacol* 2014; 155(3): 1500–7.

7. Barua CC et al. Anxiolytic effect of hydroethanolic extract of *Drymaria cordata* L Willd. *Ind J Exp Biol* 2009; 47(12): 969–73.

WILD RASPBERRY

1. Shan S et al. Evaluation of polyphenolics content and antioxidant activity in edible wild fruits. *Biomed Res Int* 2019; 2019: 1381989.

   Noratto GD et al. Red raspberry (*Rubus idaeus* L.) intake decreases oxidative stress in obese diabetic (db/db) mice. *Food Chem* 2017; 227: 305–14.

   Teng H et al. Hepatoprotective effects of raspberry (*Rubus coreanus* Miq.) seed oil and its major constituents. *Food Chem Toxicol* 2017; 110: 418–24.

   Baby B et al. Antioxidant and anticancer properties of berries. *Crit Rev Food Sci Nutr* 2018; 58(15): 2491–507.

   Aiyer S et al. Prevention of oxidative DNA damage by bioactive berry components. *Nutr Cancer* 2008; 60(S1): 36–42.

   Godevac D et al. Antioxidant properties of raspberry seed extracts on micronucleus distribution in peripheral blood lymphocytes. *Food Chem Toxicol* 2009; 47(11): 2853–9.

2. Ryan T et al. Antibacterial activity of raspberry cordial in vitro. *Res Vet Sci* 2001; 71(3): 155–9.

3. Fotschki B et al. Grinding levels of raspberry pomace affect intestinal microbial activity, lipid and glucose metabolism in Wistar rats. *Food Res Int* 2019; 120: 399–406.

   Schell J et al. Raspberries improve postprandial glucose and acute and chronic inflammation in adults with type 2 diabetes. *Ann Nutr Metab* 2019; 74(2): 165–74.

   Noratto GD et al. Red raspberry (*Rubus idaeus* L.) intake decreases oxidative stress in obese diabetic (db/db) mice. *Food Chem* 2017; 227: 305–14.

4. Jansen-Alves C et al. Rosaceae *Rubus rosifolius* Smith: nutritional, bioactive and antioxidant potential of unconventional fruit. *Nat Prod Res* 2023; 37(23): 4013–17.

5. Rambaran TF et al. Hypoglycaemic effect of the fruit extracts of two varieties of *Rubus rosifolius*. *J Food Biochem* 2020; 44(9): e13365.

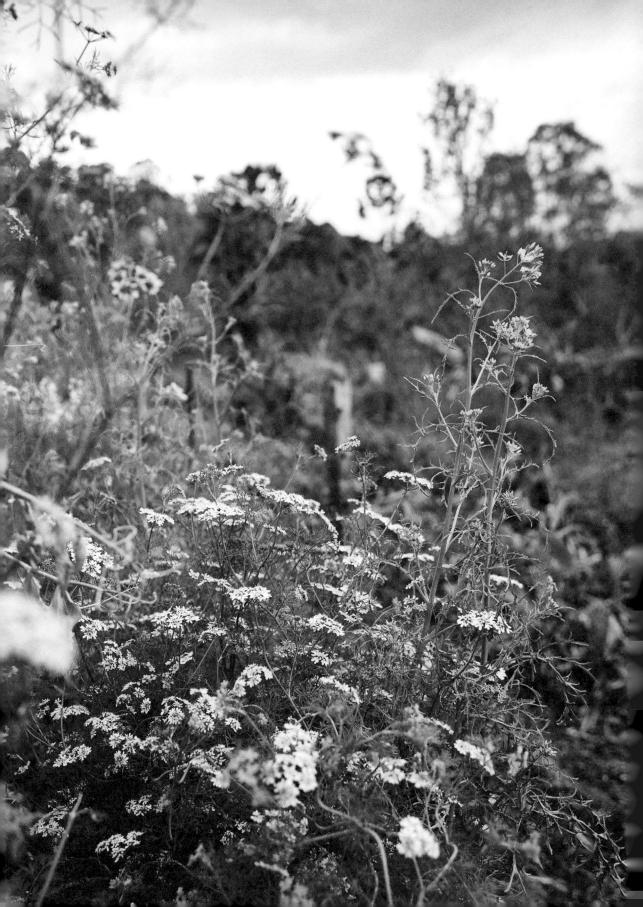

Acknowledgements

I'm so incredibly grateful for all the support I had during the making of this book. Writing a book about wild plants in less than 12 months is quite a feat: not everything is in season when you need it, so I had to call in many favours from people across the country!

Biggest thanks go to my mother, Shannon Merika, who helped forage countless plants, stayed with me for a week doing non-stop recipe testing, did weeks of editing, and supported me throughout the entire process in every possible way. Anton Vlatko, who collected endless amounts of marshmallow peas and nasturtium seeds, provided me with countless plants and always supports me in all my endeavours to share plants with the world. Lisa Delanoue, who has given me more plants than anyone over the years and has always supported every one of my herbal adventures, your garden is one of my favourite places in the world. Thanks to all the folks at Bellbunya Sustainable Community who have shared their gardens and kitchens with me over the years as I ran my Wildcraft courses — and to all the people who came to those courses. This book was born from that work.

Joanne Sanna, who put so much effort into creating the first draft of the dosage chart in the Herbal Medicine-making Fundamentals chapter. Sally Kingsford-Smith for knocking on the doors of strangers to ask for their prickly pears, and driving me for hours on treasure hunts for St John's wort, and for the *Parietaria judaica* photo on page 66. Erin Lovell Verinder for giving us the St John's wort treasure map. Aleta Bon, for foraging countless plants and bringing me all the kombucha I could drink, and for the walks and talks. Karen McElroy for inventing crispy fried ribwort and testing cobbler's pegs curry. Cat Green, for recipe testing, foraging dock and creating the best job I ever had, and for all your support with everything I do.

Thanks to Rosie and Jemima for taste-testing marshmallows and dock banana bread, and making it fun every time I come to your house. To all my recipe testers and plant providers, Meg Wall, Kristin Hamilton, Liv Grey, Jacqui Bushell, Carly Garner and Nadja Dinneen for the advice on mugwort and TCM. To Kylie Sigel and the whole family for driving miles to give me fat hen, amaranth and ribwort. To all the people who posted plants from interstate, Lilly Taylor, Caitlin Graham-Jones, Naomi Ingleton, Chris Doyle. To Pat Collins (one of my favourite herbalists) for permission to use the blackberry nightshade recipe, to Monica Davis for inspiration for the marshmallows and permission to use her recipe. To Diego Bonetto, the weedy one, for sharing the best foraging spots in Sydney and for teaching foraging with such a generous heart and for all your support. To my plant spirit teacher Pam Montgomery for the plant communication section. And Katrina Sharpe, without your beautiful photographic and layout work on Wildcraft, this book would never have happened. To Tracy Lines, for the beautiful proposal.

To the amazing team at Murdoch Books, Alexandra Payne for first believing in the project and getting it accepted. Justin Wolfers, Megan Pigott, Katri Hilden, Rob Palmer, Cath Muscat, Vanessa Austin and the one and only Jimmy Callaway, so glad I got to work with you guys.

The Wild Witches: Aleta Bon, Karen McElroy, Anne Harris and Lucia Cimino for all your love and support over a lifetime.

To my family, Ayla, Coco and Malcolm Atkins, for supporting me from the beginning of this crazy journey, to Shannon Merika and Honi Chaitanya for everything since I was born, to Petra for your courage, and to my beautiful partner John Reid for all your love and care — and to all of you for your help and support during the making of this book. I love you all, with all my heart.

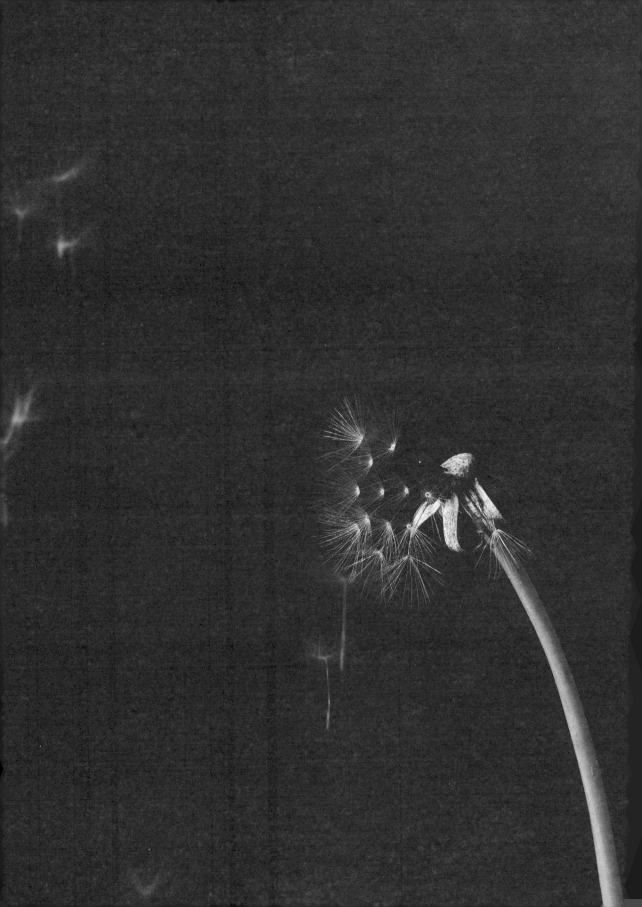

Index

A

alcohol-infused oils 31
Amaranth porridge 58
Amaranth-crusted tofu 60
anti-inflammatory remedies
    Anti-inflammatory gel 90
    Chickweed anti-inflammatory gel 119
    Chinese mugwort anti-inflammatory balm 125
    Cobbler's pegs anti-inflammatory juice 151
    Tropical chickweed anti-inflammatory juice 302
antibacterial skin juice, Cobbler's pegs 151
antifungal ointment, Cat's ear 108
Asthma weed cough syrup 70
Ayurvedic CCF tea blend 190

B

balls, Cleavers, potato & quinoa, with cleavers dipping sauce 132
balms 32–4
    Beeswax base balm 33
    Blackberry nightshade cold sore balm 80
    Chinese mugwort anti-inflammatory balm 125
    Herb robert healing balm 207
    ingredients for 32
    Lantana itch balm 212
    Vegan base balm 32
banana bread, Dock seed 170
bars, Dock scroggin fruit & nut 169
Bathua saag aloo 181
Beeswax base balm 33
Beeswax base ointment 34
Bitter salad 156
Blackberry nightshade cold sore balm 80
Blackberry nightshade jam 77
blackberry nightshade oil 80
Blackberry nightshade, nodding top & artichoke spelt pizza 78
Blue top eczema & psoriasis cream 86
Blue top poultice 88
Blue top shampoo 88
bread, Dock seed banana 170
brownies, Fat hen vegan 182
butters 46

C

cake, Nettle & blackberry forest 239
calendula oil 297
capers, Nasturtium 229
capsules 21–2
    calculating dose for 22
    Gotu kola capsules 198
    Herb robert capsules 206
carrots, Maple roast, with nodding top 248
cashew cheese 178
Cat's ear antifungal ointment 108
Cat's ear root coffee 108
cat's ear root oil 108
Cat's ear savoury pancakes 106
cheese, cashew 178
cheese, Sweet fennel cream 189
chest tonic, Head &, for excess mucus 281
Chickweed anti-inflammatory gel 119
Chickweed ice 119
Chickweed skin cream 118
Chickweed, cashew & caper toasts 116
Chickweed, cucumber & apple juice 116
chimichurri, Nodding top 246
Chinese mugwort anti-inflammatory balm 125
Chinese mugwort smudge stick 124
chutney, Fresh asthma weed 68
Cleavers coffee 134
cleavers dipping sauce 132
cleavers infused oil 135
Cleavers lymph cream 135
Cleavers, potato & quinoa balls with cleavers dipping sauce 132
Clover cupcakes with orange cashew icing 142
Clover syrup 140
Cobbler's pegs anti-inflammatory juice 151
cobbler's pegs antibacterial skin juice 151
Cobbler's pegs gel 151
Cobbler's pegs, lentil & tomato curry 148
coffees
    Cat's ear root coffee 108
    Cleavers coffee 134
    Dandelion root coffee 160

cold sore balm, Blackberry nightshade 80
cold & flu tonic, Nasturtium 228
constipation, Sow thistle, aloe & pear juice for 289
cordial, Wild raspberry 312
cough syrup, Asthma weed 70
crackers, Wild seed 172
cream cheese, Sweet fennel 189
creams 34–7
    Blue top eczema & psoriasis cream 86
    Chickweed skin cream 118
    Cleavers lymph cream 135
    common ingredients for 34–5
    Gotu kola healing cream 199
    Tropical chickweed healing cream 303
    troubleshooting 37
    Vegan herbal base cream 37–8
crispy fried ribwort leaves 276
Crispy fried ribwort with tempeh & greens on greens 276
cupcakes, Clover, with orange cashew icing 142
curries
    Bathua saag aloo 181
    Cobbler's pegs, lentil & tomato curry 148

D

dandelion dipping sauce 158
Dandelion root coffee 160
Dandelion straws 160
decoctions 22–3
Deep-fried dandelion flowers 158
Dock & cannellini bean soup 166
Dock scroggin fruit & nut bars 169
Dock seed banana bread 170
dosage chart 26–9
dressings
    golden salad dressing 226
    lemon dressing 156
    maple citrus dressing 114
drying herbs 20–1

E

eczema & psoriasis cream, Blue top 86
equipment 44–5
essences, flower 42–3
essential oils 50–1

F

Fat hen & cashew cheese tart 178
fat hen seeds, activating 182
Fat hen vegan brownies 182
fermented herbal teas 22–3
flower essences 42–3
flu tonic, Nasturtium cold & 228
Fresh aloe vera gel 38–9
Fresh asthma weed chutney 68

G

gels 47
    Anti-inflammatory gel 90
    Chickweed anti-inflammatory gel 119
    Cobbler's pegs gel 151
    Fresh aloe vera gel 38–9
    herbal gels 38–9
    Purslane gel 271
glaze, ribwort 276
glue 126
glycerine, plantain infused 98
glycetracts 24
    dosage 26–9
    dried herb ratios 24
gnocchi verdi, Nettle 237
gochujang sauce 60
golden salad dressing 226
Gotu kola capsules 198
Gotu kola healing cream 199
Gotu kola iced tea 196
gotu kola infused oil 199
Gotu kola sambal 196
Gripe water 190

H

harvesting herbs 20
Head & chest tonic for excess mucus 281
healing balms & creams
    Gotu kola healing cream 199
    Herb robert healing balm 207
    Tropical chickweed healing cream 303
Herb robert & radish salad 204
Herb robert capsules 206
Herb robert healing balm 207
herb robert infused oil 207
herbal gels *see* gels
herbs
    dosage chart 26–9
    drying 20–1
    harvesting 20
    infusing oils with 30–1
    storing 21

I

ice, Chickweed 119
iced tea, Gotu kola 196
icing, lemon & blackberry 239
icing, orange cashew 142
infused oils *see* oils
infusions 22–3
ingredients for herbal medicine-making 46–51
inhalation, Tropical chickweed 304
insect repellent & itch spray, Natural 213
itch balm, Lantana 212
itch spray, Natural insect repellent & 213

J

jams
    Blackberry nightshade jam 77
    Prickly pear jam 262
juices
    Chickweed, cucumber & apple juice 116
    Cobbler's pegs anti-inflammatory juice 151
    Sow thistle, aloe & pear juice for constipation 289
    Tropical chickweed anti-inflammatory juice 302

L

lacto-ferment pickling 229, 270
Lantana itch balm 212
lantana oil 212
lemon & blackberry icing 239
lemon dressing 156
lemonade, Oxalis 254
lemony amaranth leaves 60
Liver tonic powder 248
lung tea, Mallow 218
lymph cream, Cleavers 135

M

Mahalabia with clover syrup 140
Mallow lung tea 218
Mallow salad 218
maple citrus dressing 114
Maple roast carrots with nodding top sauce 248
marshmallows, Wild vegan 220
meditating with plants 40–1
Moxa sticks 126
mucus, Head & chest tonic for excess 281
muffins, Wild raspberry 310
mugwort oil 125

Mushroom, thyme, garlic & nettle soup 234

N

Nasturtium capers 229
Nasturtium cold & flu tonic 228
Nasturtium salad 226
Natural insect repellent & itch spray 213
Natural vegan sun lotion 296–7
Nettle & blackberry forest cake 239
Nettle gnocchi verdi 237
Nettle tea 240
Nettle tea blends 240
Nodding top chimichurri 246
nodding top sauce 248
nutrition of wildcrafted food 14

O

oils 47–8
    Alcohol-infused oils 31
    cat's ear root oil 108
    cleavers infused oil 135
    essential oils 50–1
    fast infused oil 31
    gotu kola infused oil 199
    herb robert infused oil 207
    infused blackberry nightshade oil 80
    infused calendula oil 297
    infused lantana oil 212
    infused oils 30–1
    infused St John's wort oil 297
    infused tropical chickweed oil 303
    infusing with fresh herbs 31
    mugwort oil 125
    slow-infused oil 30–1
    St John's wort infused oil 294
ointments 32–4
    Beeswax base ointment 34
    Cat's ear antifungal ointment 108
    Plantain & charcoal drawing ointment 98
    Plantain ointment 100
    Ribwort ointment 280
    St John's wort pain ointment 295
    Vegan base ointment 33–4
orange cashew icing 142
Oxalis & lime tarts 254
Oxalis lemonade 254

P

pain ointment, St John's wort 295
pancakes, Cat's ear savoury 106
pesto, Wild weed 279
Pickled purslane 270
pizza bases 78

pizza, spelt, with Blackberry night-shade, nodding top & artichoke 78
plant awareness and communication 40–1
Plantain & charcoal drawing ointment 98
plantain infused glycerine 98
Plantain ointment 100
Plantain poultice for wounds & ulcers 100
Plantain seed pudding 97
porridge, Amaranth 58
potato balls 132
poultices
　Blue top poultice 88
　Plantain poultice for wounds & ulcers 100
powders 21–2
　Liver tonic powder 248
　Wild greens powder 150
preservatives 50
Prickly pear chia pudding 263
Prickly pear jam 262
Prickly pear smoothie 262
Prickly pear with tomato, onion & chilli 260
psoriasis cream, Blue top eczema & 86
puddings
　Plantain seed pudding 97
　Prickly pear chia pudding 263
Purslane gel 271
Purslane salsa verde 269

R
raw materials for medine-making
　see ingredients
Ribwort & horseradish syrup 280
ribwort glaze 276
Ribwort ointment 280
Room & travel spray 212

S
salads
　Bitter salad 156
　Herb robert & radish salad 204
　Mallow salad 218
　Nasturtium salad 226
　Spring salad 114
salsa verde, Purslane 269
salves 32–4
sambal, Gotu kola 196
sauces
　cleavers dipping sauce 132
　dandelion dipping sauce 158
　gochujang sauce 60
　nodding top sauce 248

seeds, collecting 20
shampoo, Blue top 88
skin cream, Chickweed 118
smoothie, Prickly pear 262
smudge stick, Chinese mugwort 124
solvents 49–50
　Universal solvent 24
soups
　Dock & cannellini bean soup 166
　Mushroom, thyme, garlic & nettle soup 234
Sow thistle & jackfruit 286
Sow thistle, aloe & pear juice for constipation 289
sprays
　Natural insect repellent & itch spray 213
　Room & travel spray 212
Spring salad 114
St John's wort infused oil 294
St John's wort oil 297
St John's wort pain ointment 295
sterilising bottles and jars 23
sticks, Moxa 126
storing herbs 21
straws, Dandelion 160
sun lotion
　Natural vegan sun lotion 296–7
Sweet fennel cream cheese 189
syrups
　Asthma weed cough syrup 70
　Clover syrup 140
　Ribwort & horseradish syrup 280

T
tarts
　Fat hen & cashew cheese tart 178
　Oxalis & lime tarts 254
teas
　Ayurvedic CCF tea blend 190
　fermented hebal teas 22–3
　Gotu kola iced tea 196
　Mallow lung tea 218
　Nettle tea 240
　Nettle tea blends 240
　Wild raspberry leaf fermented tea 312

toasts, Chickweed, cashew & caper 116
tofu, Amaranth-crusted 60
tonics
　Head & chest tonic for excess mucus 281
　Liver tonic powder 248
　Nasturtium cold & flu tonic 228
travel spray, Room & 212

Tropical chickweed anti-inflammatory juice 302
Tropical chickweed healing cream 303
Tropical chickweed inhalation 304
tropical chickweed oil 303

U
ulcers, Plantain poultice for wounds & 100
Universal solvent 24

V
Vegan base balm 32
Vegan base ointment 33–4
Vegan herbal base cream 37–8
vinegar pickling 229, 270

W
water, Gripe 190
waxes 46
Wild greens powder 150
Wild raspberry cordial 312
Wild raspberry leaf fermented tea 312
Wild raspberry muffins 310
Wild seed crackers 172
Wild vegan marshmallows 220
Wild weed pesto 279
wildcrafted food nutrition 14
wildcrafting
　challenges of 15
　guidelines for sustainable 17
　safety 16
Wilted wild greens 60
wounds & ulcers, Plantain poultice for 100

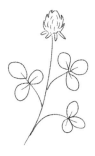

Published in 2024 by Murdoch Books, an imprint of Allen & Unwin

Murdoch Books Australia
Cammeraygal Country
83 Alexander Street
Crows Nest NSW 2065
Phone: +61 (0)2 8425 0100
murdochbooks.com.au
info@murdochbooks.com.au

Murdoch Books UK
Ormond House
26–27 Boswell Street
London WC1N 3JZ
Phone: +44 (0) 20 8785 5995
murdochbooks.co.uk
info@murdochbooks.co.uk

For corporate orders and custom publishing, contact our business development team
at salesenquiries@murdochbooks.com.au

Publisher: Alexandra Payne
Editorial manager: Justin Wolfers
Design manager: Megan Pigott
Designer and illustrator: Julia Cornelius
Editor: Katri Hilden
Photographer: Cath Muscat
Stylist: Vanessa Austin
Photoshoot chef: Jimmy Callaway
Production director: Lou Playfair

Text © Heidi Merika 2024
The moral right of the author has been asserted.
Design © Murdoch Books 2024
Photography © Cath Muscat 2024, except front cover and pages 1, 4 (top and
bottom left), 6, 7, 9, 11, 17, 39, 41, 51, 54, 64, 72, 82, 92, 95, 102, 105, 110, 113,
120, 123, 128, 136, 138, 139, 144, 146, 147, 152, 162, 164, 174, 177, 184-185, 192,
200, 203, 208, 210, 214-215, 217, 222, 224, 225, 230, 242, 244, 250, 253, 256,
259 (left), 264, 267, 272, 275, 282, 285, 290, 298, 306, 309 (left), 322 © Rob
Palmer 2024; pages 35, 131 © Jimmy Callaway 2024; page 66 © Sally Kingsford-
Smith 2024; page 85 © Heidi Merika 2024; pages 75, 309 © Alamy 2024

Murdoch Books acknowledges the Traditional Owners of the Country on which we live and work.
We pay our respects to all Aboriginal and Torres Strait Islander Elders, past and present.

ISBN 9 781 76150 009 1

A catalogue record for this
book is available from the
National Library of Australia

A catalogue record for this book is available from the British Library

Colour reproduction by Splitting Image Colour Studio Pty Ltd, Wantirna, Victoria
Printed by 1010 Printing International Limited, China

OVEN GUIDE: You may find cooking times vary depending on the oven you are using. For fan-forced ovens, as a general rule, set the
oven temperature to 20°C (35°F) lower than indicated in the recipe.

TABLESPOON MEASURES: We have used 20 ml (4 teaspoon) tablespoon measures. If you are using a 15 ml (3 teaspoon) tablespoon
add an extra teaspoon of the ingredient for each tablespoon specified.

DISCLAIMER: The information and suggestions in this book are for your consideration only and may not be suitable to your particular
circumstances. We are not recommending that people eat certain foods or follow any particular dietary advice. This is particularly so
if you have allergies or other conditions that may give rise to adverse reactions to certain foods or diets. Before undertaking any of the
suggestions in this book, therefore, we strongly recommend that you consult your own health care professional. Neither the author/s
nor the publisher accepts any liability or responsibility for any loss or damage suffered or incurred as a result of undertaking or following
any suggestions contained in this book. Individuals using or consuming the plants listed in this book do so entirely at their own risk.
Always check a reputable source to ensure that the plants you are using are non-toxic, organic, unsprayed and safe to be consumed.
The author and/or publisher cannot be held responsible for any adverse reactions.

10 9 8 7 6 5 4 3 2 1

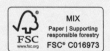

MIX
Paper | Supporting
responsible forestry
FSC® C016973

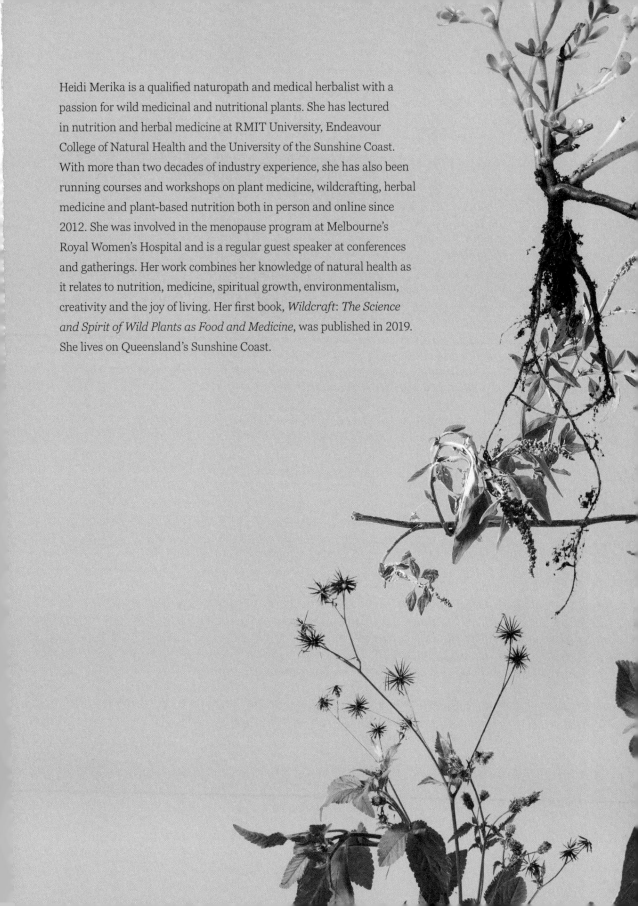

Heidi Merika is a qualified naturopath and medical herbalist with a passion for wild medicinal and nutritional plants. She has lectured in nutrition and herbal medicine at RMIT University, Endeavour College of Natural Health and the University of the Sunshine Coast. With more than two decades of industry experience, she has also been running courses and workshops on plant medicine, wildcrafting, herbal medicine and plant-based nutrition both in person and online since 2012. She was involved in the menopause program at Melbourne's Royal Women's Hospital and is a regular guest speaker at conferences and gatherings. Her work combines her knowledge of natural health as it relates to nutrition, medicine, spiritual growth, environmentalism, creativity and the joy of living. Her first book, *Wildcraft*: *The Science and Spirit of Wild Plants as Food and Medicine*, was published in 2019. She lives on Queensland's Sunshine Coast.

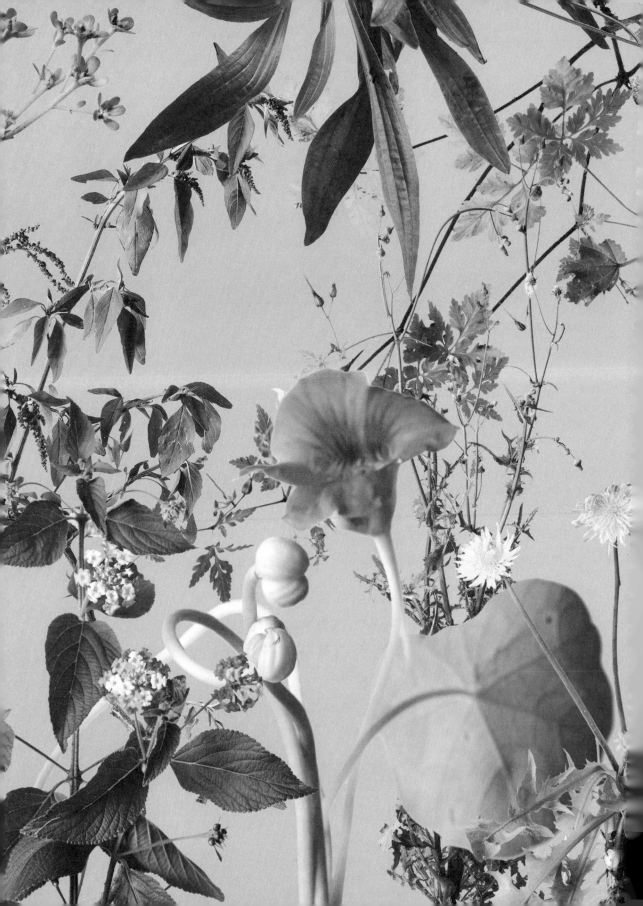